What Do Children Need to Flourish?

The Search Institute Series on Developmentally Attentive Community and Society

Series Editor
Peter L. Benson, *Search Institute, Minneapolis, Minnesota*

Series Mission
To advance interdisciplinary inquiry into the individual, system, community, and societal dynamics that promote developmental strengths; and the processes for mobilizing these dynamics on behalf of children and adolescents.

DEVELOPMENTAL ASSETS AND ASSET-BUILDING COMMUNITIES:
Implications for Research, Policy, and Practice
Edited by Richard M. Lerner and Peter L. Benson

OTHER PEOPLE'S KIDS:
Social Expectations and American Adults' Involvement with Children and Adolescents
Peter C. Scales with Peter L. Benson, Marc Mannes, Nicole R. Hintz, Eugene C. Roehlkepartain, and Theresa K. Sullivan

WHAT DO CHILDREN NEED TO FLOURISH?
Conceptualizing and Measuring Indicators of Positive Development
Edited by Kristin Anderson Moore and Laura H. Lippman

A Continuation Order Plan is available for this series. A continuation order will bring delivery of each new volume immediately upon publication. Volumes are billed only upon actual shipment. For further information please contact the publisher.

What Do Children Need to Flourish?

Conceptualizing and Measuring Indicators of Positive Development

Edited by

Kristin Anderson Moore
Child Trends
Washington, DC

and

Laura H. Lippman
Child Trends
Washington, DC

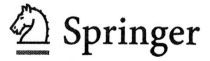 Springer

Library of Congress Cataloging-in-Publication Data

What do children need to flourish? : conceptualizing and measuring indicators of positive
    development / edited by Kristin A. Moore and Laura Lippman.
        p. cm.
    Papers presented at a conference held in Washington, D.C. in March 2003.
    Includes bibliographical references and index.
    ISBN 0-387-23061-0
    1. Child development–Evaluation–Congresses.   I. Moore, Kristin A.   II. Lippman, Laura.

HQ767.82.W43 2005
305.231–dc22

                                                                        2004059116

ISBN 0-387-23061-0   ISBN 13: 978-038-723061-0   Printed on acid-free paper.

Printed in the United States of America.   (TB/EB)

9 8 7 6 5 4 3 2 1   SPIN 150043

springeronline.com

This book is dedicated to our children

Lindsay

Eric

Brigit

and

Jonathan

May they flourish!

Preface

The Search Institute Series on Developmentally Attentive Community and Society seeks to create a forum for leading scholars from many disciplines to introduce cutting-edge theories, models, and research on the nature of positive human development and the web of community and societal factors that contribute to that development. The goal is not only to advance scholarship but also to contribute to what Lerner, Fisher, and Weinberg (2000) call a "science for and of the people" (p. 11)—research that intentionally leads to improving the lives of individuals, families, communities, and society.

What Do Children Need to Flourish? exemplifies the vision for the series. Kristin Anderson Moore and Laura H. Lippman have drawn together leading scholars to examine how this nation might begin to build national indicator systems focused on optimal development—flourishing—that offers a complementary balance to the problem-focused indicators that currently shape public dialogue, policy, funding, and most research.

This volume attests to the explosion of interest and quality scholarship in positive development that has emerged in recent decades. Much of that research and practice has been exploratory. For example, since the early 1990s, Search Institute has been actively engaged in exploring what young people need in their lives in order to grow up healthy, caring, and responsible (see Lerner & Benson, 2003). Over time, hundreds of grassroots communities and thousands of organizations have begun efforts aimed at strengthening positive development. This positive focus will not reach its full potential impact, however, until it enters the systems of national indicators that guide funding, research, policy, and practice priorities and decisions.

Thus, articulating national indicators of positive development plays a vital role not only in advancing scientific inquiry but also in supporting the development of policies, practices, and public dialogue that view development through a new, positive lens. By introducing this balance to research, dialogue, and policy setting, this volume exemplifies what Earls (1999) calls a *critical* social science—neither solely positivist nor solely interpretative—in which "the science itself is part of an act of transforming society" (p. 521). We are honored that our colleagues at Child Trends have chosen to introduce this vital work through this series.

Peter L. Benson, Ph.D.

Search Institute
Series Editor

References

Earls, F. (1999). Frontiers of research on children, youth, and families. *Journal of Community Psychology*, *27*, 517–524.

Lerner, R. M., & Benson, P. L. (Eds.). (2003). *Developmental assets and asset-building communities: Implications for research, policy, and practice.* New York: Kluwer Academic/Plenum Publishers.

Lerner, R. M., Fisher, C. B., & Weinberg, R. A. (2000). Toward a science for and of the people: Promoting civil society through the application of developmental science. *Child Development*, *71*, 11–20.

Acknowledgments

It is a pleasure to thank the sponsors who not only provided the means for us to organize and convene a conference on indicators of positive development but also collaborated with us in varied ways across a period of years. Our sponsors, in alphabetical order, are:

Administration for Children and Families, DHHS
Edna McConnell Clark Foundation
Federal Interagency Forum on Child and Family Statistics
John Templeton Foundation
MacArthur Network on Successful Pathways Through Middle Childhood
National Institute of Child Health and Human Development Family and
    Child Well-being Research Network
Office of the Assistant Secretary for Planning and Evaluation, DHHS

We would also like to acknowledge and thank our colleagues who helped organize the conference and bring this book to reality. Rosalind Johnson helped identify scholars, conceptualize the conference and book, and review draft papers. Jacquelynne Eccles provided essential help in identifying scholars who have studied education and achievement. Erik Michelsen also helped identify researchers and implement the conference. Julie Dombrowski helped to organize and then summarize the conference and to review paper revisions. Hugh McIntosh edited the papers from both a substantive and technical perspective. Mary Byers served as copy editor and prepress coordinator for the book on behalf of Search Institute.

Fanette Jones helped organize the conference logistics. The actual conference was greatly enhanced by the contributors of distinguished moderators and discussants, as well as presentations on related international work, including, in alphabetical order:

Duane Alexander
Steve Blumberg
Brett Brown
Sonia Chessen
James Connell
Pat Fagan
Dan Hart
David Johnson
Corey Keyes
Mariann Lemke

Dan Lichter
David Murphy
Mairead Reidy
Jodie Roth
Laura Salganik
Shephard Smith
Judith Torney-Purta
Katherine Wallman
Harry Wilson

We are also delighted that Peter L. Benson, director of Search Institute, participated as a contributor and, with his colleague, Eugene C. Roehlkepertain, suggested and supported turning the conference papers into a book as a part of the Search Institute Series on Developmentally Attentive Community and Society.

Finally, we would like to thank the authors of these excellent papers, who traveled to Washington, D.C., at a time when tensions due to terrorism and war were high. We share our thanks and appreciation to all of them for joining in a critical effort to examine rigorously how to conceptualize and measure the attributes that we seek in our children to help all young people flourish.

Contents

1. **Introduction and Conceptual Framework**   1
   Kristin Anderson Moore and Laura H. Lippman

Part I   Positive Formation of the Self: Character, Attitudes, Spirituality, and Identity

2. **The Values in Action Inventory of Character Strengths for Youth**   13
   Nansook Park and Christopher Peterson

3. **Adolescent Spirituality**   25
   Peter L. Benson, Peter C. Scales, Arturo Sesma Jr., and Eugene
   C. Roehlkepartain

4. **Children's Life Satisfaction**   41
   E. Scott Huebner, Shannon M. Suldo, and Robert F. Valois

5. **Measuring Hope in Children**   61
   C. R. Snyder

6. **The Ethnic Identity Scale**   75
   Adriana J. Umaña-Taylor

Part II   Healthy Habits, Positive Behaviors, and Time Use

7. **Leisure Time Activities in Middle Childhood**   95
   Sandra L. Hofferth and Sally C. Curtin

8. **Healthy Habits among Adolescents: Sleep, Exercise, Diet,
   and Body Image**   111
   Kathleen Mullan Harris, Rosalind Berkowitz King, and
   Penny Gordon-Larsen

9. **Adolescent Participation in Organized Activities**   133
   Bonnie L. Barber, Margaret R. Stone, and Jacquelynne S. Eccles

10. **Positive Interpersonal and Intrapersonal Functioning: An
    Assessment of Measures among Adolescents**   147
    Brian K. Barber

11. **A Scale of Positive Social Behaviors**   163
Sylvia R. Epps, Seoung Eun Park, Aletha C. Huston,
and Marika Ripke

Part III   Positive Relationships with Parents and Siblings

12. **The Parent–Adolescent Relationship Scale**   183
Elizabeth C. Hair, Kristin Anderson Moore, Sarah B. Garrett,
Akemi Kinukawa, Laura H. Lippman, and Erik Michelson

13. **Positive Indicators of Sibling Relationship Quality: The
Sibling Inventory of Behavior**   203
Brenda L. Volling and Alysia Y. Blandon

**Part IV   Positive Attitudes and Behaviors toward Learning
and School Environments**

14. **The Patterns of Adaptive Learning Survey**   223
Eric M. Anderman, Tim Urdan, and Robert Roeser

15. **Ability Self-Perceptions and Subjective Task Values in
Adolescents and Children**   237
Jacquelynne S. Eccles, Susan A. O'Neill, and Allan Wigfield

16. **Assessing Academic Self-Regulated Learning**   251
Christopher A. Wolters, Paul R. Pintrich, and
Stuart A. Karabenick

17. **Identifying Adaptive Classrooms: Dimensions of the
Classroom Social Environment**   271
Helen Patrick and Allison M. Ryan

18. **Connection to School**   289
Clea McNeely

19. **School Engagement**   305
Jennifer A. Fredricks, Phyllis Blumenfeld, Jeanne Friedel,
and Alison Paris

Part V   Enacting Positive Values and Behaviors in Communities

20. **Community-Based Civic Engagement**   325
Scott Keeter, Krista Jenkins, Cliff Zukin, and Molly Andolina

21. **Prosocial Orientation and Community Service**   339
    Peter C. Scales and Peter L. Benson

22. **Frugality, Generosity, and Materialism in Children and**
    Adolescents   357
    Tim Kasser

Contributors   375

Index   383

1 Introduction and Conceptual Framework

Kristin Anderson Moore and Laura H. Lippman

Child Trends

Flourishing is a strong word. It is a word with wonderful, happy, and healthy connotations, but it is still a strong word. It means something to say that we don't just want children not to use drugs or commit crimes. We don't just want children to avoid becoming dropouts and teen parents. We want children to flourish. But what does this mean?

Are children who flourish healthy, strong, and athletic? Are they children who sing and laugh? Are they children who are kind and empathic? Who are close to their parents? Who serve their communities? Who love learning and who do well in school?

And who decides what it means to be a flourishing child? Is it a matter of values? Is it a determination for economists or politicians to make? Is it a construct that adults should define? Keyes (2003, p. 294) has defined flourishing as "a state in which an individual feels positive emotion toward life and is functioning well psychologically and socially." Certainly this gets at the sense of flourishing, but we apply the term here to all domains of a child's life, including education and health, as well as social and emotional outcomes. Another concern that is frequently raised is whether flourishing can be measured. Are positive traits, attitudes, and behaviors too "soft" to be measured with precision and rigor? Is it possible that although we all think we can recognize a child who is flourishing, we cannot agree on the specifics?

We undertook this project because we thought it was time to become serious and concrete about conceptualizing and measuring positive indicators for children. Our scans indicated few measures of positive outcomes in reports on child well-being or in national surveys (Federal Interagency Forum on Child and Family Statistics, 2003; U.S. Department of Health and Human Services, 2002; Zaff, 2000). Believing that "what gets measured gets emphasized, and what gets emphasized gets measured," as stated by Arthur Schwartz, vice president for

Research and Programs in the Human Sciences at the John Templeton Foundation in his opening remarks to the conference from which this collection came, we felt it was time to cast our nets broadly and see what had been done or what could be done. Our goal was to provide strong measures of positive attributes that could be assessed and monitored at the national level. We also imagined, however, that a coherent set of positive measures would be an important addition to longitudinal research studies and that such measures would be useful to program providers conducting evaluations.

For any of these purposes, it is crucial to identify measures that are psychometrically solid. Moreover, they need to be meaningful, in a diverse national population, to children from varied social, cultural, and economic groups. In addition, it is important to consider whether and how positive indicators matter. Some want assurance that positive characteristics in children translate into higher earnings, self-sufficiency, family responsibility, and good citizenship in adulthood. Others are satisfied to be assured that children are happy and flourishing while they are children. This distinction is sometimes referred to as the debate between *well-being* and *well-becoming*. Feeling that both well-being and well-becoming are important criteria, we sought to examine whether constructs and measures predict to both contemporaneous outcomes and to outcomes in the future.

Background

An interest in positive development has characterized programs for many years. Preschool education programs, Scouts, service-learning, child-care teachers, school clubs, religious programs, and sports teams have often focused on teaching positive values, skills, and habits. The research community (with some important exceptions), on the other hand, was slower to focus on positive outcomes. This pattern may reflect the greater funding available for studies of problem behaviors from government agencies and foundations. However, a focus on positive behaviors and outcomes has gradually evolved, for a variety of reasons. One factor was undoubtedly the demand for such measures from programs and funders who support youth development and other positive development programs. If the goal of the program was to produce a positive outcome, then a positive outcome measure was needed to assess program success. Similar needs were experienced by state policy makers designing evaluations to study welfare reform and children. Policy makers wanted positive as well as negative outcomes to be examined.

Another factor was the gradual recognition that a focus on the negative is scientifically unbalanced and incomplete. In addition, as indicator reports such as *America's Children: Key National Indicators of Well-being*, produced by the Federal Interagency Forum on Child and Family Statistics (2003), and the *Kids Count Data Book*, produced by the Annie E. Casey Foundation (2003), became widely disseminated, the dearth of positive measures was noted by those producing and reading the reports. Given evidence that the public perceives the state of America's children to be worse than it really is (Guzman, Lippman, Moore, & O'Hare, 2003; Public Agenda, 1999), some raised the possibility that the focus on negative outcomes distorts the public's perception of how America's children are faring.

Another factor is the need to adapt to social change. Over the past century, modern industrial nations, including the United States, have met and responded to a wide range of threats to child health and survival. Infant mortality, for example, declined dramatically over the past century, and important improvements have occurred in the health, education, housing, and economic security of children. This is not to say that problems do not remain or that disparities do not exist, but rather that large and important improvements have occurred. With these improvements, a focus on quality-of-life issues has become more central, and such a perspective is very complementary to a focus on positive outcomes (Ben-Arieh, 1997).

Thus, for numerous reasons, researchers in various fields were coming to a common conclusion: There is a need to conceptualize and measure positive development for children and youth. However, Child Trends' review of available national databases found relatively few that included positive measures, beyond the standard measures of educational achievement and attainment, which were quite limited compared with the set of possible positive measures that could be conceptualized. Before moving ahead to develop such measures, it made sense to see what the scholarly community might have developed. Fortunately, we were able to identify a number of high-quality local and regional studies as well as some national surveys that have incorporated aspects of positive development.

To jump-start the development of positive measures, a conference was held in Washington, D.C., in March 2003, to bring together scholars working on varied aspects of positive development to share their work. Authors were commissioned to provide a literature review conceptualizing their construct and summarizing research to date and to provide information on data quality for their proposed measure. Since contributors were working with existing data in all but one case, it was not always possible for them to conduct all of the requested psychometric analyses; they were asked to assess the amount of missing data, the distribution of responses, the reliability of their measure(s), and both the concurrent and prospective validity of their measures to examine well-being and well-becoming. In addition, where possible, authors were asked to conduct analyses for major subgroups, including age, gender, race and Hispanic origin, and disability status.

Summaries of the Papers

Papers presented at the conference and included in this book cover a wide range of constructs. Part I addresses the positive formation of the self, including character, attitudes, spirituality, and identity.

Nansook Park and Christopher Peterson explore the assessment of character strengths, which builds on the Values in Action Inventory of Character Strengths for Youth. They argue that a strength should be visible in a person's thoughts, words, or actions; contribute to the good life for the self and for others, yet be valued in and of itself even if it does not produce clear benefits; not "diminish other people" but rather inspire or support them; and be cultivated by the larger society and recognized by a societal consensus regarding its importance. In addition, it should not be possible to decompose a strength into component elements. Park and Peterson also share initial conceptual and measurement work on character strengths.

Peter L. Benson, Peter C. Scales, Arturo Sesma Jr., and Eugene C. Roehlkepartain explore indicators of adolescent spirituality. They note that two commonly used measures—attendance and salience or importance—have repeatedly been found to be associated with better development and behavior among children. The explanatory power of these measures is modest, however, and Benson and his colleagues argue that it is necessary to move beyond these fairly superficial markers to explore a richer set of beliefs, values, behaviors, and community aspects of religion and spirituality. Also, they note that American culture has become increasingly diverse, and new measures are needed to capture aspects of spirituality in varied cultural and social groups. They further distinguish between "vertical" and "horizontal" themes, that is, a focus on a Supreme Being, life force, or spirit and a focus on the effect of religious or spiritual beliefs in moving adherents toward involvement with others in this world.

E. Scott Huebner, Shannon M. Suldo, and Robert F. Valois examine two brief measures of children's life satisfaction. Using these measures, children make judgments about whether they are satisfied with their lives, which is one aspect of positive mental health. One scale measures global life satisfaction, and the other examines specific domains of life satisfaction; both scales have been successfully fielded. The scales have very good internal reliability and discriminate and construct validity. The authors found that children who were more satisfied with their lives had very low levels of depression and anxiety, very positive self-concepts, and good family relationships.

C. R. Snyder presents the Children's Hope Scale (CHS). Snyder conceptualizes hope in children as an overall perception that one's goals can be met and that one has the capacity to find routes to goals (pathways thinking) and the motivation or sense of agency to pursue goals (agency thinking). Scores on the CHS have been found to correlate with perceived competency and control and to predict cognitive achievement. Also, the scale is inversely correlated with childhood depression and loneliness. The CHS has been tested on many different samples of children, some with life-threatening illnesses (e.g., cancer) as well as other disabilities for whom hope is a critical asset. Differences by gender and family income have not been found, but Snyder notes that additional research is needed to explore differences by race/ethnicity.

Adriana J. Umaña-Taylor shares work on an evolving scale of ethnic identity. She distinguishes the processes of building an ethnic identity, including exploration, resolution, and affirmation as distinct components. Evidence from diverse samples provides support for construct validity and indicates that individuals can, as hypothesized, be described as having four identity statuses:

resolved (have explored and feel committed to their ethnic identity) and affirm it positively or negatively; foreclosed (have not explored but are committed to their identity) positive or negative; moratorium (have explored but are not yet committed) positive or negative; and diffuse (have not explored and are not committed) positive or negative, with most youth feeling that they have resolved their ethnic identity and feeling positively about it.

Part II addresses measures of healthy habits, positive behaviors, and time use. Sandra L. Hofferth and Sally C. Curtin look at time use using data from the 1997 Child Development Supplement of the Panel Study of Income Dynamics. Examining time diary data in relation to outcomes for children, net of confounding influences, they identify three activities that qualify as measures of positive behavior during middle childhood: reading for pleasure, activities in a religious community, and participation in sports. Reading is associated with higher scores on a cognitive test, whereas participation in sports is related to higher achievement test scores, and time spent in church activities is related to achievement. In addition, use of computers at home was related with higher applied problem scores, and shopping was associated with higher achievement, perhaps because parents shop together with children during the middle childhood years. On the other hand, time spent doing housework was not related to positive outcomes, and therefore the authors do not recommend time spent doing housework as a positive indicator.

Kathleeen Mullan Harris, Rosalind Berkowitz King, and Penny Gordon-Larsen explore healthy habits among adolescents using the National Longitudinal Study of Adolescent Health (Add Health). They confirm that adequate sleep, consumption of fruits and vegetables, and exercise are positive indicators, while inactivity (measured by hours of TV viewing) is negative. They also examine body image and find that concordance between actual and perceived weight provides interesting insights into adolescents. They find that African American girls, while generally less likely to have healthy habits, tend to have a healthier body image, which reduces their risk for eating disorders and depression.

Bonnie L. Barber, Margaret R. Stone, and Jacquelynne S. Eccles explore participation in organized activities. Such activities include sports, clubs, arts, academic clubs, faith community, and performing arts, both in school and out of school. These authors note that asking about "any" participation yields less reporting than a more detailed checklist, and they suggest that information be obtained about time spent in activities, not just whether children participate. They also note that participation in different kinds of activities is associated with different outcomes. For example, 10th graders who participated in prosocial activities reported less alcohol and drug use, whereas those involved with team sports reported higher rates of drinking alcohol. Overall, a measure of the total number of clubs and activities was found to predict a number of positive outcomes, including less alcohol use, better psychological outcomes, a higher GPA, and more civic engagement. They also suggest that activities could usefully be collapsed by type of activity, specifically, prosocial activities, sports, and academic clubs.

Brian K. Barber distinguishes intrapersonal functioning (measured by self-esteem, perspective taking, and empathy) from interpersonal functions (measured by social initiative, peer connection, and communication with mother and father). He draws on scales that are widely used, but which have not been systematically assessed, and examines longer and shorter versions of the scales for varied subgroups. He finds that the psychometric properties of the scales across the adolescent years are strong overall and for all of the subgroups that could be tested using data for Utah students. Barber notes the need for additional tests of validity, including longitudinal analyses.

Sylvia R. Epps, Seoung Eun Park, Aletha C. Huston, and Marika Ripke examine the Positive Behavior Scale, a measure of social competence, compliance, and autonomy or self-reliance. They find the scale useful, especially the full scale rather than the subscales. Results differed for a general sample compared with a low-income sample, with teachers more positive about advantaged children but parents somewhat more positive about disadvantaged children. The measure, these authors note, appears to be appropriate across social and ethnic groups and can be used for both parents and teachers.

Part III explores measures of positive relationships with parents and siblings.

Elizabeth C. Hair, Kristin Anderson Moore, Sarah B. Garrett, Akemi Kinukawa, Laura H. Lippman, and Erik Michelson explore parent–child relationships. They analyze a scale that Child Trends provided to the National Longitudinal Survey of Youth, 1997 cohort. Adolescents aged 12–14 were asked a set of eight questions regarding the supportiveness of their mother and their father, both resident and nonresident, for example, their enjoyment of spending time with the parents, and how often their parent praised or criticized them. The authors examine longer and shorter subscales among varied subpopulations, and they conduct multivariate analyses assessing whether the parent–child relationship predicts to better outcomes in the future. Analyses indicate that the scale enjoys good reliability and validity and is associated with a lower incidence of delinquency, substance use, sexual activity, and suspension, and with better grades, even taking account of numerous confounding influences. The one caveat is that positive parent–child relationships are less protective of low-income and minority adolescents than those from higher income and White families. (Many of the associations are in the expected direction, but fall short of being statistically significant.) It is particularly noteworthy that these data were obtained from adolescents, not from parents, and indicate that most young adolescents feel positively about their parents.

Brenda L. Volling and Alysia Y. Blandon address sibling relationships. They point out that people who have siblings typically spend more of their lifetime with those siblings than with any other person. Despite the importance and longevity of this relationship, little research has addressed children's relationships with their sibling. In their study of families with preschool children, Volling and Blandon examine the Sibling Inventory of Behavior as expanded by Hetherington and Clingempeel for research with preadolescents and adolescents. Although the scale seems to have good psychometrics, the authors note that it would benefit from being tested in larger and more diverse samples.

Part IV addresses positive attitudes and behaviors toward learning and the school environment.

Eric M. Anderman, Tim Urdan, and Robert Roeser discuss the Patterns of Adaptive Learning Survey (PALS), which measures the achievement goals of mastery, performance, and performance avoidance. Mastery is being able to exhibit competence in understanding material or performing a task; performance is demonstrating something to others; and performance avoidance is avoiding a potential display of a lack of competence. These achievement goal measures have been used by numerous researchers with middle school, high school, and college samples. The authors find that the measures have strong predictive and concurrent validity, although they are not strongly predictive of academic achievement.

Jacquelynne S. Eccles, Susan A. O'Neill, and Allan Wigfield have developed scales measuring self-perception of ability and subjective task values. They conceptualize value importance as having four aspects: Attainment value is succeeding in one's core values; intrinsic value is how much enjoyment and pleasure one gets from a task; utility value is how instrumental a task is in reaching one's goals; and cost value is what is lost from engaging in an activity. The scales enjoy high predictive validity and reliability, and they explain links between gender and achievement in English and math.

Christopher A. Wolters, Paul R. Pintrich, and Stuart A. Karabenick present another way of conceptualizing how learners assess their academic goals and align their actions to them in their chapter on assessing self-regulated academic learning. The authors developed the Motivated Strategies for Learning Questionnaire (MSLQ) to measure the three self-regulated learning strategies: cognition, including rehearsal, elaboration, and organization; motivation, including rewarding oneself, environmental structuring, and self-talk; and behaviors that regulate time, effort, and seeking help. The MSLQ has been used in middle school, high school, and college samples, and predicts academic achievement.

Helen Patrick and Allison M. Ryan have developed measures of student perceptions of their classroom social environment, including teacher support, and teacher promotion of mutual respect among students, student task-related interactions, and performance goals. The survey was administered to three samples of students from fifth through eighth grade, and independent observers of the classroom environment were also used to compare with student reports. The measures had good face validity and internal consistency, and the teacher support measure had strong within-class correlation. The measures correlated in expected directions with indices of motivation and engagement in the classroom, but long-term outcomes are as yet unstudied and unknown.

Clea McNeely evaluates existing measures of school connectedness in the National Longitudinal Study of Adolescent Health (Add Health) as potential positive indicators. The measures tap the two subdomains of students' feelings of social belonging at the school and their feelings about their relationships with their teachers. Interestingly, NcNeely found that despite the attention that broad measures of school connectedness are getting, the measure of social belonging, when tested separately, is less predictive of positive outcomes than was the measure of a positive student–teacher relationship. The measure of social belonging, however, had better psychometric properties.

Jennifer A. Fredricks, Phyllis Blumenfeld, Jeanne Friedel, and Alison Paris develop survey and interview measures of behavioral, emotional, and cognitive engagement in school. They administered two sets of surveys to inner-city elementary school students and their teachers in two waves, and found that student and teacher responses correlated with each other, particularly in the area of behavior. The measures had adequate reliability and concurrent validity, but without long-term outcome data, they were unable to test prospective validity. A unique feature of their study is in-depth interviews with a subset of students to identify themes underlying levels of school engagement, showing a wide variety of sources of disengagement.

Part V takes the discussion from positive attitudes and behaviors to enacting positive values in communities.

Community-based civic engagement is the subject of a program of research directed by Scott Keeter, working with Krista Jenkins, Cliff Zukin, and Molly Andolina. Addressing concerns about low rates of voting among contemporary youth, Keeter and his colleagues distinguish three constructs: informal group activity to solve community problems; volunteering; and group membership, which includes both belonging and donating money and also being actively involved. They find that, while those who engage in one activity are more likely to do the others, the associations are not high. Also, these are complex constructs and the level of reporting varies depending upon the question. Keeter et al. suggest asking an initial "gatekeeper" question that allows respondents to provide a socially desirable answer. They then follow with a question about activities during the past 12 months. Like other researchers, they recognize that asking about all possible types of involvement directly increases the number of activities reported but requires considerably more time.

Peter C. Scales and Peter L. Benson share work done by Search Institute on prosocial orientation and community service. They conclude that their seven-item measure of prosocial orientation, which includes both attitudes and behavioral intentions, is a solid measure but that it should be tested among more diverse populations.

Tim Kasser developed original items commissioned for the 2003 conference on frugality, generosity, and materialism for use with children and adolescents. He used brief four-item measures in each of these areas on a sample of students in 5th through 12th grade, which proved to be reliable. Frugality correlated with positive outcomes such as self-esteem, positive environmental behaviors, and with less risk behavior. In addition to those outcomes, generous students reported being happier, whereas materialistic students were less happy, more anxious, had lower self-esteem, and engaged in fewer positive environmental behaviors. These measures break new ground but need to be tested on larger and more diverse samples, along with measures of long-term outcomes to establish their prospective validity.

Next Steps

A number of themes emerged across these chapters. In general, the authors found solid empirical evidence that the positive traits, attitudes, and behaviors being examined can, indeed, be measured rigorously. Authors were not, however, Pollyannaish in their enthusiasm. They noted important caveats and even rejected some of the constructs that were considered. For example, doing housework was not found to be related to better development for children, so it was not recommended as a positive indicator.

As the authors themselves consistently acknowledge, virtually all of the measures need further work. Measures were generally developed for use in a research study. Developing positive indicators for monitoring child well-being was not even on the radar for most authors. Accordingly, many scales are rather long and the language has not been tested for children of different ages and varied social and cultural groups. It is particularly important that scales be tested among low-income as well as higher income children, and among children from varied cultural backgrounds. The few instances in which this was done suggest that differences are possible. At this point, it is not clear whether such differences reflect on the usefulness of the scales or simply reflect different social environments and risks.

Another important question is whether the various scales are redundant. Might there be a general positive or prosocial factor that underlies at least some of the scales? These scales are derived from different databases collected by different researchers in different places. Therefore, we are not yet able to put several scales into the same analysis to see whether some of the scales overlap or are redundant. In addition, most measures need to be shortened and then examined among adolescents from varied social, economic, age, and racial/ethnic groups.

Given these concerns, it will be necessary to refine these measures with cognitive testing, focus groups, and pretests among diverse samples, and with additional analyses. Nevertheless, the work shared in these chapters offers a body of evidence that rigorous measures of positive development are available, and that they are related to and sometimes predict to numerous outcomes valued by society. These authors suggest that ongoing work to conceptualize and measure positive constructs is a worthy step toward understanding and enhancing children's prospects for flourishing.

References

Annie E. Casey Foundation. (2003). *Kids count data book: State profiles of child well-being.* Baltimore, MD: Author.

Ben-Arieh, A. (1997). Introduction: Measuring and monitoring the state of children. In A. Ben-Arieh & H. Wintersberger (Eds.), *Monitoring and measuring the state of children: Beyond survival* (Eurosocial Report 62). Vienna, Austria: European Centre for Social Welfare Policy and Research.

Federal Interagency Forum on Child and Family Statistics. (2003). *America's children: Key national indicators of well-being.* Washington, DC: U.S. Government Printing Office.

Guzman, L., Lippman, L., Moore, K. A., & O'Hare, W. (2003). *How children are doing: The mismatch between public perception and statistical reality* (Child Trends Research Brief, publication #2003-12). Washington, DC: Child Trends.

Keyes, C. L. M. (2003). Complete mental health: An agenda for the 21st century. In C. L. M. Keyes & J. Haidt (Eds.), *Flourishing: Positive psychology and the life well-lived.* Washington, DC: American Psychological Association.

Public Agenda. (1999). *Kids these days '99: What Americans really think about the next generation.* New York: Public Agenda.

U.S. Department of Health and Human Services, Office of the Assistant Secretary for Planning and Evaluation. (2002). *Trends in the well-being of America's children and youth, 2002.* Washington, DC: Author.

Zaff, J. (2000). *Positive indicators in national surveys.* Washington, DC: Child Trends.

I   Positive Formation of the Self: Character, Attitudes, Spirituality, and Identity

2 The Values in Action Inventory of Character Strengths for Youth

Nansook Park

University of Rhode Island

Christopher Peterson

University of Michigan

Raising virtuous children is an ultimate goal not only of parents and educators but also of societies. Across different eras and cultures, identifying character strengths (virtues) and cultivating them in children and youth have been among the chief interests of philosophers, theologians, and educators. With few exceptions, these topics have been neglected by psychologists. However, the emerging field of positive psychology specifically emphasizes building the good life by identifying individual strengths of character and fostering them (Seligman, 2002). Character strengths are now receiving attention from psychologists interested in positive youth development. Initial findings suggest that such strengths may contribute to a variety of positive outcomes, as well as work as a buffer against many negative outcomes, including psychological disorders (Peterson & Seligman, in press).

What is character, and how can we measure it? In recent years, we have made a serious effort to answer these questions scientifically (e.g., Peterson & Park, 2003; Peterson, Park, & Seligman, in press). We began with the following assertions. First, good character is neither unitary nor discrete. Rather, character is made up of a family of positive traits—individual differences that exist in degrees and are manifest in a range of thoughts, feelings, and actions. Second, good character is not outside the realm of self-commentary and certainly not a mystery to those in one's immediate social circle. Third, many of the core components of good character are already present as individual differences among young children. However, the manifestations of character nonetheless change across the life span. These conclusions have important implications for assessment.

As a family of traits, character needs to be measured with an appropriately broad strategy. There is no reason for a researcher to refrain from assessing a single component of good character—kindness or wisdom, for example. But it would be misleading to then treat this single component as the whole of character. We believe that researchers interested in character per se must assess it in its breadth. Good character can only be captured by a set of components that vary across people.

As individual differences that exist in degrees, the components of character must be assessed in ways that allow gradations. Politicians and everyday citizens alike may talk about character as present versus absent (e.g., "Character must be restored to government"), but such statements are rhetorical and at odds with a considered definition of good character. We need to be cautious about searching for single indicators of good character or even single indicators of a component of good character. Some indicators are important in their own right and can be assessed with simple yes/no questions: for example, sexual abstinence or sobriety among teenagers. But we should regard these behaviors as indicative of themselves and not infallible signs of prudence as a trait and certainly not of good character in its broad sense. If our interest lies beyond specific behaviors, the best we can do as researchers is to ask about a range of behaviors and look for common threads.

Especially in a culturally diverse society like the contemporary United States, there is good reason for researchers interested in character and its components to focus on widely valued positive traits and not those that we have dubbed culture-bound (Peterson & Seligman, in press). Individuality and competition, for example, are valued traits in some cultures but not others, and a measure of character that privileges these traits to the exclusion of more universally valued traits is likely to lack generality and thus validity.

Most philosophers emphasize that moral activity involves choosing virtue in light of a justifiable life plan (Yearley, 1990). This characterization means that people can reflect on their own strengths of character and talk about them to others. People may of course be misled and/or misleading, but character is not, in principle, outside the realm of self-commentary. Self-report surveys are therefore one reasonable way to assess the components of character.

Legitimate concerns about the pitfalls of self-report and the validity threat posed by "social desirability" also exist (Crowne & Marlowe, 1964). The premise of these concerns is worth examining. We seem to be quite willing, as researchers and practitioners, to trust what individuals say about their problems. With notable exceptions (such as substance abuse and eating disorders, in which denial is part and parcel of the problem), the preferred way to measure psychological disorder relies on self-report, either by symptom questionnaires or structured interviews. So why not ascertain good character in the same way? Character strengths are not contaminated by a response set of social desirability; they *are* socially desirable, especially when reported with fidelity.

In order to improve the validity of assessment, additional or alternative strategies are needed, such as reports from knowledgeable informants (family members, friends, and teachers), observations, and scenario methods. Different strategies of assessment should converge, and we have found in our research that they indeed do, so long as we give informants the option of saying that they have not had the opportunity to observe the component in question.

Even very young children possess character strengths such as curiosity and persistence, although self-report questionnaires to measure them are obviously not useful. Some character strengths may be rooted in temperament differences such as sociability, and they take on moral meaning very early in life. Other components of good character—open-mindedness and fairness, for example—require a degree of cognitive maturation (see Kohlberg, 1981, 1984; Piaget, 1932). How young is too young to show good character? This is an empirical question, and one of our intended projects is to devise methods for assessing the components of good character among young children by relying on observations and parental reports. For practical reasons, our assessment work to date has extended only to 10-year-olds who are able to complete self-report questionnaires.

Although we are interested in the long-term developmental trajectory of good character, it is not plausible to use the same measures across the life span. Adolescents may show their bravery by the type of clothes they wear or their willingness to befriend otherwise ostracized classmates. Adults, in contrast, may show their bravery by dissenting from the majority in town meetings or by blowing the whistle on wrongdoing at work. There is continuity in the psychological meaning of these acts, although the behaviors differ across developmental stages. We need parallel measures across the life span that are at the same time developmentally appropriate. In our project, we devised surveys that use developmentally appropriate questions but measure the same components of character among youth and adults.

Values in Action Classification

Our work on good character has been self-consciously conducted under the umbrella provided by the field of positive psychology, which calls for as much focus on strength as on weakness, as much interest in building the best things in life as in repairing the worst, and as much concern with fulfilling the lives of healthy people as healing the wounds of the distressed (Seligman, 2002). The most critical tools for positive psychologists are a vocabulary for speaking about the good life and assessment strategies for investigating its components. As noted, we have focused our attention on positive traits—strengths of character such as curiosity, kindness, and hope. What are the most important of these, and how can they be measured as individual differences?

Our project—the Values in Action (VIA) Classification of Strengths—aims at completing what the *Diagnostic and Statistical Manual* of the American Psychiatric Association (1987) has begun, by focusing generally on what is right about people and specifically on the strengths of character that make the good life possible (Peterson & Seligman, in press). We are following the example of *DSM-III-R* and its collateral creations by proposing a classification scheme and devising assessments for its entries.

The project first identified consensual components of character and then devised ways to assess these components as individual differences. We generated the entries for the VIA Classification by reviewing pertinent contemporary and historical literatures—from psychiatry, youth development, character education, religion, ethics, philosophy, organizational studies, and psychology—that addressed good character. From the many candidate strengths identified, we winnowed the list by combining redundancies and applying the following criteria:

- *A strength needs to be manifest in the range of an individual's behavior— thoughts, feelings, and/or actions—in such a way that it can be assessed.* In other words, a character strength should be traitlike in the sense of having a degree of generality across situations and stability over time.
- *A strength contributes to various fulfillments that comprise the good life for the self and for others.* Although strengths and virtues no doubt determine how an individual copes with adversity, our focus is on how they fulfill an individual. Strengths allow the individual to achieve more than the absence of distress and disorder. They break through the zero point of psychology's traditional concern with disease, disorder, and failure to address quality-of-life outcomes.
- *Although strengths can and do produce desirable outcomes, each strength is morally valued in its own right, even in the absence of obvious beneficial outcomes.* To say that a strength is morally valued is an important qualification, because there exist individual differences that are widely valued and contribute to fulfillment but still fall outside of our classification. Consider intelligence or athletic prowess. These talents are valued more for their tangible consequences (acclaim, wealth) than are strengths of character. Someone who "does nothing" with a talent like high intelligence or physical dexterity courts eventual disdain. In contrast, we never hear the criticism that a person did nothing with her hope or authenticity. Talents and abilities can be squandered, but strengths of character cannot.
- *The display of a character strength by one person does not diminish other people in the vicinity but rather elevates them.* Onlookers are impressed, inspired, and encouraged by their observation of virtuous action. Admiration is created but not jealousy, because character strengths are the sorts of characteristics to which all can, and do, aspire.
- As suggested by Erikson's (1963) discussion of psychosocial stages and the virtues that result from their satisfactory resolutions, the larger society provides institutions and associated rituals for cultivating strengths and virtues. *These can be thought of as simulations: trial runs that allow children and adolescents to display and develop a valued characteristic in a safe (as-if) context in which guidance is explicit.*
- *Yet another criterion for a character strength is the existence of consensually recognized paragons of virtue.* Paragons of character display what Allport (1961) called a cardinal trait, and the ease with which we can think of paragons in our own social circles gives the lie to the claim that virtuous people are either phony or boring (Wolf, 1982).

- *A final criterion is that the character strength is arguably unidimensional and not able to be decomposed into other strengths in the classification.* For example, the character strength of tolerance meets most of the other criteria enumerated but is a blend of judgment, kindness, and fairness. The character strength of responsibility seems to result from integrity, persistence, and teamwork. And so on.

When we applied these criteria to the candidate strengths we identified through literature searches and brainstorming, we ended up with 24 positive traits organized under six broad virtues (see Appendix). In some cases, the classification of a given strength under a core virtue can be debated. Regardless, we have measured only the more specific strengths, although we plan eventually to test this hierarchical classification empirically with appropriate multivariate techniques. If the data suggest that a given strength belongs elsewhere because of its co-occurrence with other strengths, the classification system will be modified accordingly.

Character Strengths among Youth

What distinguishes the VIA Classification from previous attempts to articulate the components of good character is its simultaneous concern with broad-based assessment. The assessment strategy we have most extensively developed to date entails self-report surveys that can be completed by respondents in a single session. We have devised several versions of a self-report questionnaire for youth, the *VIA Inventory of Strengths for Youth* (*VIA-Youth*).We experimented with different item formats and phrasings before arriving at the current inventory, which contains 189 items (7 to 9 items for each of the 24 strengths, in nonsystematic order). The character strength of persistence, for example, is measured with items such as "When I start a project, I always finish it." Kindness is measured with items such as "I often do nice things for others without being asked." Respondents use a 5-point scale to indicate whether the item is *very much like me* (5) or *not like me at all* (1). Each scale includes one or more reverse-scored items.

Previous and current versions of the *VIA-Youth* have been completed by more than 1,400 middle and high school students of varying ethnicities and socioeconomic levels in seven states (Alabama, California, Nebraska, New Jersey, Ohio, Pennsylvania, and Texas). These inventories were administered in a group format during regular class times by the regular classroom teachers, who read the instructions aloud to students and answered their questions. Students completed the survey in 40 to 45 minutes.

A recent study with high school students provides promising evidence of the reliability and validity of the *VIA-Youth*. Along with measures of subjective well-being, the most recent version of the *VIA-Youth* was completed by 306 students in two different Philadelphia public schools (46% 8th graders, 30% 9th graders, and 24% 10th graders). The sample was evenly divided between males and females. Fifty-three percent identified themselves as African American, 27%

Table 1. Psychometrics of VIA-Youth Scales

	Number of items	Cronbach's alpha	Mean (SD)
1. Wisdom and knowledge			
Creativity	7	0.86	3.72 (0.80)
Curiosity	7	0.76	3.73 (0.74)
Judgment/critical thinking	8	0.85	3.61 (0.76)
Love of learning	8	0.87	3.63 (0.86)
Perspective	8	0.84	3.66 (0.78)
2. Courage			
Bravery	8	0.78	3.62 (0.71)
Industry/perseverance	8	0.82	3.75 (0.79)
Authenticity/honesty	8	0.75	3.41 (0.76)
Zest	7	0.73	3.67 (0.73)
3. Humanity			
Love/intimacy	7	0.85	4.00 (0.86)
Kindness	8	0.81	3.83 (0.77)
Social intelligence	8	0.77	3.71 (0.70)
4. Justice			
Teamwork/citizenship	8	0.78	3.69 (0.73)
Fairness	8	0.74	3.66 (0.72)
Leadership	7	0.84	3.48 (0.86)
5. Temperance			
Forgiveness/mercy	7	0.76	3.24 (0.78)
Modesty/humility	8	0.73	3.51 (0.70)
Prudence	8	0.70	3.27 (0.69)
Self-control/self-regulation	9	0.66	3.23 (0.67)
6. Transcendence			
Awe/appreciation	7	0.82	3.59 (0.95)
Gratitude	7	0.85	4.14 (0.75)
Hope	7	0.82	3.88 (0.77)
Playfulness	7	0.81	3.91 (0.79)
Spirituality	7	0.85	3.37 (1.06)

as White, 8% as Latino, 5% as Asian American, 1% as Native American, and 6% as "other."

Overall, mean scores for all character strengths were in the positive range but still showed variation (Table 1). Most scales had moderate to satisfactory Cronbach's alphas (.66 to .87), although the strengths of temperance proved more difficult to measure reliably than other strengths. The results showed gender differences. Girls scored higher than boys on a number of the strengths (e.g., appreciation of beauty, open-mindedness, gratitude, kindness, love, perspective, spirituality; all $ps < .05$). Interestingly, boys never scored higher than girls, a finding in need of an explanation. Age differences were also observed. In general, 10th graders scored higher than 8th graders on most of the strengths, although 10th graders showed a slight decrease in the strengths of temperance and spirituality (all $ps < .05$). There were no meaningful ethnic differences on any of the scales except for spirituality, where non-White students (especially African Americans) scored higher than White students ($p < .001$).

The results also support the validity of the *VIA-Youth*. Students' subjective well-being correlated with most of the interpersonal strengths, a finding consistent with results from our studies of adults ($ps < .001$). Strengths of temperance predicted grades in English, math, and science courses, even when ability test scores were controlled ($ps < .01$).

Principal component analysis of scale scores using varimax rotation suggested a four-factor solution—not surprisingly, a somewhat simpler structure than the five- or six-factor solution we usually find for adults (Peterson et al., in press). We tentatively identified three of these factors as being akin to basic traits captured in the Big Five taxonomy of personality—conscientiousness (prudence, self-control, persistence), openness to experience (creativity, curiosity, zest), and agreeableness (kindness, fairness, forgiveness)—plus a fourth factor comprised mainly of St. Paul's theological virtues (spirituality, hope, love). As we develop the *VIA-Youth* further and obtain larger samples, additional exploratory and confirmatory factor analyses both of individual items and scale scores are needed to confirm this solution.

Studies with previous versions of the *VIA-Youth* further support the validity of the scale (Dahlsgaard, Davis, Peterson, & Seligman, 2002). Students' self-nominations of strengths correlated with the majority of the corresponding scale scores on the *VIA-Youth*. Teacher nominations of student strengths correlated with the corresponding student scale scores for about half of the strengths—those manifest in everyday behavior as opposed to those requiring specific occasions (like an experience of fear or threat for the display of courage). Also, teacher ratings of student popularity correlated with interpersonal strengths.

Conclusions

Almost all of the strengths in the VIA Classification have been subjected to empirical research using various strategies of assessment (Peterson & Seligman, in press). Despite likely links, however, these lines of research have been conducted in isolation from one another, in part because an efficient battery of strength measures has not existed. The *VIA-Youth* allows 24 different strengths to be assessed comprehensively and efficiently, making possible research that looks at the joint and interactive effects of different character strengths.

Furthermore, the *VIA-Youth* measures allow an investigator to control for one strength while ascertaining the correlates or consequences of another. Conclusions can thereby be drawn more clearly. For example, a researcher using these measures would be able to say that spirituality has (or does not have) consequences beyond the contributions of associated strengths such as hope, a conclusion not possible if only measures of spirituality are used in the study.

The *VIA-Youth* measures can be used in applied research to evaluate prevention and intervention programs for positive youth development. Roth and Brooks-Gunn (2003) reported that character building is the second most frequently cited goal of youth development programs. Despite growing interest in character education curricula and wellness promotion programs, empirical validation of their effectiveness is scant. In some cases, strengths of character are the explicit outcome of interest, and in other cases, one or another character strength is proposed as a mediator or moderator of the effects of the intervention on other outcomes. The availability of our character measures will allow such interventions to be rigorously evaluated and perhaps will lead to the discovery of unanticipated effects of interventions. Eventually, this information will provide a concrete basis for designing effective youth development programs.

In addition, the *VIA-Youth* may have some utility—theoretical and practical—when scored ipsatively. That is, its scales not only allow comparisons and contrasts of character strength scores among individuals and groups, they also can be used to identify an individual's "signature strengths" relative to his or her other strengths (Seligman, 2002).

Although we have concluded that the measures we have developed are efficient, they are not as instantaneous as exit interviews, and they would be expensive if used with state or national samples. Our surveys take time to complete, and younger respondents require supervision to prevent breakoff effects due to wandering attention. As we noted, *VIA-Youth* is not designed for practitioners looking for single indicators of character strengths. Character strengths are sufficiently complex that a single-indicator approach to their assessment poses serious limitations. Anyone interested in assessing character strengths needs to appreciate that there is no shortcut to measuring character.

Self-report seems to be a valid way of measuring psychological constructs, but we still have lingering concerns about social desirability with the *VIA-Youth*. A youth development leader might inadvertently "teach to the test." Also, survey methods based on self-report have obvious limitations for measuring character strengths among very young children or children with certain disabilities. Accordingly, in order to improve validity, assessment should include alternative methods such as informant reports and observations. Structured interviews to measure character strengths also deserve attention.

Finally, although we have argued that the character strengths in the VIA Classification are ubiquitously valued—perhaps universally so—there is a need to test this argument with cross-national and cross-cultural data. We have so far surveyed respondents from almost 50 different nations about character strengths that are most valued. Such results will tell us which strengths should ultimately be included in the final version of our classification.

Authors' Note

We appreciate the feedback on this chapter provided at the Indicators of Positive Development Conference on March 12–13, 2003, in Washington, DC, especially by Daniel Hart. With gratitude, we acknowledge the encouragement and support of the Manuel D. and Rhoda Mayerson Foundation in creating the Values in Action Institute, a nonprofit organization dedicated to the development of a scientific knowledge base of human strengths. And we thank Katherine Dahlsgaard, Angela Duckworth, Martin Seligman, and Jennifer Yu for their help. Address correspondence to Christopher Peterson, Department of Psychology, University of Michigan, 525 East University, Ann Arbor, MI 48109-1109 (chrispet@umich.edu).

Appendix

VIA Classification of Character Strengths

1. **Wisdom and knowledge**—cognitive strengths that entail the acquisition and use of knowledge.
   - *Creativity*: Thinking of novel and productive ways to do things; includes artistic achievement but is not limited to it.
   - *Curiosity*: Taking an interest in all of ongoing experience; finding all subjects and topics fascinating; exploring and discovering.
   - *Judgment/critical thinking*: Thinking things through and examining them from all sides; *not* jumping to conclusions; being able to change one's mind in light of evidence; weighing all evidence fairly.
   - *Love of learning*: Mastering new skills, topics, and bodies of knowledge, whether on one's own or formally; obviously related to the strength of curiosity but goes beyond it to describe the tendency to add *systematically* to what one knows.
   - *Perspective*: Being able to provide wise counsel to others; having ways of looking at the world that make sense to the self and to other people.
2. **Courage**—emotional strengths that involve the exercise of will to accomplish goals in the face of opposition, external or internal.
   - *Bravery*: *Not* shrinking from threat, challenge, difficulty, or pain; speaking up for what is right even if there is opposition; acting on convictions even if unpopular; includes physical bravery but is not limited to it.
   - *Industry/perseverance*: Finishing what one starts; persisting in a course of action in spite of obstacles; "getting it out the door"; taking pleasure in completing tasks.
   - *Authenticity/honesty*: Speaking the truth but, more broadly, presenting oneself in a genuine way; being without pretense; taking responsibility for one's feelings and actions.
   - *Zest*: Approaching life with excitement and energy; *not* doing things halfway or halfheartedly; living life as an adventure; feeling alive and activated.
3. **Humanity**—interpersonal strengths that involve "tending" and "befriending" others (Taylor et al., 2000).
   - *Kindness*: Doing favors and good deeds for others; helping them; taking care of them.
   - *Love/intimacy*: Valuing close relations with others, in particular those in which sharing and caring are reciprocated; being close to people.
   - *Social intelligence*: Being aware of the motives and feelings of other people and the self; knowing what to do to fit into different social situations; knowing what makes other people tick.
4. **Justice**—civic strengths that underlie healthy community life.
   - *Teamwork/citizenship*: Working well as member of a group or team; being loyal to the group; doing one's share.
   - *Fairness*: Treating all people the same according to notions of fairness and justice; *not* letting personal feelings bias decisions about others; giving everyone a fair chance.
   - *Leadership*: Encouraging one's group to get things done and, at the same time, encouraging good relations within the group; organizing group activities and seeing that they happen.

5. **Temperance**—strengths that protect against excess.
   - *Forgiveness/mercy*: Forgiving those who have done wrong; giving people a second chance; *not* being vengeful.
   - *Modesty/humility*: Letting one's accomplishments speak for themselves; *not* seeking the spotlight; *not* regarding oneself as more special than one is.
   - *Prudence*: Being careful about one's choices; *not* taking undue risks; *not* saying or doing things that might later be regretted.
   - *Self-control/self-regulation*: Regulating what one feels and does; being disciplined; controlling one's appetites and emotions.
6. **Transcendence**—strengths that forge connections to the larger universe and provide meaning.
   - *Awe/appreciation of beauty and excellence*: Noticing and appreciating beauty, excellence, and/or skilled performance in all domains of life, from nature to art to mathematics to science to everyday experience.
   - *Gratitude*: Being aware of and thankful for the good things that happen; taking time to express thanks.
   - *Hope*: Expecting the best in the future and working to achieve it; believing that a good future is something that can be brought about.
   - *Playfulness*: Liking to laugh and tease; bringing smiles to other people; seeing the light side; making (not necessarily telling) jokes.
   - *Spirituality*: Having coherent beliefs about the higher purpose and meaning of the universe; knowing where one fits within the larger scheme; having beliefs about the meaning of life that shape conduct and provide comfort.

References

Allport, G. W. (1961). *Pattern and growth in personality*. New York: Holt, Rinehart, & Winston.

American Psychiatric Association. (1987). *Diagnostic and statistical manual of mental disorders* (3rd ed., Rev.). Washington, DC: Author.

Crowne, D. P., & Marlowe, D. (1964). *The approval motive: Studies in evaluative dependence*. New York: Wiley.

Dahlsgaard, K., Davis, D., Peterson, C., & Seligman, M. E. P. (2002, October 4). *Is virtue more than its own reward?* Poster presented at the First Positive Psychology International Summit (Washington, DC).

Erikson, E. (1963). *Childhood and society* (2nd ed.). New York: Norton.

Kohlberg, L. (1981). *Essays on moral development: Vol. 1. The philosophy of moral development*. New York: Harper & Row.

Kohlberg, L. (1984). *Essays on moral development: Vol. 2. The nature and validity of moral stages*. San Francisco: Harper & Row.

Peterson, C., & Park, N. (2003). Positive psychology as the even-handed positive psychologist views it. *Psychological Inquiry, 14*, 141–146.

Peterson, C., Park, N., & Seligman, M. E. P. (in press). Assessment of character strengths. In G. P. Koocher, J. C. Norcross, & S. S. Hill III (Eds.), *Psychologists' desk reference* (2nd ed.). New York: Oxford University Press.

Peterson, C., & Seligman, M. E. P. (2004). *Character strengths and virtues: A classification manual and handbook*. New York: Oxford University Press; Washington, DC: American Psychological Association.

Piaget, J. (1932). *Moral judgment of the child*. New York: Harcourt, Brace.

Roth, J. L., & Brooks-Gunn, J. (2003). Youth development programs: Risk, prevention, and policy. *Journal of Adolescent Health, 32*, 170–182.

Seligman, M. E. P. (2002). *Authentic happiness*. New York: Free Press.

Taylor, S. E., Klein, L. C., Lewis, B. P., Gruenewald, T. L., Gurung, R. A. R., & Updegraff, J. A. (2000). Biobehavioral responses to stress in females: Tend-and-befriend, not fight-or-flight. *Psychological Review, 107,* 422–429.

Wolf, S. (1982). Moral saints. *Journal of Philosophy, 79,* 419–439.

Yearley, L. H. (1990). *Mencius and Aquinas: Theories of virtue and conceptions of courage.* Albany: State University of New York Press.

3 Adolescent Spirituality

Peter L. Benson, Peter C. Scales, Arturo Sesma Jr., and Eugene C. Roehlkepartain

Search Institute

Interest in adolescent religious and spiritual development has risen sharply in recent years. Several major and recent reviews of positive youth development have moved this domain to center stage, positioning the spiritual religious domain as a developmental resource that lessens risk behavior and enhances positive outcomes (Bridges & Moore, 2002; Donahue & Benson, 1995; National Research Council and Institute of Medicine, 2002; Scales & Leffert, 1999). Moreover, there is substantial interest at the local and national level in "faith-based initiatives."

Although this dimension of adolescent development holds promise for inclusion in a pantheon of positive indicators, the selection or development of appropriate measures requires responses to several critical issues. One, of course, has to do with the definitional distinctions between the concepts of religion and spirituality. The research tradition strongly emphasizes the former. In that regard, the dominant measures used in quantitative studies are the degree of importance respondents attach to religion and the frequency of participation in religious communities (i.e., worship attendance at a mosque, synagogue, church, or other type of congregation).

These two measures are, one could argue, fairly superficial approaches to a domain that has a potentially rich array of belief, value, behavior, and communal dimensions. Any attempt to propose indicators worthy of serious attention must both begin with a thorough examination of the utility of these cursory measures and also look for potential measures that get more deeply inside the spiritual/religious domain. In addition, there is the issue of inclusivity. Much of the extant research has utilized samples of Christians in fairly conventional (i.e., institutional) settings. Accordingly, many of the efforts to measure deeper themes and dimensions utilize items and scales tailored to these samples. If there is any trend that describes the American spiritual/religious landscape, it is the growth and spread of new religious beliefs, practices, forms, and movements (Eck, 2001). Hence, a critical measurement issue has to do with how to capture this rich diversity of spiritual and religious energy.

The American Context

Although it varies in form and level of intensity, a high level of religious/spiritual engagement has been documented across cultures and in different societies. A Gallup International Association (1999) poll of 50,000 adults in 60 countries found that, on average, 87% of respondents consider themselves part of a religion, 63% indicate that God is highly important in their lives (between 7 and 10 on a 10-point scale), and 75% believe in either a personal God or "some sort of spirit or life force." There is wide variability across cultures in specific beliefs about religious or spiritual matters and in whether people participate in religious activities with significantly lower levels of religious involvement on some continents than religious affiliation or spiritual beliefs. Yet the overall patterns reinforce the idea that spirituality remains an important part of life around the globe, with some of the strongest commitments being evident in developing nations.

Also, self-reported religious/spiritual engagement by North Americans is far above the international average. A 2003 Gallup Poll in the United States showed that 61% of adults said religion was "very important" in their lives, with another 24% reporting it as "fairly important" (Gallup Poll News Service, 2004). Many have written about the high and persistent engagement percentages in the United States, particularly in comparison to Western Europe (Eck, 2001; Kerestes & Youniss, 2003; Wuthnow, 1994). This American pattern of engagement has remained fairly constant across the past several decades, in spite of sociological predictions that processes of modernization and secularization would lead to a significant withering of religious interest (Berger, 1999).

What has shifted, of course, is the diversity of religious forms. Harvard professor Diana Eck captures this theme in the title of her recent book, *A New Religious America: How a "Christian Country" Has Become the World's Most Religiously Diverse Nation* (Eck, 2001). This is the story of the rapid rise of Muslim, Hindu, and Buddhist communities. A second transformation of religious engagement is the rapid rise of Pentecostalism in the United States (and throughout Latin America and Africa). Finally, there is the growing number of American adults (and, one presumes, young people) who consider themselves "spiritual, but not religious" (Fuller, 2001; Smith, Faris, Denton, & Regnerus, 2003). Each of these changes provides additional challenge for developing indicators that capture the breadth and depth of religious/spiritual sentiment.

In a nation where religious/spiritual engagement is so normative, it is confounding that the field of psychology has by and large marginalized the inquiry of the development and consequences of the religious/spiritual impulse. Many scholars have documented the relative lack of research attention in mainstream psychology (Gorsuch, 1988; Paloutzian, 1996), within the study of adolescence

(Benson, Donahue, & Erickson, 1989; Bridges & Moore, 2002; Smith et al., 2003), and in child development (Nye, 1999). In addition, it should be noted that the highly touted volume, *A Psychology of Human Strengths: Fundamental Questions and Future Directions for a Positive Psychology*, recently published by the American Psychological Association (Aspinwall & Staudinger, 2003), pays no noticeable attention to religion or spirituality as human strength or predictor of strength. There is a persistent pattern here: When it comes to religion and spirituality, mainstream psychology keeps its distance.

The Religious Landscape of Adolescence

There are, nevertheless, a number of studies published in a variety of fields (social psychology, social work, sociology, the psychology of religion, sociology of religion, medicine, religious studies, education, public health) that constitute a body of knowledge from which we can learn. In building toward recommendations for measurement of spirituality/religion, we look first at literature on adolescence, relying heavily on two sources of data: One consists of ongoing national studies that include religiosity measures. These include Monitoring the Future and the National Longitudinal Study of Adolescent Health. The other is an aggregated sample of 217,277 students in grades 6–12 in public and alternative schools who completed the *Search Institute Profiles of Student Life: Attitudes and Behaviors* survey in the 1999–2000 school year. This self-selected sample—including urban, suburban, and rural schools—has been weighted to reflect the 1990 census data for community size and race/ethnicity. New analyses of this data set are used in this paper to probe into greater detail on the predictive utility of religiosity among adolescents, with a particular eye to testing how well patterns of relationships hold across demographic subgroups.[1]

Spiritual/Religious Engagement during Adolescence

The ongoing Monitoring the Future study (Bachman, Johnston, & O'Malley, 2000) shows that the religious engagement of American adolescents is both stable and changing. In the senior high school class of 2000, 83.7% reported affiliation with a religious denomination or tradition. Though affiliation is still dominated by Christian denominations, trends across 20 years (1976–1996) of Monitoring the Future studies show increases in the percentages of youth affiliating with non-Christian traditions (Smith, Denton, Faris, & Regnerus, 2002).

Several reexaminations of Monitoring the Future annual surveys of high school students show fairly high stability in both affiliation and self-reported religious service attendance across time (Donahue & Benson, 1995; Smith et al.,

---

[1] Greater details about this survey instrument and the concepts of developmental assets, thriving behavior, and risk behavior can be found in a series of publications (Benson, Scales, Leffert, & Roehlkepartain, 1999; Leffert et al., 1998; Scales, Benson, Leffert, & Blyth, 2000).

2002). From 1976 to 1996, only small declines were observed in both indicators (Smith et al., 2002). However, the major point is that, on general measures of engagement, the vast majority of American adolescents report affiliation and at least occasional service attendance.

Using the two most commonly used indicators of religious/spiritual engagement (importance or salience, and attendance), a comparison of two large sample studies conducted in 1999–2000 suggests that more than half of high school seniors are engaged at a meaningfully high level. Comparing seniors in 2000 via Monitoring the Future and seniors in 1999–2000 via the Search Institute (SI) composite data set across several hundred communities shows that both studies place frequent participation in a religious institution at about 50%, and both find the self-report of religion/spirituality as quite or very important to be above 50%.

The SI composite data set from 1999–2000 allows us to extend this descriptive portrait to grades 6 through 12, gender, race/ethnicity, city size, and maternal education. In this data set, religious attendance is measured with the question: "During an average week, how many hours do you spend going to groups, programs, or services at a church, synagogue, mosque, or other religions or spiritual place?" Response options are 0, 1, 2, 3–5, 6–10, and 11 or more. Religious importance (salience) is measured with the question: "How important is each of the following to you in your life: Being religious or spiritual?" There are five response options: *not important, somewhat important, not sure, quite important, very important*. Six findings by demographic groupings are reported here:

Grade Trends. Both religious participation and importance decline with grade: 70% of 6th-grade students reported 1 hour or more per week of participation, falling to 54% among 12th graders, with a fairly linear downward trend. However, the percentage reporting that religion or spirituality is "quite" or "very" important remained more stable across grades: grade 6, 55%; grade 7, 57%; grade 8, 55%; grade 9, 54%; grade 10, 53%; grade 11, 56%; and grade 12, 53%. There was, though, a slight increase in the percentage reporting that being religious or spiritual is "not important," from 10% in grade 6 to 16% in grade 12.

Gender Differences. As shown in many studies (Benson, 1992; Bridges & Moore, 2002; Donahue & Benson, 1995), females report higher levels of religious/spiritual engagement than males. In the SI composite data set, 65% of girls reported 1 hour or more per week of religious attendance, whereas 59% of boys reported that level of attendance. A small difference was also found for importance, with 58% of girls saying religion/spirituality is "quite" or "very" important compared with 52% of boys.

Race/Ethnicity. The major finding here is that the highest rates for participation and importance are reported by African American youth. This has been documented in a number of other studies (Benson et al., 1989; Benson & Donahue, 1989; Swanson, Spencer, Dell'Angelo, Harpalani, & Spencer, 2002).

City Size. The SI composite data set showed little variation in participation and importance rates across five categories of population size.

Maternal Education. This demographic item provides a glimpse of the relationship of religious engagement to socioeconomic status (SES), given the assumption that maternal education is a proxy for family income. Among studies of adults, religious engagement and SES tend to be inversely related. In this composite data set, however, we see some evidence for religious participation increasing with maternal education. For example, religious attendance of 1 hour or more per week was reported by 57.1% of youth whose mothers have a grade school education or less and by 68.7% of youth whose mothers have a graduate or professional education.

Salience and Attendance Combined. Although attendance and importance (or salience) are commonly used indicators, we have not seen any previous attempt to look at how responses to these two items combine. At a descriptive level, and in anticipation of questions about what items to recommend for a "spirituality index," it is useful to discover how these items interrelate, beyond the fact that the correlation between them is .47 ($N = 216,383$) in the SI composite data set. Since one of the two items (attendance) has an institutional face, and the other (importance) more directly taps salience or commitment, it seems likely that there will be cases both where adolescents are institutionally active but report low importance (a combination that could emerge where teenagers are compelled by parents to attend) and where the reverse is true (that is, high importance, low attendance). This category represents what some presume to be in the United States a growing form of spiritual expression (i.e., importance)— and perhaps even an active life of practice—outside religious institutions or communal expressions of spirituality.

To describe these categories of religious/spiritual engagement, we created two binary variables: low/high importance and low/high attendance. For the religious/spiritual importance item, *not important, somewhat important,* and *not sure* are coded as low, whereas *quite important* and *very important* are coded as high. For the attendance item, 0 hours per week is coded as low; 1 hour or more per week is coded as high.

Results are shown in Table 1. For the total sample ($N = 216,383$), 44.6% are high/high and 27.7% are low/low. As expected, particularly during adolescence, there is a sizable percentage (18%) that combine high attendance with low importance. There are multiple explanations for this phenomenon. As noted earlier, this could be the result of parental pressure. Equally probable, however, is that the social/friendship aspect of participation is the primary motivator for some young people's attendance in programs, activities, and services, not

Table 1. Percentage Reporting Importance and/or Participation, by Gender, Grade, and Race/Ethnicity[a]

| | | | Low | Low | High | High | High on importance |
| | Religious/spiritual importance: | | Low | Low | High | High | |
	Participation in religious community:		Low	High	Low	High	and/or participation
		N	%	%	%	%	%
Total		216,383	27.7	18.0	9.7	44.6	72.3
Gender	Male	102,377	30.7	18.1	10.0	41.2	69.3
	Female	112,406	24.9	17.9	9.6	47.6	75.1
Grade	6	25,822	21.6	24.1	8.5	45.8	79.4
	7	27,395	22.7	21.2	8.6	47.5	77.3
	8	47,314	25.3	19.9	8.8	45.9	74.7
	9	30,108	28.8	17.6	10.2	43.4	71.2
	10	37,497	31.7	15.8	10.4	42.1	68.3
	11	29,000	30.5	13.1	11.0	45.3	69.5
	12	18,903	34.6	12.9	11.5	41.1	65.4
Race/ ethnicity	Native American	2,085	34.2	22.0	12.3	31.4	65.8
	Asian/Pacific Islander	6,485	30.4	17.5	16.3	35.9	69.6
	African American	29,395	17.1	18.9	12.8	51.1	82.9
	Hispanic	22,716	26.3	19.8	14.7	39.1	73.7
	White	147,073	29.6	17.5	8.0	44.9	70.4
	Biracial	8,628	29.8	17.8	11.3	41.2	70.2

Source: Search Institute (2003). Unpublished tabulations.
[a] For the religious/spiritual importance item, not important, somewhat important, and not sure are coded as low; quite important and very important are coded as high. For the attendance items, 0 hours of attendance at programs or services per week is coded as low; 1 hour or more is coded as high.

necessarily religious or spiritual importance. Finally, some youth spend time in religious institutions participating in youth programs that may or may not have an explicitly religious or spiritual theme. An after-school tutoring program, for example, may be based in a congregation's facility but be largely secular in orientation. In addition, about 1 in 10 of the young people in this sample (9.7%) attach high importance to religion/spirituality, yet report no attendance, with percentages ranging from 8.5% in grade 6 to 11.5% in grade 12.

We also combined percentages for youth high on one or both items to yield a global indicator of religious/spiritual engagement. Overall, 72.3% of the total sample met this condition (high on one or both). This combination puts into perspective the normative nature of religious/spiritual engagement in the United States. That is, nearly three of four adolescents in this 6th- to 12th-grade sample evidence either importance or attendance (or both). Although the national representativeness of the SI composite sample cannot be directly ascertained, as noted above, the SI sample and the Monitoring the Future sample (which is drawn to be representative of American high schools) are quite equivalent on these two indicators of engagement.

In further describing American adolescents, these two findings are important: Two-thirds or more of youth in each race/ethnicity category are "high" on one or both indicators. The percentages move from a low of 65.8% for Native Americans to 82.9% for African Americans. Also, the type composed of high importance/low institutional attendance is more common for each category of minority youth (e.g., Hispanic, Black, Native American, Asian, biracial) than it is for Whites.

Developmental Patterns

Few longitudinal studies exist to describe how religious/spiritual engagement changes during adolescence (Bridges & Moore, 2002). Although all theorists expect adolescence to be a time of tradition testing, there are few data other than cross-sectional studies (e.g., Monitoring the Future and the SI composite data set) that can speak to developmental trajectories. However, an ongoing longitudinal study employing the *Search Institute Profiles of Student Life: Attitudes and Behaviors* instrument provides an initial and tentative look at these patterns. The sample consists of 370 students who completed the survey in fall 1997 (grades 6, 7, or 8), fall 1998, and fall 2001. All students attend school in a fairly heterogeneous suburb of a midwestern metropolitan area. For the total sample, 35.5% remained low on religious importance from 1997 to 2001, and 31.1% stayed high during that time. Another 20% changed from high to low across the 4 years, and 13% changed from low to high. By this fairly global measure, the data suggest that overall, about two-thirds of youth stay constant in religious importance across 4 years, while one-third experience a shift (either low to high or high to low). Patterns for boys and girls are similar.

Predicting Developmental Outcomes

Numerous studies have shown that religion/spirituality functions as a protective factor, inoculating youth against health-compromising behavior. These relationships have been summarized in a number of reviews (Benson et al., 1989; Benson, Roehlkepartain, & Rude, 2003; Bridges & Moore, 2002; Donahue & Benson, 1995; Kerestes & Youniss, 2003). What we tend to see across dozens of studies are low but significant zero-order correlations between measures of salience and attendance and multiple indicators of risk behavior (e.g., substance use, violence, and onset of sexual activity). As an overall generalization, these studies—which also use multivariate procedures to control for key demographics (such as age, gender, and race)—tend to find significant but very modest effects for religion, as measured by salience and attendance.

The large SI data set permits analyses that can extend this line of inquiry on the predictive and explanatory power of salience and attendance. We are particularly interested in how well these relationships generalize across race/ethnicity and gender and to the concept of thriving. Table 2 describes 10 types of risk behavior and 8 types of thriving that are measured in this composite data set. Table 3 reveals several important patterns as we examine zero-order correlations of salience and attendance with these 18 indicators. All of the relationships are in the hypothesized direction (that is, salience and attendance are

Table 2. Definitions of Risk Behavior Patterns and Thriving Indicators

Risk Behavior

Alcohol	Has had alcohol three or more times in the past month or got drunk once or more in the past two weeks.
Tobacco	Smokes one or more cigarettes every day or uses chewing tobacco frequently.
Illicit drugs	Used illicit drugs three or more times in the past year.
Sexual activity	Has had sexual intercourse three or more times in a lifetime.
Depression/suicide	Is frequently depressed and/or has attempted suicide.
Antisocial behavior	Has been involved in three or more incidents of shoplifting, trouble with police, or vandalism in the past year.
Violence	Has engaged in three or more acts of fighting, hitting, injuring a person, carrying or using a weapon, or threatening physical harm in the past year.
School problems	Has skipped two or more days in the past month and/or has below a C average.
Driving and drinking	Has driven after drinking or ridden with a drinking driver three or more times in the past year.
Gambling	Has gambled three or more times in the past year.

Thriving Indicator

Succeeds in school	Self-reported grades are A's or mostly A's.
Helps others	Helps friends or neighbors one or more hours per week.
Values diversity	Places high importance on getting to know people of other racial/ethnic groups.
Maintains good health	Pays attention to healthy nutrition and exercise.
Exhibits leadership	Has been a leader of a group or organization in the last 12 months.
Resists danger	Avoids doing things that are dangerous.
Controls impulses	Self-reports tendency to "save money for something special..."
Overcomes adversity	Self-reports ability to navigate through hardship.

related *negatively* to risk and *positively* to thriving). Nearly all the correlations are extremely modest. These patterns generalize to gender and race/ethnicity subgroups. Finally, predictions appear to be stronger for thriving than for risk behaviors.

We ran three-step regression models (grade and gender, salience and attendance, interaction of salience and attendance) on the overall longitudinal study sample ($N = 370$) described earlier, generally finding that salience and attendance account for roughly 3% to 5% of the variance on many of the risk and thriving measures. Although these are modest effects, they both replicate the kinds of effect sizes for religion measures in the National Longitudinal Study on Adolescent Health (Resnick et al., 1997) and roughly equal the effects shown for other protective factors such as self-esteem and parental presence.

We are also interested in exploring the degree to which the salience and attendance measures interact. Preliminarily, we note that the two dimensions have an additive effect as shown in Table 4.

What accounts for the constant and generalizable relationship between the two religion/spirituality measures and both risk behavior and thriving? A fairly recent line of inquiry supports the hypothesis that developmental assets mediate

Table 3. Correlations of Religious/Spiritual Importance and Participation with Risk Behaviors and Thriving Indicators, by Gender and Race/Ethnicity

| | Total Sample | | Gender | | | | Race/Ethnicity | | | | | | | | | |
| | | | Male | | Female | | Native American | | Asian | | Black | | Hispanic | | White | |
	I	P	I	P	I	P	I	P	I	P	I	P	I	P	I	P
Risk Behaviors																
Alcohol	-17	-15	-16	-13	-18	-16	-11	-11	-08	-06	-10	-09	-14	-10	-18	-16
Antisocial behavior	-17	-10	-16	-08	-16	-09	-14	-07	-07	-04	-15	-08	-15	-04	-19	-12
Driving and drinking	-12	-12	-12	-11	-13	-12	-07	-07	-04	-06	-07	-08	-12	-09	-14	-13
Depression/suicide	-08	-04	-07	-04	-11	-07	-04	02	-01	-01	-02	01	-05	-02	-10	-06
Illicit drugs	-17	-14	-16	-13	-17	-15	-10	-12	-07	-05	-12	-12	-15	-10	-18	-15
Gambling	-09	-08	-08	-07	-07	-05	-04	-07	-06	-05	-07	-07	-07	-05	-11	-09
School problems	-17	-13	-16	-14	-16	-12	-13	-13	-04	-07	-15	-12	-16	-10	-20	-17
Sexual activity	-13	-12	-11	-09	-14	14	-11	-11	-04	-06	-07	-11	-09	-07	-17	-16
Tobacco	-14	-13	-12	-11	-17	-15	-12	-09	-05	-03	-08	-08	-11	-07	-15	-14
Violence	-12	-06	-11	-05	-11	-04	-07	-05	-03	-01	-12	-05	-12	-04	-15	-09
Thriving Indicators																
Resists danger	14	11	11	08	13	11	07	10	09	02	10	08	08	05	13	09
Values diversity	23	12	24	14	19	09	26	13	21	07	20	11	23	10	22	12
Maintains good health	16	15	19	16	14	14	16	13	10	10	06	10	13	14	19	15
Controls impulses	10	09	11	09	10	8	13	11	09	05	07	08	11	09	11	09
Helps others	06	19	07	20	04	17	07	25	07	24	06	27	06	20	06	17
Exhibits leadership	14	20	13	20	15	20	11	15	10	19	12	18	08	17	15	21
Overcomes adversity	05	04	04	02	07	06	-02	-05	00	02	05	02	03	01	06	05
Succeeds in school	15	12	14	13	15	10	12	12	03	07	15	12	15	10	19	16

Note: I = degree of importance on religion/spirituality; P = hours per week participating in programs and services in a religious community.
Source: Search Institute (2003). Unpublished tabulations.

*Table 4. Relationship of Importance and Participation to Risk Behaviors
and Thriving Indicators*

Religious/Spiritual Importance:	Low	Low	High	High
Participation in Religious Community:	Low	High	Low	High
	%	%	%	%
Risk Behaviors				
Alcohol	31.7	23.9	24.3	15.9
Antisocial behavior	26.4	22.0	20.6	13.4
Driving and drinking	21.9	16.3	20.0	12.0
Depression/suicide	27.7	24.3	25.9	19.0
Illicit drugs	24.4	14.7	19.0	9.2
Gambling	20.2	16.4	19.4	13.5
School problems	28.4	22.7	25.7	14.6
Sexual activity	24.3	16.2	23.2	12.5
Tobacco	19.2	10.9	14.0	6.7
Violence	38.3	34.9	34.8	26.5
Thriving Indicators				
Values diversity	53.0	57.8	70.0	69.6
Resists danger	18.7	22.4	25.8	27.3
Maintains good health	44.8	54.3	53.1	63.0
Controls impulses	41.0	44.2	45.3	50.3
Helps others	75.0	85.5	73.4	86.6
Exhibits leadership	58.2	69.5	58.3	77.0
Overcomes adversity	68.2	68.4	67.9	74.7
Succeeds in school	17.3	18.0	16.3	28.2

Note: N = 217,277.
Source: Search Institute (2003). Unpublished tabulations.

the influence of religion.[2] That is, religious contexts afford the kind of asset-building resources—such as intergenerational relationships, caring neighborhood, adult role models—known to facilitate positive development (Benson et al., 2003; Wagener, Furrow, King, Leffert, & Benson, 2003). For example, in Search Institute's large data set, the correlation among attendance at religious services or programs and the developmental assets is a moderate .38 for external assets and .26 for the internal assets, and both external and internal assets are moderately negatively related to risk behaviors and positively related to thriving behaviors (correlations between .47 and .60).

A recent analysis using ordinary least squares regression provides strong evidence that religious engagement does enhance the developmental asset landscape (Wagener et al., 2003). A related study, using a national sample of 614 adolescents (ages 12 to 17 years), provides strong evidence that frequency of attendance is related to positive engagement with adults outside of one's family

---

[2] For a review of the categories of developmental assets—support, empowerment, boundaries and expectations, constructive use of time, commitment to learning, positive values, social competencies, and positive identity—see Benson, 1997; Benson, Leffert, Scales, & Blyth, 1998; and, linked to the religious context, Roehlkepartain, 1998.

(Scales, Benson, & Mannes, 2003). Such networks of adult relationships can be powerful influences on both risk behaviors and thriving (Scales & Leffert, 1999).[3]

Beyond Salience and Attendance

Based on analyses of two indicators (importance or salience, and participation) of the religious/spirituality domain, several conclusions seem warranted. The two are connected to gender and grade in ways that theory predicts. The two individually (and perhaps additively) predict many important measures of developmental success, serving simultaneously as protective factors (risk indicators) and enhancement factors (thriving indicators). These effects generalize across gender and race/ethnicity. Further, religious/spiritual importance, attendance, or both are clearly quite normative for American adolescents. Hence, it is suggested that this religious/spiritual dimension belongs in any comprehensive attempt to measure developmental resources and/or developmental success.

Nevertheless, the predictive and explanatory power of these two religion/spirituality indices is very modest. It is not difficult to posit some of the factors that might suppress the relationships. Particularly salient is that the items are so global they mask what could be great variation in depth, belief, ideology, and experience. Single items on attendance, for example, tell nothing about quality, relationships, climate, or developmental attentiveness within places and programs. Similarly, global importance/salience items mask considerable variability in worldview, belief, value, and behavioral intent.

By analogy, imagine an item that asks, "Do you identify with a political party?" It is reasonable to expect that citizens who do identify with a party demonstrate small increases in civic engagement and related forms of connectedness compared with those who do not identify. If we also know which political worldview (e.g., Democrat, Republican, Green) a person holds, the predictive power would be greatly enhanced. In contrast, however, one's specific religious affiliation (Catholic, Jewish, Baptist, etc.)—another common measure of religiousness—is typically not a strong predictor of one's specific beliefs, practices, or behaviors (Matthews et al., 1999; McCullough, Larson, Koenig, & Lerner, 1999).

The critical question is how to deepen measurement within the spiritual/religious domain so that we can better capture the dynamics that enhance developmental success. Several criteria should guide this effort. One is about inclusivity. That is, indices of spiritual/religious life cannot assume, in a religiously diverse culture, a particular religious ideology. They cannot assume monotheism (that is, a creator God as found in Christian, Jewish, and Muslim traditions). And

---

[3] Several recent publications build on this research to suggest strategies for enhancing the developmental impact of religious communities of multiple faiths (e.g., Roehlkepartain, 1998; Roehlkepartain, 2003a; Roehlkepartain, 2003b; Roehlkepartain & Scales, 1995).

they cannot assume any particular ideology about diversity, eschatology, human nature, spiritual transformation (e.g., conversion), or particular practices.

A second criterion is that any new measure of this domain ought to enhance prediction of developmental outcomes beyond what is predicted by importance and attendance items. Although there is a long tradition, particularly within psychology of religion research, to develop multidimensional measures of personal theology and worldview, we are best served by searching for or developing a unidimensional scale composed of multiple items that provide high variability along a single continuum.

There is a body of research that demonstrates that various dimensions of religious belief can have a sizable influence on behavior—beyond the impact of attendance and salience (Benson & Williams, 1986). However, such dimensions apply only to those who are already connected to a specific religious tradition. Hence, although this approach is promising for developing a "deeper" measure capable of meeting criterion 2, it violates criterion 1.

Third, new measures must be concise enough to be practical for use in multiple instruments and studies. Finally, there are land mines that need to be understood and navigated around before a new spiritual/religious index receives full public support (e.g., active parental consent, as well as concerns about separation of church and state and the establishment of religion).

It is beyond the scope of this chapter to propose a multi-item scale that meets all of these criteria. If we were to propose such a scale, it would not only include items such as the importance and attendance indicators analyzed in this study, but also capture greater depth.

Significant conceptual, definitional, and measurement work needs to be done to move measurement to a next stage. Moving to greater depth in measurement requires a sustained effort to define and disentangle the constructs of spirituality and religion. Although many have tried, consensus on these definitions proves elusive.

The vast majority of researchers agree that spirituality has multiple domains. For example, Scott (as cited in Zinnbauer, Pargament, & Scott, 1999) analyzed the content of scientific definitions of religiousness and spirituality published in the last half of the 20th century. Although she found no consensus or even dominant approaches, Scott identified nine content categories in definitions of spirituality: experiences of connectedness or relationship; processes leading to greater connectedness; behavioral responses to something (either sacred or secular); systems of thought or beliefs; traditional institutional structures; pleasurable states of being; beliefs in the sacred, transcendent, and so forth; attempts at or capacities for transcendence; and existential questions. In another study, MacDonald (2000) analyzed 20 measures of spirituality, identifying five "robust dimensions of spirituality" (p. 185): cognitive orientation, an experiential/phenomenological dimension, existential well-being, paranormal beliefs, and religiousness.

Because of its multidimensionality, spirituality does not fit neatly inside any particular domain of social science. Hill et al. (2000) noted that religion and spirituality inherently involve developmental, social-psychological phenomena, cognitive phenomena, affective and emotional phenomena, and personality. They note that "few phenomena may be as integral across life span development as religious or spiritual concerns" (p. 53). Further, Piedmont (1999) presents evidence that spirituality may be an independent dimension of personality. Thus a multidisciplinary approach is essential to develop a comprehensive understanding of the domain.

A persistent and important definitional, measurement, and philosophical challenge is distinguishing spirituality from religiosity and distinguishing spiritual development from religious development. Is spirituality little more than a "politically correct" term for religiousness? Are spirituality and religiousness unique, polarized domains? Is one embedded within the other? How are they related and distinct? The answers to those questions depend, of course, on how one defines both religion and spirituality.

Furthermore, in the same way that spirituality is itself complex and multidimensional, so is religion (Hood, Spilka, Hunsberger, & Gorsuch, 1996). Pargament (1997) defined religion broadly as "a search for significance in ways related to the sacred" (p. 34). Koenig, McCullough, and Larson (2001) defined religion more specifically as "an organized system of beliefs, practices, rituals, and symbols designed (a) to facilitate closeness to the sacred or transcendent (God, higher power, or ultimate truth/reality) and (b) to foster an understanding of one's relationship and responsibility to others in living together in community" (p. 18). In examining the relationship between religion and spirituality, Reich (1996) identified four possibilities: religion and spirituality as synonymous or fused; one as a subdomain of the other; religion and spirituality as separate domains; and religion and spirituality as distinct but overlapping domains.

There is considerable evidence (largely from studies of adults) that people experience religion and spirituality as overlapping but not synonymous domains. For example, a nationally representative sample of 1,422 U.S. adults who responded to a special ballot on religion and spirituality as part of the 1998 General Social Survey found high correlation (.63) between self-perceptions of religiosity and spirituality (Shahabi et al., 2002). Similarly, Marler and Hadaway (2002) examined data from several national U.S. studies (again, of adults) that examined this question and concluded that

> the relationship between "being religious" and "being spiritual" is not a zero-sum. In fact, these data demonstrate that "being religious" and "being spiritual" are most often seen as distinct but interdependent concepts. . . . Indeed, the most significant finding about the relationship between "being religious" and "being spiritual" is that most Americans see themselves as both. (p. 297)

The explosion of interest in spirituality as a legitimate arena of scientific inquiry is promising. It is also complex, and no clear consensus about definitions is on the horizon. Furthermore, a scan of published studies using "spirituality" measures located no data that show strong predictive or explanatory relationships with risk behavior or thriving.

One other line of inquiry needs to be included to ascertain possibilities for items and indicators that meet the criteria, described earlier. There is a body of literature that explores how and to what degree religious sentiment (in whatever form) compels (or implores) one to be engaged in the world. In general terms, this is the distinction between "vertical" and "horizontal" themes. Vertical refers to the degree to which one honors/listens to/affirms/accepts the sacred dimension of experience (whether this is understood as God, Allah, life force, or spirit). The horizontal dimension refers to the degree to which spiritual/religious belief pushes one toward a compassionate engagement in the world. Several studies of American adolescents show that these two dimensions—individually and in combination—are stronger predictors of risk and thriving than are measures of importance or attendance (Benson, Donahue, & Erickson, 1993; Benson, Williams, & Johnson, 1987; Benson, Yeager, Wood, Guerra, & Manno, 1986). The salient dimension that cuts across these vertical and horizontal dimensions is the degree to which one's spiritual-religious engagement is about "me" or "we": that is, does spirituality/religion function to promote individualism or community?

This and other research traditions on religious themes and dynamics are fertile territories for locating possible indicators that discriminate and predict. It is too early, however, to definitively name and advocate for a particular set of indicators that simultaneously honor diversity in orientation and add explanatory power for developmental success. However, emerging initiatives (e.g., Roehlkepartain, King, Wagener, & Benson, in preparation) hold promise for developing the kinds of conceptual clarity, advances in measurement, and predictive studies that will and should inform this search for inclusive and impactful indicators.

References

Aspinwall, L. G., & Standinger, U. M. (2003). *A psychology of human strengths: Fundamental questions and future directions for a positive psychology.* Washington, DC: American Psychological Association.

Bachman, J., Johnston, L. D., & O'Malley, P. M. (2000). *Monitoring the future.* Ann Arbor: University of Michigan, Institute for Social Research.

Benson, P. L. (1992). Patterns of religious development in adolescence and adulthood. *Psychologists Interested in Religious Issues Newsletter (APA Division 36), 17*(2), 2–9.

Benson, P. L. (1997). *All kids are our kids: What communities must do to raise caring and responsible children and adolescents.* San Francisco: Jossey-Bass.

Benson, P. L., & Donahue, M. J. (1989). Ten-year trends in at-risk behavior: A national study of Black adolescents. *Journal of Adolescent Research, 4*(2), 125–139.

Benson, P. L., Donahue, M. J., & Erickson, J. A. (1989). Adolescence and religion: A review of the literature from 1970 to 1986. *Research in the Social Scientific Study of Religion, 1,* 153–181.

Benson, P. L., Donahue, M. J., &. Erickson, J. A. (1993). The faith maturity scale: Conceptualization, measurement, and empirical validation. *Research in the Social Scientific Study of Religion, 5,* 1–26.

Benson, P. L., Leffert, N., Scales, P. C., & Blyth, D. A. (1998). Beyond the "village" rhetoric: Creating healthy communities for children and adolescents. *Applied Developmental Science, 2*(3), 138–159.

Benson, P. L., Roehlkepartain, E. C., & Rude, S. P. (2003). Spiritual development in childhood and adolescence: Toward a field of inquiry. *Applied Developmental Science, 7*(3), 205–213.

Benson, P. L., Scales, P. C., Leffert, N., & Roehlkepartain, E. C. (1999). *A fragile foundation: The state of developmental assets among American youth.* Minneapolis: Search Institute.

Benson, P. L., & Williams, D. L. (1986). *Religion on Capitol Hill: Myths and realities.* New York: Oxford University Press.

Benson, P. L., Williams, D., & Johnson, A. (1987). *The quicksilver years: The hopes and fears of early adolescence.* San Francisco: Harper & Row.

Benson, P. L., Yeager, R. J., Wood, P. K., Guerra, M. J., & Manno, B. V. (1986). *Catholic high schools: Their impact on low-income students.* Washington, DC: National Catholic Educational Association.

Berger, P. (1999). *The desecularization of the world: Resurgent religion and world politics.* Grand Rapids, MI: Eerdmans.

Bridges, L. J., & Moore, K. A. (2002). *Religion and spirituality in childhood and adolescence.* Washington, DC: Child Trends.

Donahue, M. J., & Benson P. L. (1995). Religion and the well-being of adolescents. *Journal of Social Issues, 51*(2), 145–160.

Eck, D. L. (2001). *A new religious America: How a "Christian country" has become the world's most religiously diverse nation.* San Francisco: Harper.

Fuller, R. C. (2001). *Spiritual, but not religious: Understanding unchurched America.* New York: Oxford University Press.

Gallup International Association. (1999). *Gallup international millennium survey.* Accessed on September 9, 2002, from www.gallup-international.com/surveys1.htm.

Gallup News Service (2004, March 2). American public opinion about religion. *Focus on Religion.* Accessed on March 4, 2004, from www.gallup.com.

Gorusch, R. L. (1988). Psychology of religion. *Annual Review of Psychology, 39,* 201–221.

Hill, P. C., Pargament, K. I., Hood, R. W., McCullough, M. E., Swyers, J. P., Larson, D. B., et al. (2000). Conceptualizing religion and spirituality: Points of commonality, points of departure. *Journal for the Theory of Social Behavior, 30*(1), 52–77.

Hood, R. W., Spilka, B., Hunsberger, B., & Gorsuch, R. (1996). *The psychology of religion: An empirical approach* (2nd ed.). New York: Guilford Press.

Kerestes, M., & Youniss, J. E. (2003). Rediscovering the importance of religion in adolescent development. In R. M. Lerner, F. Jacobs, & D. Wertlieb (Eds.), *Handbook of applied developmental science: Vol. 1. Applying developmental science for youth and families.* Thousand Oaks, CA: Sage.

Koenig, H. G., McCullough, M. E., & Larson, D. B. (2001). *Handbook of religion and health.* Oxford: Oxford University Press.

Leffert, N., Benson, P. L., Scales, P. C., Sharma, A. R., Drake, D. R., & Blyth, D. A. (1998). Developmental assets: Measurement and prediction of risk behaviors among adolescence. *Applied Developmental Science, 2*(4), 209–230.

MacDonald, D. A. (2000). Spirituality: Description, measurement, and relation to the five factor model of personality. *Journal of Personality, 68*(1), 157–197.

Marler, P. L., & Hadaway, C. K. (2002). "Being religious" or "being spiritual" in America: A zero-sum proposition. *Journal for the Scientific Study of Religion, 41*(2), 288–300.

Matthews, D. A., McCollough, M. E., Swyers, J. P., Milano, M. G., Larson, D. B., & Koenig, H. G. (1999). Religious commitment and health status. *Archives of Family Medicine, 8,* 476.

McCollough, M. E., Larson, D. B., Koenig, H. G., & Lerner, R. (1999). The mismeasurement of religion: A systematic review of mortality research. *Mortality, 4,* 182–194.

National Research Council and Institute of Medicine. (2002). *Community programs to promote youth development.* Washington, DC: National Academy Press.

Nye, R. M. (1999). Relational consciousness and the spiritual lives of children: Convergence with children's theory of mind. In K. H. Reich, F. K. Oser, & W. G. Scarlett (Eds.), *Psychological studies on spiritual and religious development: Vol. 2. Being human: The case of religion* (pp. 57–82). Lengerich, Germany: Pabst Science Publishers.

Paloutzian, R. F. (1996). *Invitation to the psychology of religion* (2nd ed.). Needham Heights, MA: Allyn and Bacon.

Pargament, K. I. (1997). *The psychology of religion and coping: Theory, research, practice.* New York: Guilford Press.

Piedmont, R. L. (1999). Does spirituality represent the sixth factor of personality? Spiritual transcendence and the five-factor model. *Journal of Personality, 67*(6), 985–1013.

Reich, K. H. (1996). A logic-based typology of science and theology. *Journal of Interdisciplinary Studies, 8*(1–2), 149–167.

Resnick, M. D., Bearman, P. S., Blum, R. W., Bauman, K. E., Harris, K. M., Jones, J., et al. (1997). Protecting adolescents from harm: Findings from the National Longitudinal Study on Adolescent Health. *Journal of the American Medical Association, 278*(10), 823–832.

Roehlkepartain, E. C. (1998). *Building assets in congregations: A practical guide for helping youth grow up healthy.* Minneapolis: Search Institute.

Roehlkepartain, E. C. (2003a). Building strengths, deepening faith: Understanding and enhancing youth development in Protestant congregations. In R. M. Lerner, F. Jacobs, & D. Wertlieb (Eds.), *Handbook of applied developmental science: Vol. 3. Promoting positive youth and family development* (pp. 515–534). Thousand Oaks, CA: Sage.

Roehlkepartain, E. C. (2003b). Making room at the table for everyone: Interfaith engagement in positive child and adolescent development. In R. M. Lerner, F. Jacobs, & D. Wertlieb (Eds.), *Handbook of applied developmental science: Vol. 3. Promoting positive youth and family development* (pp. 535–563). Thousand Oaks, CA: Sage.

Roehlkepartain, E. C., King, P. E., Wagener, L. M., & Benson, P. L. (Eds.). (in preparation). *The handbook of spiritual development in childhood and adolescence.* Thousand Oaks, CA: Sage.

Roehlkepartain, E. C., & Scales, P. C. (1995). *Youth development in congregations: An exploration of the potential and barriers.* Minneapolis: Search Institute.

Scales, P. C., Benson, P. L., Leffert, N., & Blyth, D. A. (2000). Contribution of developmental assets to the prediction of thriving among adolescents. *Applied Developmental Science, 4*(1), 27–46.

Scales, P. C., Benson, P. L., & Mannes, M. (2003). *The impact of adolescents' prosocial orientation on reported engagement with unrelated adults.* Manuscript submitted for publication.

Scales, P. C., & Leffert, N. (1999). *Developmental assets: A synthesis of the scientific research on adolescent development.* Minneapolis: Search Institute.

Shahabi, L., Powell, L. H., Musick, M. A., Pargament, K. I., Thoresen, C. F., Williams, D., et al. (2002). Correlates of self-perceptions of spirituality in American adults. *Annals of Behavioral Medicine, 24*(1), 59–68.

Smith, C., Denton, M. L., Faris, R., & Regnerus, M. (2002). Mapping American adolescent religious participation. *Journal for the Scientific Study of Religion, 41*(4), 597–612.

Smith, C., Faris, R., Denton, M. L., & Regnerus, M. (2003). Mapping American adolescent subjective religiosity and attitudes of alienation towards religion: A research report. *Sociology of Religion, 64,* 111–133.

Swanson, D. P., Spencer, M. B., Dell'Angelo, T., Harpalani, V., & Spencer, T. R. (2002, Fall). Identity processes and the positive development of African Americans: An explanatory framework. *New Directions for Youth Development,* 73–100.

Wagener, L. M., Furrow, J. L., King, P. E., Leffert, N., & Benson, P. (2003). Religion and developmental resources. *Review of Religious Research, 44*(3), 271–284.

Wuthnow, R. (1994). *Producing the sacred: An essay on public religion.* Urbana: University of Illinois Press.

Zinnbauer, B. J., Pargament, K. I., & Scott, A. B. (1999). The emerging meanings of religiousness and spirituality: Problems and prospects. *Journal of Personality, 67*(6), 889–919.

4 Children's Life Satisfaction

E. Scott Huebner, Shannon M. Suldo, and Robert F. Valois

University of South Carolina

Psychology has long focused on the study of psychopathological conditions. In contrast, positive psychologists have argued for the complementary study of wellness, including the nature and development of key human strengths (Seligman & Csikszentmihalyi, 2000). Although a taxonomy of human strengths has been suggested (Seligman, 2002), research is just beginning in this area, particularly studies devoted to identifying, understanding, and promoting important strengths in children and youth. The first purpose of this chapter is to suggest that one crucial, personal strength that merits study among children and adolescents is *life satisfaction*. Although research on child and adolescent life satisfaction is scant relative to that on adults, a body of literature is emerging that supports its meaningfulness and relevance to the promotion of positive well-being and the prevention of psychopathology in children and adolescents (see Huebner, Suldo, Smith, & McKnight, 2004). The second purpose of this chapter is to review research on two measures of life satisfaction, the Students' Life Satisfaction Scale (SLSS: Huebner, 1991a) and the Brief Multidimensional Students' Life Satisfaction Scale (BMSLSS: Seligson, Huebner, & Valois, 2003), both of which are appropriate for use with youth in large-scale survey research. The final purpose of this chapter is to delineate recommendations for future research needed to further validate the two measures.

Life satisfaction has been defined as a person's subjective, global evaluation of the positivity of her/his life as a whole or with specific life domains (e.g., family life, school experiences) (Diener, Suh, Lucas, & Smith, 1999). Life satisfaction scales encompass judgments ranging from very negative (e.g., terrible) to neutral to very positive (e.g., delighted). Thus, life satisfaction scales reflect conceptualizations of positive well-being that extend beyond merely the absence of dissatisfaction. In support of distinction between positive and negative well-being indicators, Greenspoon and Saklofske (2001) have demonstrated the usefulness of a dual-factor model of child mental health, in which life satisfaction is the key indicator of positive psychological well-being.

Life satisfaction research with adults has shown that positive levels of life satisfaction are *not* just an epiphenomenon, that is, a simple by-product of positive life experiences, personality characteristics, and so forth. Rather, many benefits accrue to those who typically experience high levels of life satisfaction. These benefits include positive outcomes in intrapersonal, interpersonal, vocational, health, and educational arenas (see King, Lyubormirsky, & Diener, 2003). Low levels of life satisfaction are similarly predictive of a variety of negative outcomes, including mental and physical health problems (see Frisch, 2000, for a review).

Research with children has been restricted mostly to studies of correlates of life satisfaction. An impressive array of correlates has been revealed, including a variety of risk behaviors (e.g., alcohol and drug use, aggressive and violent behavior, sexual activities), psychopathological symptoms (depression, anxiety, low self-efficacy, loneliness), and physical health indices (e.g., eating behavior, exercise) (see Huebner et al., in press, for a review). Although there has been little research on the consequences of individual differences in life satisfaction among children and youth, recent research in our lab has shown that life satisfaction links stressful life events and psychopathological behavior in adolescents. Studies have revealed that global life satisfaction mediates the impact of stressful life events (McKnight, Huebner, & Suldo, 2002) and parenting behavior (Suldo & Huebner, 2004) on adolescent problem behavior. Furthermore, a longitudinal study (Suldo & Huebner, in press) showed that initial life satisfaction reports of adolescents moderated the relationship between their experiences of stressful life events and their later externalizing behavior. That is, adolescents with high levels of life satisfaction showed significantly less subsequent externalizing behavior in the face of adverse life events relative to students who were dissatisfied with their lives. Thus, life satisfaction appears to operate as an intrapersonal strength that helps buffer against the development of psychopathology in the face of increasing stressful life events. Taken together, research to date demonstrates that assessment of levels of life satisfaction in children and youth provides important information in and of itself, and also provides important information regarding risk for subsequent psychological problems.

There exist roughly a half dozen life satisfaction scales suitable for use with children and/or adolescents. However, most of these measures are too lengthy or impractical for large-scale group administration. On the other hand, two instruments, the SLSS and BMSLSS, are sufficiently brief, appropriate for children, and demonstrate adequate reliability and validity; these measures are useful in large-scale surveys, longitudinal studies, experience sampling studies, and other studies in which time constraints limit the number of items that can be administered. These instruments will be reviewed below.

Review of Students' Life Satisfaction Scale

The SLSS is a seven-item self-report measure that has been used with children ages 8–18. The items require respondents to rate their satisfaction with respect to items that are domain-free (e.g., "My *life* is better than most kids" vs. "My *family life* is better than most kids"). The original version of the scale consisted of 10 items; the scale was subsequently reduced to 7 items based on item analysis data and reliability estimates (Huebner, 1991a). Additional positive and negative affect items were included and used to clarify the boundaries of the construct tapped by the SLSS, through the provision of evidence of discriminant validity vis-à-vis other subjective well-being variables (Huebner, 1991c).

Early studies of the SLSS used a response format composed of a 4-point frequency scale, with 1 = *never*, 2 = *sometimes*, 3 = *often*, and 4 = *always*. More recent studies have employed a 6-point extent format, with 1 = *strongly disagree*, 2 = *moderately disagree*, 3 = *mildly disagree*, 4 = *mildly agree*, 5 = *moderately agree*, and 6 = *strongly agree*. One study has suggested caution with respect to the assumption of comparability of scores across the two formats (Gilman & Huebner, 1997).

Samples

The SLSS has been employed in studies involving samples of students ranging in age from 8 to 18 years. Samples from independent studies that employed the SLSS include the following: 254 students ages 7–14 and 329 children ages 8–14, both from a midwestern state (Huebner, 1991a); 79 students from grades 5–7 in a midwestern state; 222 students from grades 8–12 in a southern state (Dew & Huebner, 1994); 321 students from grades 9–12 in a southern state (Huebner, Funk, & Gilman, 2000); and 1,201 students from grades 6–12 in a southern state (McKnight et al., 2002; Suldo & Huebner, 2004). Additional samples of clinical populations have included students referred for psychoeducational evaluations and at-risk programs (Huebner & Alderman, 1993), and adjudicated adolescents (Crenshaw, 1998). Other clinical samples involve students with identified exceptionalities, such as children with learning disabilities (McCullough & Huebner, 2003), emotional disturbance (Huebner & Alderman, 1993), and gifted students (Ash & Huebner, 1998).

All aforementioned studies have employed the SLSS as a continuous measure in investigating the relationships between life satisfaction and various constructs and outcomes. To date, empirical guidelines for "cut points" that might classify children into optimal/adequate/risk levels of life satisfaction have not been established. Future researchers may be interested in following methodology set forth by Gambone, Klem, and Connell (2002) that facilitated the identification of *thresholds* "at which youth's chances for success on later elements increase dramatically" (p. 11), thus identifying palpable levels of variables for which practitioners concerned with public policy and/or intervention and prevention programs could strive to meet. To date, only one study (Suldo & Huebner, in press) has analyzed SLSS scores on a dichotomy. In this case, classifying children into initial levels of high versus low life satisfaction based on their mean SLSS score allowed these researchers to predict different developmental outcomes in the groups' reactions to stressful life events. This study used a cut point of 4.0, with the low life satisfaction group made up of students with mean scores between 1 and 3.9, and mean scores at or above 4.0 indicating high life satisfaction. Future research employing more sophisticated methodology (i.e., conditional probabilities) may be useful in identifying optimal and, conversely, risk levels of life satisfaction that would predict dramatic changes in future levels of psychosocial variables of interest.

Distribution of Responses

Extant research with the SLSS demonstrates that students' mean SLSS scores typically contain substantial variability among the six response options, with the average score consistently in the positive range of life satisfaction. For instance, in Suldo and Huebner's (2004) sample of 1,188 adolescents, the mean SLSS score was 4.21 (range: 1–6) with a standard deviation of 1.14. As further evidence of response variability, more than a quarter of the sample possessed mean SLSS scores in the bottom half of the range, indicating dissatisfaction with their lives. Although the distribution of responses among the 1,188 subjects had a slight negative skew (−0.61) and was slightly platykurtic (−0.26), these values are within acceptable limits (i.e., between −1.0 and +1.0), demonstrating acceptable levels of skewness and kurtosis and, therefore, a normal distribution of scores on the SLSS.

Reliability

Coefficient alphas in the .70–.80 range have consistently been reported across all age groups (see Table 1). For example, Huebner (1991a) reported an

Table 1. Studies of Coefficient Alphas of the Students' Life Satisfaction Scale (SLSS) with Children and/or Adolescents

Study	Participants	Coefficient alpha
Griffin & Huebner, 2000 (one item removed from the scale)	49 severely emotionally disabled students, grades 6–8, and 49 students matched, but without a severe emotional disability	SED (.75) Non-SED (.79)
Huebner, Funk, & Gilman 2000	321 students, grades 9–12 at Time 1; 99 students, grades 10–12 at Time 2	Time 1 (.84) Time 2 (.79)
Gilman & Huebner, 1997	84 students, grades 6–8	6-point extent scale (.84) 4-point frequency scale (.82)
Terry & Huebner, 1995	183 students, grades 3–5	.73
Dew & Huebner, 1994	222 students, grades 8–12	.86
Huebner, 1991b	79 students, grades 5–7	.82
Huebner, 1991a	254 students, grades 3–8	.84

alpha of .82 in a sample of students in grades 4–8 in a midwestern U.S. state, and Dew and Huebner (1994) reported an alpha of .86 in a sample of students in grades 9–12 in a southeastern U.S. state. Furthermore, comparisons of alpha coefficients for African American and Caucasian adolescents revealed cross-group comparability (Huebner & Dew, 1993). Similar internal consistency coefficients for the SLSS have been obtained with students in South Korea (Park, Huebner, Laughlin, Valois, & Gilman, 2004) and Spain (Casas, Alsinet, Rossich, Huebner, & Laughlin, 2001).

Test–retest reliability has also been established with correlations of .76, .64, and .53 across 1–2 weeks (Terry & Huebner, 1995), 1-month (Gilman & Huebner, 1997), and 1-year (Huebner, Funk et al., 2000) time intervals, respectively.

Validity

Factor Structure

The SLSS items have been subjected to factor analyses in several studies, all of which have supported a one-factor structure for the instrument (Dew & Huebner, 1994; Gilman & Huebner, 1997; Huebner, 1991a). Comparisons across African American and Caucasian students have revealed factorial equivalence for adolescents (Huebner & Dew, 1993) and preadolescents (Huebner, 1994). Conjoint factor analyses of the SLSS with self-concept measures have supported discriminant validity as well (Huebner, 1995; Huebner, Gilman, & Laughlin, 1999; Terry & Huebner, 1995).

Relationships with Other Life Satisfaction Measures

SLSS scores demonstrate significant associations with parent estimates of their child's life satisfaction. Dew and Huebner (1994) obtained a correlation of .48 between self- and parent reports of high school students. Similarly, Gilman and Huebner (1997) obtained a correlation of .54 between middle school students and their parents. These correlations are comparable to similar self-other reports of life satisfaction for adults.

SLSS scores also display appropriate correlations with other life satisfaction self-report measures. These measures include the Perceived Life Satisfaction Scale ($r = .58$), the Piers-Harris Happiness subscale ($r = .53$), Andrews and Withey one-item scale ($r = .62$), and DOTS-R Mood scale ($r = .34$) (Huebner, 1991a).

Criterion-Related Validity

Construct validity of SLSS reports has been supported by a wide-ranging nomological network of related variables, as illustrated in Table 2. Life satisfaction is not an isolated variable, but is related to a variety of important life outcomes (see Huebner et al., in press, for a review). For example, as noted previously, SLSS reports of children and youth are inversely related to important maladaptive psychosocial conditions, such as depression, anxiety, social stress,

Table 2. Studies of Correlates of the Students' Life Satisfaction Scale (SLSS) with Children and/or Adolescents

Study	Participants	Correlates
Ash & Huebner, 2001	152 students, grades 9–12	Locus of control (−.46) **Life Stressors:** Family (−.33) Friends (−.36) Health (−.18) Home and money (−.40) Parents (−.33) School (−.41) Sibling (−.17) Boyfriend/girlfriend (−.19) Negative life events (−.46) **Social Resources:** Family (.22) Friends (.26) Parents (.23) School (.24) Sibling (.18) Positive life events (.20)
Dew & Huebner, 1994	222 students, grades 8–12	Locus of control (−.52) Global self-esteem (.52) **Self-Concept Areas:** Physical abilities (.15) Physical appearance (.19) Opposite-sex peer relations (.33) Same-sex peer relations (.29) Honesty-trustworthiness (.38) Parent relations (.62) Emotional stability (.48) General self (.52) Math (.17) General school (.25)
Fogle, Huebner, & Laughlin, 2002	160 students, grades 6–8	Social self-efficacy (.29) Extraversion (.22) Neuroticism (−.33)
Gilman & Huebner, 1997	99 students, grades 6–8 at Time 1; 84 students, grades 6–8 (4 weeks later) at Time 2	**Time 1:** Self-report academic self-concept (.31) Parent-report academic self-concept (.35) Parent-report life satisfaction (.54) **Time 2:** Grade (−.24) **Self-Concept Areas:** Math (.30) Physical appearance (.31) General self (.57) Honesty-trustworthiness (.37) Physical abilities (.30) Verbal (.35) Emotional stability (.43) Parental relations (.54)

Table 2. (Continued)

Study	Participants	Correlates
		General school (.50)
		Opposite-sex relations (.45)
		Same-sex relations (.27)
		Global self-concept (.58)
Huebner, 1991a	254 students, grades 3–8	General self-concept (.53)
		Happiness (.53)
		Anxiety (.38)
		Mood (.34)
		Happiness item (.36)
		Life satisfaction item (.62)
Huebner, 1991b	79 students, grades 5–7	Anxiety (−.51)
		Locus of control (−.48)
		Extraversion (.23)
		Neuroticism (−.46)
		Self-esteem (.65)
Huebner et al., 2000	166 students, grades 10–12	**Clinical Scales:**
		Locus of control (−.39)
		Depression (−.39)
		Anxiety (−.33)
		Social stress (−.50)
		Atypicality (−.35)
		Adaptive:
		Self-esteem (.22)
		Relations with parents (.38)
		Interpersonal relations (.25)
Huebner, Gilman, and Laughlin, 1999	290 students, grades 6–8 (Study 1); 183 students, grades 3–5 (Study 2)	**Self-Concept Areas (Study 1):**
		Physical abilities (.22)
		Physical appearance (.38)
		Opposite-sex peer relations (.26)
		Same-sex peer relations (.38)
		Honesty-trustworthiness (.37)
		Parent relations (.61)
		Emotional stability (.44)
		General self (.52)
		Math (.30)
		Verbal (.27)
		General school (.37)
		Demographics:
		Sex (.17)
		Self-Concept Areas (Study 2):
		Physical abilities (.31)
		Physical appearance (.30)
		Peer relations (.41)
		Parent relations (.56)
		Reading (.29)
		Math (.34)
		General school (.36)
		General self (.47)

(continued)

Table 2. (Continued)

Study	Participants	Correlates
McCullough, Huebner, & Laughlin, 2000	92 students, grades 9–12	Positive daily events (.39) Negative daily events (−.34) Positive major events (.30) Negative major events (−.22) Self-concept (.45) Positive affect (.44) Negative affect (−.28)
McKnight et al.	1,201 students, grades 6–12	Stressful life events (−.23) Neuroticism (−.39) Externalizing behavior (−.37) Internalizing behavior (−.50)
Rigby & Huebner, 2003	212 students, grades 9–12	Emotional stability (.29) Attributions good events (.40) Attributions bad events (−.23)
Suldo & Huebner, in press-b	1,045 students, grades 6–11 at Time 1 816 students, grades 7–12 at Time 2 (1 year later)	**Time 1 (concurrent):** Stressful life events (−.22) Externalizing behavior (−.37) Internalizing behavior (−.49) **Time 2 (concurrent):** Stressful life events (−.23) Externalizing behavior (−.37) Internalizing behavior (−.48) **Time 2 (delayed):** Stressful life events (−.17) Externalizing behavior (−.30) Internalizing behavior (−.37)
Suldo & Huebner, in press-a	1,201 students, grades 6–12	Parental supervision (.21) Parental social support (.49) Parental autonomy granting (.17) Externalizing behavior (−.38) Internalizing behavior (−.49)
Terry & Huebner, 1995	183 students, grades 3–5	**Self-Concept Areas:** Physical abilities (.30) Physical appearance (.26) Reading (.23) Math (.31) Peers (.40) Parent (.53) General school (.32) General self (.45)

loneliness, and aggressive behaviors. Additionally, negative environmental experiences, including acute life events (e.g., death of a parent) and daily hassles (e.g., chronic family discord) are associated negatively with SLSS scores. However, positive life experiences are associated positively with SLSS scores. Finally, SLSS scores have also been related positively to personality characteristics, such as temperament (extraversion), adaptive cognitive attributions, self-efficacy, and participation in meaningful activities. Taken together, the pattern of associations suggests substantial concurrent validity.

Discriminant Validity

SLSS reports have been distinguished from several constructs with which life satisfaction is not expected to relate. First, SLSS scores have weak correlations with social desirability responding (Huebner, 1991a). Second, SLSS scores are not significantly related to IQ scores (Huebner & Alderman, 1993) or school grades (Huebner, 1991b). Finally, using conjoint factor analysis procedures, SLSS scores have been differentiated from measures of positive and negative affect (Huebner, 1991c; Huebner & Dew, 1996).

Discriminative validity studies have also been conducted, with SLSS scores distinguishing appropriately among various known groups. Compared to normal students, SLSS scores are lower for students with emotional disorders (Huebner & Alderman, 1993) and adjudicated adolescents (Crenshaw, 1998). Consistent with studies in which SLSS scores are unrelated to school grades and/or IQ scores, MSLSS scores did not distinguish between normal students and gifted students (Ash & Huebner, 1998) or students with learning disabilities (McCullough & Huebner, 2003).

Predictive Validity

Finally, predictive validity studies have been supportive of the SLSS. Using zero-order correlational analyses, Huebner, Funk et al. (2000) reported in a study of 99 adolescents that SLSS scores significantly predicted social stress, depression, and anxiety scores 1 year later. Furthermore, using hierarchical multiple regression analyses, Suldo and Huebner (in press) demonstrated that Time 1 SLSS scores of 816 adolescent students predicted externalizing behavior 1 year later, even after controlling for Time 1 externalizing behavior scores. Finally, and most important, Suldo and Huebner found support for a moderational model of the influence of life satisfaction on the relationship between adverse life events and externalizing behavior of adolescents 1 year later. Specifically, adolescents with positive Time 1 SLSS scores (in contrast to youth who reported dissatisfaction with their lives) were less likely to develop subsequent externalizing behavior problems in the face of adverse life events. Taken together, the predictive validity studies show that life satisfaction, as measured by the SLSS, operates as a protective strength that buffers against the effects of adverse life events in adolescence.

Demographics and the SLSS

SLSS scores have shown meager relationships with demographic variables in studies of students in the United States (see Gilman & Huebner, 2003, for a review). These variables have included age, gender, ethnicity, and socioeconomic status (SES). It should be noted that studies with very low SES students (e.g., homeless students) have yet to be undertaken. The mean life satisfaction score of students from each demographic group is consistently positive (i.e., above the neutral point), suggesting that most children and youth are satisfied with their lives in general. These findings are consistent with studies of adults in the United States and many other countries, suggesting that the baseline for life satisfaction is positive, that is, among people whose basic needs (e.g., food, clothing, shelter) have been met.

Summary

More than a decade of research supports the SLSS as a brief, psychometrically sound measure of global life satisfaction for students from grades 3 to 12. Predictive validity studies suggest that the SLSS predicts important mental health behaviors independently and interactively with measures of stressful life events. The SLSS has been used effectively with a variety of student populations, including students with emotional disabilities and learning disabilities, as well as gifted students. However, difficulties have been encountered in using the SLSS with adolescents with mild mental disabilities (Brantley, Huebner, & Nagle, 2002), despite the fact that the students were able to reliably respond to a multidimensional life satisfaction measure. Major limitations of the SLSS include (a) lack of a nationally representative sample, (b) repetitive wording of the items, and (c) the need for further research with students with cognitive impairments (e.g., children with mental disabilities).

Perhaps the major limitation of the SLSS is that it measures only satisfaction with life as a whole. The scale does not allow for the assessment of satisfaction across various important domains of interest to children and youth, such as satisfaction with family, friends, and school. Multidimensional measures, which assess satisfaction with multiple life domains, would offer a more differentiated picture of the perceived quality of life of children and youth. For example, although a large statewide sample of high school students in a U.S. southeastern state revealed generally positive global life satisfaction scores, scores across five specific domains (family, friends, school, self, living environment) were more variable, with substantial dissatisfaction observed among students' reports of satisfaction with their school experiences in particular (Huebner, Drane, & Valois, 2000). Such differences in levels of life satisfaction illustrate the incremental validity of multidimensional measures of life satisfaction. Thus, in the next section, research findings for a brief, multidimensional measure of life satisfaction for children and youth (i.e., the Brief Multidimensional Students' Life Satisfaction Scale) will be reviewed.

Review of Brief Multidimensional Students' Life Satisfaction Scale

The BMSLSS is a five-item self-report measure developed to assess children's and adolescents' satisfaction with respect to the areas of life most pertinent during youth development. Specifically, students are instructed to rate their satisfaction with their family life, friendships, school experiences, self, and then living environment. Response options are on a 7-point scale (Andrews & Withey, 1976) that ranges from 1 = *terrible* to 7 = *delighted*. All studies to date have employed subjects' mean response to the five items as a continuous variable in data analyses. The BMSLSS was initially created for inclusion in the 1997 South Carolina Youth Risk Behavior Survey (YRBS) of the Centers for Disease Control, administered to over 5,500 public school students from 63 high schools (Huebner, Drane, et al., 2000). An additional item, measuring students' satisfaction with their overall life, was included in initial data collection opportunities to provide preliminary validation information about the relationship of the BMSLSS to global life satisfaction.

Samples

Since its inception, the BMSLSS has been employed in studies of middle and high school students who reside in the southeastern United States. In addition to the aforementioned sample of students in grades 9–12, the BMSLSS was used in a study of 2,502 students in grades 6–8 (Huebner, Suldo, Valois, & Drane, 2002). Later, independent samples of 221 students in grades 6–8 and 46 high school students completed the BMSLSS during preliminary validation studies of the measure (Seligson et al., 2003). The BMSLSS, still in its early years of development and use, clearly has not yet received the research attention afforded the senior SLSS. However, it is notable that the sampling procedures used in the larger studies assured a diversified, representative sample composed of large numbers of adolescents from all SES levels and ethnic backgrounds in South Carolina.

Distribution of Responses

Similar to the SLSS, the BMSLSS affords considerable variability in regard to the distribution of mean scores (note: response options are 1 = *terrible*; 2 = *unhappy*; 3 = *mostly dissatisfied*; 4 = *mixed* [about equally satisfied and dissatisfied]; 5 = *mostly satisfied*; 6 = *pleased*; 7 = *delighted*) (cf. Andrews & Withey, 1976). Data from the 1997 South Carolina YRBS (see Huebner, Drane, et al., 2000) indicated that most students report positive feelings toward the important domains in their life; specifically, the mean BMSLSS score was in the positive range ($M = 4.97$; $SD = 1.25$; range: 1–7). Moreover, slightly more than a quarter of the sample reported mean BMSLSS scores in the "mixed" range or below. Skew and kurtosis values of the BMSLSS were also within acceptable limits (skew = −0.98; kurtosis = .88) and thus demonstrated that while the distribution of scores is slightly negatively skewed and leptokurtic, the BMSLSS possesses a relatively normal distribution.

Reliability

Coefficient alphas for the total score (the sum of respondents' ratings across the five items) have been reported at .75 for middle school students and .81 for high school students (Seligson et al., 2003; Zullig, Valois, Huebner, Oeltmann, & Drane, 2001). Zullig et al. report that alpha coefficients ranging from .80 to .85 were continually yielded following the removal of any single item from the BMSLSS. In sum, preliminary data with young and late adolescents indicate that the internal consistency of the BMSLSS meets acceptable levels for research purposes when used with secondary school students.

Validity

Construct Validity

The BMSLSS was designed to tap the same dimensions of life measured in the lengthier and well-researched Multidimensional Students' Life Satisfaction Scale (MSLSS: Huebner, 1994). The MSLSS is based on a hierarchical model of life satisfaction with general life satisfaction at the apex, along with the five lower order domains (i.e., family, friends, school, etc.). Confirmatory factor analyses have supported the hierarchical model underlying the MSLSS (see Huebner, Laughlin, Ash, & Gilman, 1998).

Construct validity of the BMSLSS has been supported in two ways. First, the meaningfulness of the general or total life satisfaction score has been assessed. Specifically, BMSLSS reports of 221 middle school students were subjected to principal axis factor analysis. Only one factor displayed an eigenvalue greater than 1, and the results of the scree test also suggested that only one factor was meaningful. This single factor accounted for 50% of the total variance. BMSLSS items and corresponding factor loadings are presented in Table 3. Using a factor loading cutoff of .40, all five items were found to load satisfactorily on the first factor.

Item-total correlations have also been reported with the middle school sample (Seligson et al., 2003). Coefficients ranged from .65 to .73.

Second, the construct validity of the five one-item domain based scores for the BMSLSS has been supported by multitrait-multimethod (MTMM)

Table 3. Factor Loadings from Principal Axis
Factor Analysis of BMSLSS (N = 221)

Factor 1	Item/Domain
.66	Family
.65	Friend
.62	Living environment
.60	School
.53	Self

correlation matrix comparisons of the total domain scores from the MSLSS with the single items on the BMSLSS using Campbell and Fiske's (1959) procedures (see Seligson et al., 2003). In all cases, correlations between the measures' corresponding domains were substantially higher than intercorrelations among the BMSLSS domains, as well as between different domains of the BMSLSS and MSLSS (e.g., MSLSS family domain, BMSLSS friend item). This pattern was produced in separate analyses of middle and high school samples; interestingly, higher convergent validity coefficients were found in the group of older students.

In sum, statistical analyses support the hierarchical structure of the BMSLSS. The scale contains a higher-order domain of general life satisfaction, in addition to differentiable lower-order domains (in this case, items). Thus, the BMSLSS affords researchers both a brief measure of adolescents' satisfaction in the areas of life historically deemed important during adolescence as well as a total score that provides a meaningful overall picture of adolescents' life satisfaction.

Relationships with Other Life Satisfaction Measures

Acceptable correlations have been obtained between the BMSLSS total score and other validated measures of life satisfaction, such as the MSLSS total score ($r = .66$) and the SLSS ($r = .62$).

Criterion-Related Validity

Extant research with the BMSLSS has demonstrated concurrent validity through significant relationships with multiple behaviors central to the health of adolescents. For example, adolescents' BMSLSS reports have shown concurrent, negative relationships with their alcohol, tobacco, and other drug use (Valois, Zullig, Huebner, Oeltmann & Drane, 2001), violent and aggressive risk behaviors, such as physical fighting and carrying a weapon (Zullig et al., 2001), sexual risk-taking behaviors (Valois, Zullig, Huebner, Kammermann, & Drane, 2002), inappropriate dieting behaviors (Valois, Zullig, Huebner, & Drane, 2003a), suicidal ideation and behavior (Valois, Zullig, Huebner, & Drane, 2004), and lack of physical activity (Valois, Zullig, Huebner, & Drane, in press).

Discriminant Validity

Similar to the SLSS, BMSLSS reports yield a low correlation with indicators of social desirability (Seligson et al., 2003). In addition, the BMSLSS shows weak relationships with health-related quality-of-life scales (Valois, 2003). Despite the high associations often found between the components of subjective well-being (i.e., positive affect, negative affect, and life satisfaction), the BMSLSS distinguished life satisfaction from affect through yielding only moderate correlations with the PANAS-C Positive Affect scale ($r = .43$) and Negative Affect scale ($r = -.27$).

Predictive Validity

Initial evidence of the predictive validity of the BMSLSS is promising. In an ethnically diverse sample of more than 1,000 Florida middle school students, Farrell, Valois, Meyer, and Tidwell (2004) reported statistically significant prospective correlations between the BMSLSS (note: the aforementioned item measuring global life satisfaction was included in analyses) and the four subscales of the Problem Behavior Frequency Scales (Farrell, Kung, White, & Valois, 2000), which were administered at the beginning of the sample's 6th- and 8th-grade years. The following Pearson product-moment correlations were found between initial BMSLSS scores and problem behavior subscales measured 2 years later: Violent Behavior Frequency ($r = -.20$), Delinquent Behavior Frequency ($r = -.22$), Drug Frequency ($r = -.23$), and Peer Provocation ($r = -.27$). These correlations were likely attenuated as a result of the nature of the study, as approximately one half of the sample participated in a violence prevention program (Responding in Peaceful and Positive Ways) during the time interval. Nevertheless, the results were consistent with expected predictions in that higher levels of student dissatisfaction predicted higher levels of future problem behaviors, including aggression, drug use, and peer problems.

Demographics and the BMSLSS

Just as the research with measures of global life satisfaction (e.g., SLSS) has found that mean scores are remarkably similar across children of various races, ages, and gender, in general the BMSLSS total score produces comparable mean levels across demographic groups of adolescents. Even in large samples that maximize statistical sensitivity, the BMSLSS total score yields similar means between males and females in grades 6–12 (Huebner et al., 2002; Huebner, Suldo, Valois, Drane, & Zullig, 2004). Similarly, no significant differences have been found between mean BMSLSS scores of African American and Caucasian middle school students. While one study found that Caucasian students in high school provide higher BMSLSS reports than their African American classmates, the effect size of this finding was small (.08), and both groups' mean rating was in the positive range (Huebner et al., 2000b). BMSLSS scores also vary little among adolescents of different age levels. For instance, Huebner et al. (2004) found no significant differences in BMSLSS scores in adolescents in grades 9–12. Although a survey of several thousand middle school students found that students in 6th grade provided slightly higher BMSLSS scores than their 7th- and 8th-grade counterparts (Huebner et al., 2002), it should be noted that mean BMSLSS scores are in the positive range for all students in grades 6–12. Given the remarkable similarity of average BMSLSS ratings among adolescents of various races, genders, and age groups, it appears that the BMSLSS total score is one measure of positive youth development that is not strongly influenced by demographic differences within the United States.

In contrast to findings pertinent to general life satisfaction, research employing multidimensional measures has yielded more complex results. For instance,

Huebner, Drane, et al.'s (2000) study of the BMSLSS with high school students indicated demographic differences within *domains* of satisfaction. Specifically, Caucasian students reported higher satisfaction than African American students on items assessing satisfaction with friends, living environment, and self. Gender differences were also found; specifically, female students reported higher levels of satisfaction than males in regard to their friends, school, and self. Thus, the BMSLSS has the potential to provide more complex information than measures that only yield a global level of life satisfaction.

Summary

The BMSLSS is a brief measure of life satisfaction in youth that gathers data concerning children and adolescents' satisfaction in important domains of their life that, taken together, provide a more complete picture of youth's overall well-being. The scale has been used successfully with students in grades 6–12, and research is currently under way to explore its suitability for younger children. Initial studies involving middle and high school students provide preliminary support of the psychometric properties of the BMSLSS. Moreover, the concurrent and predictive utility of the BMSLSS has been demonstrated through its relationships with important behavior outcomes in youth, such as substance use and risky violent behaviors. While the potential of the BMSLSS is evident, at present the scale should be used with caution because of the limitations inherent to its relative youth. Areas that should be addressed in future research include: (a) securing a nationally representative sample, (b) assessing psychometric properties with elementary level students and students with disabilities, and (c) conducting additional prospective studies.

Clearly, the BMSLSS is in the formative stage of development. Our lab is currently involved in administering the measure to children in elementary school (grades 3–5), and including the BMSLSS in longitudinal studies. Given the comprehensive picture of childrens' and adolescents' life satisfaction provided through use of the BMSLSS, we are optimistic that it can provide a crucial contribution to large national and international databases evaluating students' overall subjective well-being as well as pinpointing specific areas of life that may serve as protective or risk factors. In addition, the straightforward, concrete wording of the items lends itself well to large-scale surveys in which data are often analyzed (and disseminated) at the item level.

Conclusion

Both the SLSS and BMSLSS provide developmentally appropriate measures of positive subjective well-being of children and youth. Although both measures would benefit from further validation work, both offer promising evidence related to their psychometric properties. Each measure predicts important mental health outcomes. The SLSS has received considerable research attention and emphasizes the respondents' own standards of evaluation. The BMSLSS has received less research attention, but the preliminary evidence is very promising, especially with middle school and high school age students. The choice of which measure to use will involve the research interests of particular investigators. When unidimensional appraisals of satisfaction with life as a whole are desired, the SLSS should be the instrument of choice. When researchers would like to gather appraisals of satisfaction across multiple, important domains, the BMSLSS should be useful.

The findings of the available research with these life satisfaction measures underscore the usefulness of subjective indicators of quality of life of children and youth. Objective conditions (e.g., SES, ethnicity) do not significantly predict perceived quality-of-life judgments; thus a more differentiated understanding of the conditions of children's lives requires collecting both objective and subjective quality-of-life information. Furthermore, the finding that adolescent global life satisfaction reports appear to serve as a moderator for externalizing behavior problems and a mediator of internalizing behavior problems suggests that the inclusion of positive measures of well-being, along with the more traditional measures of negative outcomes, is needed to acquire a comprehensive portrait of adaptation. National assessments of the well-being of children and youth would benefit from the addition of life satisfaction measures to complement the pathology-based measures.

Appendix

Items in Life Satisfaction Measures

Students' Life Satisfaction Scale (SLSS)

1. My life is going well
2. My life is just right
3. I would like to change many things in my life[a]
4. I wish I had a different kind of life[a]
5. I have a good life
6. I have what I want in life
7. My life is better than most kids

Note: Response options are a 6-point Likert scale: *strongly disagree, moderately disagree, mildly disagree, mildly agree, moderately agree, strongly agree.*
[a] Items are reverse-scored.

Brief Multidimensional Students' Life Satisfaction Scale (BMSLSS)

1. I would describe my satisfaction with my family life as:
2. I would describe my satisfaction with my friendships as:
3. I would describe my satisfaction with my school experience as:
4. I would describe my satisfaction with myself as:
5. I would describe my satisfaction with where I live as:

Note: Response options are a 7-point scale: *terrible, unhappy, mostly dissatisfied, mixed* (about equally satisfied and dissatisfied), *mostly satisfied, pleased, delighted.*

References

Andrews, F. M., & Withey, S. B. (1976). *Social indicators of well-being: Americans' perceptions of life quality.* New York: Plenum.

Ash, C., & Huebner, E. S. (1998). Life satisfaction reports of gifted middle-school children. *School Psychology Quarterly, 13,* 310–321.

Ash, C., & Huebner, E. S. (2001). Environmental reports and life satisfaction reports of adolescents: A test of cognitive mediation. *School Psychology International, 22,* 320–336.

Brantley, A., Huebner, E. S., & Nagle, R. J. (2002). Multidimensional life satisfaction reports of adolescents with mild mental disabilities. *Mental Retardation, 40,* 321–329.

Campbell, D. T., & Fiske, D. W. (1959). Convergent and discriminant validation by the multitrait-multimethod matrix. *Psychological Bulletin, 56,* 81–105.

Casas, F., Alsinet, C., Rossich, M., Huebner, E. S., & Laughlin, J. E. (2001). Cross-cultural investigation of the Multidimensional Students' Life Satisfaction Scale with Spanish adolescents. In F. Casas & C. Saurina (Eds.), *Proceedings of the III Conference of International Society for Quality of Life Studies* (pp. 359–366). Girona, Spain: University of Girona Press.

Crenshaw, M. (1998). *Adjudicated violent youth, adjudicated non-violent youth vs. non-adjudicated, non-violent youth on selected psychological measures.* Unpublished master's thesis, University of South Carolina.

Dew, T., & Huebner, E. S. (1994). Adolescents' perceived quality of life: An exploratory investigation. *Journal of School Psychology, 33,* 185–199.

Diener, E., Suh, E. M., Lucas, R. E., & Smith, H. L. (1999). Subjective well-being: Three decades of progress. *Psychological Bulletin, 125,* 276–302.

Farrell, A. D., Kung, E. M., White, K. S., & Valois, R. F. (2000). The structure of self-reported aggression, drug use, and delinquent behaviors during early adolescence. *Journal of Clinical Child Psychology, 29,* 282–292.

Farrell, A. D., Valois, R. F., Meyer, A. L., & Tidwell, R. P. (2004). Impact of the RIPP Violence Prevention Program on rural middle school students. *Journal of Primary Prevention, 24,* 143–167.

Fogle, L., Huebner, E. S., & Laughlin, J. E. (2002). The relationship between temperament and life satisfaction in early adolescence: Cognitive and behavioral mediation models. *Journal of Happiness Studies, 3,* 373–392.

Frisch, M. B. (2000). Improving mental and physical health care through quality of life therapy and assessment. In E. Diener & D. R. Rahtz (Eds.), *Advances in quality of life theory and research* (pp. 207–241). London: Kluwer Academic Publishers.

Gambone, M. A., Klem, A. M., & Connell, J. P. (2002). *Finding out what matters for youth: Testing key links in a community action framework for youth development.* Philadelphia: Youth Development Strategies, Inc., and Institute for Research and Reform in Education.

Gilman, R., & Huebner, E. S. (1997). Children's reports of their life satisfaction. *School Psychology International, 18,* 229–243.

Gilman, R., & Huebner, E. S. (2003). A review of life satisfaction research with children and adolescents. *School Psychology Quarterly, 18,* 192–205.

Greenspoon, P. J., & Saklofske, D. H. (2001). Toward an integration of subjective well-being and psychopathology. *Social Indicators Research, 54,* 81–108.

Griffin, M., & Huebner, E. S. (2000). Multidimensional life satisfaction reports of students with serious emotional disturbance. *Journal of Psychoeducational Assessment, 18,* 111–124.

Huebner, E. S. (1991a). Initial development of the Students' Life Satisfaction Scale. *School Psychology International, 12,* 231–240.

Huebner, E. S. (1991b). Correlates of life satisfaction in children. *School Psychology Quarterly, 6,* 103–111.

Huebner, E. S. (1991c). Further validation of the Student's Life Satisfaction Scale: Independence of satisfaction and affect ratings. *Journal of Psychoeducational Assessment, 9,* 363–368.

Huebner, E. S. (1994). Preliminary development and validation of a multidimensional life satisfaction scale for children. *Psychological Assessment, 6,* 149–158.

Huebner, E. S. (1995). The Students' Life Satisfaction Scale: An assessment of psychometric properties with Black and White elementary school students. *Social Indicators Research, 34,* 315–323.

Huebner E. S., & Alderman, G. L. (1993). Convergent and discriminant validation of a children's life satisfaction scale: Its relationship to self- and teacher-reported psychological problems and school functioning. *Social Indicators Research, 30,* 71–82.

Huebner, E. S., & Dew, T. (1993). An evaluation of racial bias in a life satisfaction scale. *Psychology in the Schools, 30,* 305–309.

Huebner, E. S., & Dew, T. (1996). The interrelationships of positive affect, negative affect and life satisfaction in an adolescent sample. *Social Indicators Research, 38,* 129–137.

Huebner, E. S., Drane, J. W., & Valois, R. F. (2000). Levels and demographic correlates of adolescent life satisfaction reports. *School Psychology International, 21,* 281–292.

Huebner, E. S., Funk, B. A., & Gilman, R. (2000). Cross-sectional and longitudinal psychosocial correlates of adolescent life satisfaction reports. *Canadian Journal of School Psychology, 16,* 53–64.

Huebner, E. S., Gilman, R., & Laughlin, J. E. (1999). A multimethod investigation of the multi-dimensionality of children's well-being reports: Discriminant validity of life satisfaction and self-esteem. *Social Indicators Research, 46,* 1–22.

Huebner, E. S., Laughlin, J. F., Ash, C., & Gilman, R. (1998). Further validation of the Multidimensional Students' Life Satisfaction Scale. *Journal of Psychoeducational Assessment, 16,* 118–134.

Huebner, E. S., Suldo, S. M., Smith, L. C., & McKnight, C. G. (2004). Life satisfaction in children and youth: Empirical foundations and implications for school psychologists. *Psychology in the Schools, 41,* 81–94.

Huebner, E. S., Suldo, S. M., Valois, R. F., & Drane, J. W. (2002). *Brief Multidimensional Students' Life Satisfaction Scale (BMSLSS): Normative data for middle school students.* Manuscript submitted for review.

Huebner, E. S., Suldo, S. M., Valois, R. F., Drane, J. W., & Zullig, K. (2004). Brief Multidimensional Students' Life Satisfaction Scale (BMSLSS): Gender, race, and grade effects for a high school sample. *Psychological Reports, 94,* 351–356.

King, L., Lyubormirsky, S., & Diener, E. (2003). *The benefits of happiness.* Manuscript submitted for publication.

McCullough, G., & Huebner, E. S. (2003). Life satisfaction of adolescents with learning disabilities and normally achieving adolescents. *Journal of Psychoeducational Assessment, 21,* 311–324.

McCullough, G., Huebner, E. S., & Laughlin, J. E. (2000). Life events, self-concept, and adolescents' positive subjective well-being. *Psychology in the Schools, 37,* 281–290.

McKnight, C. G., Huebner, E. S., & Suldo, S. M. (2002). Relationships among stressful life events, temperament, problem behavior, and global life satisfaction in adolescents. *Psychology in the Schools, 39,* 677–687.

Park, N., & Huebner, E. S., Laughlin, J. E., Valois, R. F., & Gilman, R. (2004) . A cross-cultural comparison of the dimensions of child and adolescent life satisfaction reports. *Social Indicators Research, 66,* 61–79.

Rigby, B., & Huebner, E. S. (in press). Do causal attributions mediate the relationship between personality characteristics and life satisfaction in adolescence? *Psychology in the Schools.*

Seligman, M. E. P. (2002). *Authentic happiness.* New York: Free Press.

Seligman, M. E., & Csikszentmihalyi, M. (2000). Positive psychology: An introduction. *American Psychologist, 55,* 5–14.

Seligson, J. L., Huebner, E. S., & Valois, R. F. (2003). Preliminary validation of the Brief Multidimensional Students' Life Satisfaction Scale (BMSLSS). *Social Indicators Research, 61,* 121–145.

Suldo, S. M., & Huebner, E. S. (2004). The role of life satisfaction in the relationship between authoritative parenting dimension and adolescent problem behavior. *Social Indicators Research, 66,* 165–195.

Suldo, S. M., & Huebner, E. S. (in press). Does life satisfaction moderate the effects of stressful life events on psychopathological behavior in adolescence? *School Psychology Quarterly.*

Terry, T., & Huebner, E. S. (1995). The relationship between self-concept and life satisfaction in children. *Social Indicators Research, 35,* 39–52.

Valois, R. F. (2003). Unpublished data [Zero-order correlations between life satisfaction and health-related quality of life].

Valois, R. F., Zullig, K. J., Huebner, E. S., & Drane, J. W. (2001). Relationship between life satisfaction and violent behaviors among adolescents. *American Journal of Health Behavior, 25,* 353–366.

Valois, R. F., Zullig, K. J., Huebner, E. S., & Drane, J. W. (2003a). Relationship between perceived life satisfaction and dieting behavior among public high school adolescents. *Eating Disorders: The Journal of Treatment and Prevention, 11,* 271–288.

Valois, R. F., Zullig, K. J., Huebner, E. S., & Drane, J. W. (in press). Life satisfaction and physical activity behaviors among public high school adolescents. *Journal of School Health.*

Valois, R. F., Zullig, K. J., Huebner, E. S., & Drane, J. W. (2004). Relationship between life satisfaction and suicidal ideation and behaviors among adolescents. *Social Indicators Research, 6,* 81–105.

Valois, R. F., Zullig, K. J., Huebner, E. S., Kammermann, S. K., & Drane, J. W. (2002). Relationship between life satisfaction and sexual risk-taking behaviors among public high school adolescents. *Journal of Child and Family Studies, 11,* 437–440.

Zullig, K. J., Valois, R. F., Huebner, E .S., Oeltmann, J. E., & Drane, W. J. (2001). Relationship between perceived life satisfaction and adolescent substance use. *Journal of Adolescent Health, 29,* 279–288.

5 Measuring Hope in Children

C. R. Snyder

University of Kansas, Lawrence

Many times, I have heard people say something akin to the idea that hope is our children's chance for a better future. Appealing as this sentiment may be, however, very little psychological theory and research has addressed the topic of children's hope. The only related research has been that by Kazdin and his colleagues (1983), who described children's *hopelessness* in terms of negative expectancies toward oneself and one's future. Using this hopelessness definition, Kazdin's group developed the Hopelessness Scale for Children, and this instrument has been used to study the suicidal intentions of children with severe psychological problems (see Snyder, 1994, chapter 4). As such, the Hopelessness Scale for Children reflects the pathology viewpoint that prevailed from the 1950s through the 1990s, and this approach differs from the more recent positive psychology approach for the study of adults (Snyder & Lopez, 2002) and children (Roberts, Brown, Johnson, & Reinke, 2002). Along these latter lines, my colleagues and I have construed hope in general, and children's hope in particular, in terms of positive expectancies. Our work in developing this theory of hope and its related measures for children is the focus of this chapter.

We started by observing that many previous scholars had conceptualized hope as an *overall perception that one's goals can be met* (e.g., Menninger, 1959; Stotland, 1969). Likewise, we were influenced by the research on adults' (e.g., Pervin, 1989) and children's goal-directed thinking (e.g., Dodge, 1986). Springing from these sources of influence, our model and measures of hope were predicated on the assumption that adults and children are goal directed in their thinking and that such thinking can be understood according to the associated components of *pathways* and *agency*.

We define hope as a cognitive set involving the self-perceptions that one can produce routes to desired goals (pathways), along with the motivation to pursue those goals (agency). Both components, as well as their respective anchoring in goal formation, must be assessed together to obtain an overall sense of a

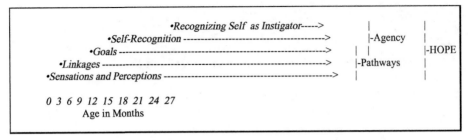

Figure 1. *Cognitive Building Blocks of Hope in the Infant-to-Toddler Stage*

child's hope. As shown in Figure 1, pathways thinking involves the perceptual recognition of external stimuli, the acquisition of temporal linkages between events, and the formation of goals. Acquired somewhat later temporally, agency thinking reflects the recognition of self, the recognition of the self as the source of actions, and the formation of goals. When aggregated, these goal-directed pathways and agency thoughts define hope in this model.

A brief elaboration of each of the processes in Figure 1 will help clarify the underpinnings of hope (see Snyder, 1994, chapter 3). In regard to sensations and perceptions, the newborn inputs stimulation so as to mentally code it with meaning. Examples include the identification of mother relative to other people through the auditory (Stevenson, Ver Hoeve, Roach, & Leavitt, 1986), olfactory (Schaal, as cited in Berger, 1991, p. 158), and visual sensory channels (Barrera & Maurer, 1981). Newborns also quickly learn the temporal connection of events because their survival depends on such "this follows that" chronologies (Schulman, 1991). From birth onward, newborns refine these abilities to form such linkages as they anticipate and plan for events (Kopp, 1989). The aforementioned perception and linkage learning leads to the infant's pointing to desired objects (from 3 to 12 months; Stevenson & Newman, 1986). This pointing behavior signals the infant's ability to single out one goal and even recruit an adult's help to obtain it (Bates, Camaioni, & Volterra, 1975). Taken together, pathways thinking involves "what's out there" perceptions and the temporal "this follows that" linkages as the infant focuses on selected goals.

So far, however, the infant does not have a sense that she is the instigational agent (thus the term agency) of action toward goals. The next processes to be acquired, therefore, involve agency thinking. Learning to identify oneself is necessary for an eventual sense of agency. Such self-recognition increases over the first several months of life and is clearly in place by 12 to 18 months (Kaplan, 1978). Markers of this "psychological birth" include the toddler's being able to identify himself in a mirror, the correct usage of the personal pronoun "I," and toddler statements about inner feelings and thoughts (Bretherton & Beeghly, 1982). Along with such unfolding self-awareness, toddlers also realize around 21 months that they are the ones making things happen. In this regard, the earliest verbal referents that toddlers make pertain to volitions and capacities (e.g., "I can ..."; Corrigan, 1978). These thoughts about selfhood, along with the insight that one is the author of actions aimed at reaching desired goals, form agency thoughts. As seen in Figure 1, goal-directed thinking is shared in both pathways and agency thinking.

To understand this definition more fully, it is necessary to consider children's thoughts about themselves when they run into goal blockages. Early research showed that children get upset when encountering goal impediments (Barker, Dembo, & Lewin, 1941). According to hope theory, such impediments should elicit negative emotions, and, conversely, the successful pursuit of goals should produce positive emotions (Snyder, 1994). In other words, perceptions about goal pursuits cause certain emotions, and our research supports this contention (Snyder et al., 1996).

The foundation of hope is set by age 2 years, and lacking some profound later childhood stressor, the level of hope would be expected to remain stable as the child navigates the preschool, middle, and adolescent years. Even though toddlers are relatively set in their hopeful thinking, they still lack the necessary language skills to respond accurately to self-report measures. These requisite language skills for responding to simple questions about themselves should be in place, however, by the second or third grade. Accordingly, we set out to develop a self-report hope scale for children ages 7 to 15 years.

Children's Hope Scale

Development of the Children's Hope Scale (CHS) began with discussion of more than 40 items by my research group, which eventually agreed upon 6 items that best reflected pathways thinking and 6 others that best reflected agency thinking. The pathways items tapped content involved with finding ways to reach goals under ordinary and blocked circumstances. The agency items tapped content reflecting an active, "doing" orientation. The 12 items were then read by 25 children (ages 7–15 years) in a pilot study, as well as by 10 of the researchers' children, who were asked to mark their responses on a continuum ranging from 1 (*none of the time*) to 6 (*all of the time*). Using the children's feedback, we developed simplified forms of the items.

This initial 12-item version of the CHS was given to 372 fourth through sixth graders in the public schools of Edmond, Oklahoma (OK pre sample). Factor analysis of the data (using principal components analysis with varimax rotations and a requested two-factor solution) found three agency and three pathway items with weak or equivocal loadings on the two factors, and these items were discarded. The remaining six items formed the final CHS (see Appendix).

To cross-validate the factor structure, the six-item CHS was given to the same Oklahoma sample 1 month later (OK post sample) and then to five other samples:

- 91 children, ages 8–17 years, with sickle-cell anemia, arthritis, or cancer who took the CHS at the beginning (MO pre sample) and end of a 1-week summer camp in Missouri (MO post sample);

- 170 boys, ages 7–13 years, with attention-deficit/hyperactivity disorder diagnoses who attended a summer treatment program in Pennsylvania (PA1 sample);
- 74 nonreferred boys similar in age to the boys in the other Pennsylvania sample (PA2 sample);
- 143 children, ages 8–16 years, previously treated for cancer in Texas;
- 322 children, ages 9–13 years, who attended public schools in Kansas.

Factor analysis showed that the three pathways items typically loaded on one factor more highly, whereas the three agency items loaded more highly on the other. Generally, the pathways items loaded most heavily on the first factor in half of the administrations, and the agency items loaded most heavily on the first factor in the other half of the administrations. Occasionally, an individual item loaded incorrectly, but overall the items loaded on the appropriate factor in 42 out of 48 instances (87.5%). Thus, the pathways and agency items are distinguishable in the children's responses. Furthermore, the eigenvalues and variances accounted for supported the robustness of each factor. For example, the median variance accounted for was 36.0% (range: 29.0%–58.1%) for the first factor, 26.4% (range: 11.3%–31.5%) for the second factor, and 63.4% for both (range: 56.4%–69.4%). In addition, the agency and pathways components correlated positively and significantly with each other in the various samples.

Psychometric Properties

The CHS scores from our six samples were negatively skewed, indicating that most children scored toward the high end of the response continuum. Means ranged from a low of 25.41 to a high of 27.03, with a median mean of 25.89 (Table 2). When total mean scores are translated to the average response on each item, a mean of 4.30 results, suggesting that children described their hope level on each item as being between "a lot of the time" and "most of the time." Analyses by subgroups, where possible, showed no significant differences in CHS scores in terms of gender or race/ethnicity. Neither age nor family income correlated with CHS scores.

Overall, the response data showed good variability and reliability. Coefficients of variability for the CHS ranged from .12 to .24, with a median of .19 (Table 2). For all samples, Cronbach's alphas were greater than .70, and item-remainder coefficients ranged from .27 to .68, with a median of .54 ($ps < .01$). In the two instances where the CHS was readministered, test-retest correlations were highly significant ($p < .001$). In the Oklahoma sample, r (359) equaled .71 when retesting after 1 month, and in the Missouri sample, r (89) equaled .73 when retesting after 1 week.

Concurrent Validity

The CHS has performed well in several tests of concurrent validity. In one test, we hypothesized that people, such as parents, who are familiar with particular children should be able to accurately rate their hope levels. Accordingly, the parents of the schoolchildren in the Oklahoma sample were asked to use a modified CHS to rate how each of the six items described their children's thought processes. Parents' ratings correlated positively with their children's actual CHS (OK pre sample) scores, r (264) = .38, p < .01. Additionally, the parents of children at the summer camps in Missouri also predicted their children's CHS (MO pre sample) scores, r (89) = .50, p < .01, as did the camp counselors, who had interacted with the children for only 5 days, r (89) = .21, p < .05.

In another assessment of concurrent validity, we gave children in four samples (OK pre sample, Kansas sample, and both Pennsylvania samples) the Self-Perception Profile for Children (Harter, 1985), which taps self-perceptions in the areas of scholastics, social acceptance, athletics, physical appearance, behavioral conduct, and global self-worth. CHS scores correlated positively and significantly with these six subscales, with only one exception (physical appearance in the Pennsylvania nonpatient sample) in 24 correlations.

Because of the positive expectations regarding goals in the CHS, positive correlations should result with variables tapping a sense of control. We tested this idea using Nowicki and Strickland's (1973) Locus of Control scale. Scores on this scale were correlated with CHS scores in three samples, yielding the following results: Oklahoma children (OK pre sample), r (337) = −.33, p < .001; Pennsylvania patients, r (35) = −.35, p < .05, and Pennsylvania nonpatients, r (45) = −.29, p < .05.[1] Also in these latter two samples, we used Connell's (1985) Multidimensional Measure of Children's Perceptions of Control, which measures control perceptions in cognitive, social, and physical domains. Correlations of this measure with the CHS showed that higher hope related to personal control (internal factors) for all three domains but did not relate strongly to control attributed to powerful others (external factors).

According to hope theory, children and adults who face repeated goal blockages and unsuccessful attempts to circumvent such impediments should be more prone to depression (Snyder, 1994). As such, the perception that one cannot reach desired goals should exacerbate depressive processes. Thus, high CHS scores should relate to lower reported depression. To test this notion, the Child Depression Inventory (Kovacs, 1985) was given to the Oklahoma (OK pre) and both Pennsylvania samples. As expected, CHS scores correlated negatively with the depression scores, r (345) = −.48, p < .001; r (109) = −.19, p < .05; and r (71) = −.40, p < .001, respectively.

Effective thinking about goal-related matters often involves other people. Thus, higher-hope children should report less loneliness, as have young adults (Snyder, 1994). To test this concurrent validity with children, we gave the Asher loneliness questionnaire (Asher & Wheeler, 1985) and the Network and Attachment Loneliness Scale (Hoza & Beery, 1993) to the two Pennsylvania samples. CHS scores correlated negatively with overall loneliness indices in the patient sample, r (110) = −.20, p < .04; attachment loneliness, rs (66) = −.28 and −.32, ps < .03, respectively, as well as in the nonpatient sample: overall loneliness, r

---

[1] Lower Nowicki-Strickland scores reflect more internality.

$(72) = -.38, p < .01$; attachment loneliness, rs $(71) = -.26$ and $-.30$, ps $< .03$, respectively.

Other Types of Validity

Children's capacities to form goals and use pathways effectively to pursue those goals should facilitate the learning of school information. As a test of this predictive validity, CHS scores obtained on the Oklahoma (OK pre) sample were correlated with their scores 6 months later on the Iowa Test of Basic Skills (ITBS; Hieronymous & Hoover, 1985), which taps general cognitive skills (word analysis, vocabulary, reading, language, word study, and mathematics; Lane, 1992). CHS scores significantly predicted the ITBS cumulative percentile scores, $r(100) = .50, p < .001$.

Discriminant validity demonstrates that there are other indices that bear only very small relationships with a new measure. In regard to the CHS, we believed that it was not tapping the same construct as the Hopelessness Scale (Kazdin et al., 1983). To test this idea, we gave both scales to patients and non-patients in the two Pennsylvania samples. The correlations were negative but not statistically significant, r $(35) = -.18$ and r $(13) = -.24$, respectively. Sharing only 3% to 6% of variance, the positive, hopeful, goal-directed thinking tapped by the CHS is not synonymous with the negative expectancies of the Hopelessness Scale.

In a second test of discriminant validity, we expected that the responses to a new scale should not be explicable in terms of socially desirable responding. We therefore administered the Children's Social Desirability Questionnaire (Crandall, Crandall, & Katkovsky, 1965) to the sample of Kansas school children, finding a positive but small relation between that scale and the CHS, r $(303) = .21, p < .001$.

Yet another aspect of scale development is incremental validity, which is the degree to which a new scale enhances predictions of a criterion variable beyond scores from previously available measures. For example, do the CHS scores augment the prediction of achievement scores beyond perceived self-worth scores? Using ITBS scores as the criterion variable, we entered scores from the global self-worth subscale of the Self-Perception Profile for Children into a hierarchical multiple regression at step 1, yielding an R^2 of .04 ($p < .05$). The addition of CHS scores to the model at step 2 generated an incremental change in R^2 of .22 ($p < .001$). In another regression with ITBS scores as the criterion variable, Nowicki-Strickland Locus of Control scores entered at step 1 resulted in an R^2 of .20 ($p < .001$), and the addition of CHS scores to the model in step 2 produced a positive change in R^2 of .35 ($p < .001$). Both of these analyses demonstrate the incremental validity of the CHS.

Status of the Children's Hope Scale

Across samples of children from differing geographical locations, the pathways and agency CHS subscales have been found to be factorially identifiable and robust. Extracted total variances of 40% to 50% reflect factor structures with substantial impacts (see Gorsuch, 1983), and the CHS always surpassed this criterion (Table 1). These two distinguishable components of hopeful thinking emerged within an overall measure that displayed internal consistency via both Cronbach's alphas and item-remainder coefficients (Table 2). Self-report scales with internal reliabilities of at least .70 are deemed acceptable for research purposes (Nunnally, 1978), and the CHS repeatedly met this standard. Also, the Cronbach's alphas and item-remainder coefficients for the CHS are of high magnitudes similar to those for the adult Hope Scale (Snyder et al., 1991). As such, 7- to 15-year-old children do not appear to be limited by cognitive inconsistencies in responding to the CHS.

Furthermore, despite the fact that the two components were factorally identifiable, they also displayed relationships of .47 to .70, sharing variances of 22% to 49% (Table 1). Although other researchers are examining the pathways and agency scores separately, we do not support this practice because of (a) the theoretical foundation suggesting that both thoughts must be added in order to measure the full hope construct, (b) the ample relationships between the components, and (c) the lack of internal reliability for scales with only three items.

The CHS was developed to tap enduring goal-directed thinking, and the test–retests conducted at 1- and 4-week intervals supported this posited stability. These test–retest correlations are of a magnitude comparable to those found for the adult Hope Scale (median r of .75; Snyder, Harris, et al., 1991). Additional work is needed, however, to test the stability of the CHS over several months and perhaps even years.

That scores on the CHS appear to be stable over time does not preclude, however, the existence of variability among individuals in responding to scale. In fact, the coefficients of variability reveal that the CHS does elicit varying responses *across different children* (Table 2). That is, within each sample, there were children reporting low, medium, and high degrees of hope. Such variability of responses across research participants is important in scale development because it suggests sensitivity to individual differences; moreover, this variability across respondents increases the likelihood that a given scale will manifest relationships with other measures. The .19 coefficient of variability for the CHS is comparable in magnitude to that for the adult Hope Scale (Snyder et al., 1991).

No differences in CHS scores appeared in relation to age in the present studies. Recall our earlier assumption that once the level of hope is established in toddlerhood, there should not be any major subsequent changes. Of course, major decrements in hopeful thinking still are possible should the child encounter severe traumatic events. It is important to note, however, that we cannot make longitudinal inferences from the cross-sectional age cohorts sampled in our various studies. Thus, future research should plot the changes in CHS scores *of the same children* over the course of their middle childhood and adolescent years.

In the present samples of children, as well as in all studies measuring hope in adults, *significant gender differences have never emerged*. Perhaps there truly are no gender differences in hopeful thinking. It may be, however, that the boys and girls in the present studies were thinking about different goals. If a strong gender bias still is operating in the lives of children in the present samples,

Table 1. Factor Analyses on Children's Hope Scale (CHS) Items across Six Samples

| | Sample | | | | | | | | | | | | | | | |
| | OK pre[a] | | OK post[b] | | MO pre[c] | | MO post[d] | | PA1[e] | | PA2[f] | | TX[g] | | KS[h] | |
Factor #	1	2	1	2	1	2	1	2	1	2	1	2	1	2	1	2
Agency item																
1	0.85	0.09	0.87	0.14	0.04	0.86	0.06	0.93	0.77	0.02	0.81	-0.03	0.13	0.84	0.26	0.86
3	0.74	0.28	0.79	0.29	0.61	0.42	0.47	0.68	0.71	0.13	0.81	0.09	0.40	0.58	0.34	0.80
5	0.64	0.21	0.57	0.39	0.34	0.69	0.59	0.37	0.18	0.78	0.56	0.37	0.13	0.74	0.67	0.37
Pathways item																
2	0.02	0.85	0.15	0.80	0.76	0.14	0.70	0.10	0.59	0.30	-0.06	0.92	0.77	0.07	0.78	0.21
4	0.32	0.52	0.43	0.65	0.84	0.12	0.71	0.36	0.69	0.40	0.50	0.67	0.68	0.21	0.73	0.34
6	0.41	0.65	0.24	0.76	0.54	0.54	0.83	0.79	0.13	0.82	0.72	0.19	0.69	0.22	0.81	0.25
Eigenvalue	2.65	0.86	3.06	0.78	2.91	0.85	2.98	0.89	2.56	0.87	2.74	1.11	1.74	1.70	3.49	0.70
% Variance accounted for	32.5	25.9	32.6	31.5	34.2	28.5	37.7	26.8	42.7	14.6	45.7	18.5	29	28.2	58.1	11.3
Correlation of agency-pathways*	0.52		0.61		0.61		0.64		0.59		0.47		0.47		0.7	

[a] OK pre = 197 boys and 175 girls, ages 9–14 years, from the 4th through 6th grade in Edmond, OK, public schools.

[b] OK post = 196 boys and 173 girls from the Edmond, OK, schools who retook the CHS after a 1-month interval.

[c] MO pre = 48 boys and 43 girls, ages 9–17 years, who took the CHS at the beginning of 1-week summer camps for children with arthritis, sickle-cell anemia, or cancer, near Kansas City, MO.

[d] MO post = the same 48 boys and 43 girls 1 week after the beginning of the Missouri camps.

[e] PA1 = 170 boys, ages 7–13 years, diagnosed with attention-deficit/hyperactivity disorder who attended a summer program run by the Western Psychiatric Institute and Clinic in Pittsburgh, PA.

[f] PA2 = 74 nonreferred control boys who were similar in age to the PA1 group above.

[g] TX = 70 boys and 73 girls, ages 8–16 years, who were or had been under treatment for cancer at the University of Texas M. D. Anderson Cancer Center.

[h] KS = 154 boys and 168 girls, ages 9–13 years, from the Overland Park and Lawrence, KS, public schools.

* For all agency-pathways correlations, $p < .001$.

Table 2. Psychometric Properties of Children's Hope Scale Total Scores across Six Samples

Measure	Sample[a]							
	OK pre	OK post	MO pre	MO post	PA1	PA2	TX	KS
Mean	25.41	27.03	25.93	26.39	25.49	25.98	25.84	25.71
Standard deviation	4.99	4.51	5.23	5.05	3.63	3.01	5.01	6.11
Coefficient of variability	0.20	0.17	0.20	0.19	0.14	0.12	0.19	0.24
Alpha	0.74	0.81	0.79	0.80	0.73	0.75	0.72	0.86
Item-remainder coefficient[b]	.38/.57	.51/.62	.43/.61	.43/.65	.38/.61	.27/.62	.42/.50	.61/.68

[a] See Table 1 for descriptions of samples.
[b] Value pairs represent ranges.

perhaps the girls relative to the boys may have "settled" for less prestigious or less challenging goals (see Snyder, 1994). In this sense, both girls and boys may be equally high in pathways and agency thoughts *for the goals that they perceive as being "appropriate" for their gender.* In future research with the CHS, therefore, it will be helpful to ask girls and boys about the actual goals that they are conjuring for themselves.

The lack of racial differences in hope was testable in only one sample (the Texas one), and the means were not statistically different. In the only other reported study of CHS scores and race, Callahan (2000) found that African Americans were highest and Caucasians second highest at the intermediate and middle school years; at the high school level, Caucasians were highest. Moreover, Native American students were third highest, and Hispanic students were lowest in CHS scores throughout the various levels. Obviously, other samples will be necessary before speculating about racial differences, or lack thereof, in CHS scores.

Family income was not related to the scores on the CHS. In this regard, elevated hope should develop in environments where children are given sufficient care and attention, and affluence per se probably does not serve as a proxy for such environments. If the primary caregiver has enough time and energy to foster a child's hopeful thinking, then family income may not have a major impact upon hope. In previous research we have found that high- as compared to low-hope adults reported that their caregiver spent much more time with them when they were growing up (Snyder, 1994). Although wealthier child-rearing environments have more money available for taking care of children, it may be that this seeming advantage is counterbalanced by the fact that the caregiver parents are personally unavailable to the children because the parents are engrossed in career or work activities.

The various CHS results generally support concurrent validation. First, it appears that observers can rate a child's hope with some degree of success. Second, the scores on the CHS exhibited the predicted negative correlations with depression and loneliness. Elsewhere, we have written that higher hope is learned in a trusting, supportive atmosphere where interpersonal relationships are a part of many goal-directed activities (Snyder, Cheavens, & Sympson, 1997). On this latter issue, children's higher CHS scores also have correlated significantly with greater parental support (Hodgkins, 2001). Furthermore, we have found empirical support for high hope being related to secure attachments (Shorey, Snyder, Yang, & Lewin, in press) and greater satisfaction with interpersonal relationships (Snyder, 2002).

Children's hopeful thinking is built upon a foundation of perceived proficiency at pursuing goals. The pathways and agency components bear similarities to what Skinner (1992) has called strategy and capacity, respectively. These latter components, according to Skinner, are the bases of children's perceptions of control. On this point, various validational results attest to the fact that higher CHS scores were related to greater self-reported competency ratings. Also, the higher-hope children perceive that they, instead of external sources, were in control in their lives. Overall, the children who score high as compared to low on the CHS are likely to think about themselves as being linked to positive outcomes, thereby validating a central premise of hope theory.

The CHS also manifested discriminant validity in that its scores correlated positively and yet minimally with socially desirable responding. Although the magnitude of this particular relationship is small, it has been suggested that high hope may at times reflect a slight, positive self-bias; moreover, it has been reasoned that such a slight hopeful bias is adaptive (see Snyder, 1989). On this latter point, research with the CHS has shown that the positive biases of higher-hope children are slight and are bounded by reality constraints (Hinton-Nelson, Roberts, & Snyder, 1996; Kliewer & Lewis, 1995).

Thus, any slight bias that high-hope children may have does not appear to be harmful, and in fact, as one data set suggests, higher hope is related to a positive outcome in terms of performance on the achievement test. Beyond predicting school-related achievement, the CHS scores augmented the perceived competency-based and locus of control predictions. Obviously, however, much additional research is needed to test the longitudinal predictive capabilities of the CHS in a variety of arenas. Such research already has revealed that the adult Hope Scale can be used to make fairly robust predictions in academics, athletics, and health (Snyder, 2002).

One area that has yet to receive much research attention to date involves the role of hope in treatments for children. A study reported by McNeal (1998) found that CHS scores increased reliably for a sample of children who underwent residential treatment for acting out inappropriately. It is impossible to make any inferences based on this study, however, because there was no comparison group of children who did not receive treatment. We have suggested that hope may be a common factor in psychotherapy with adults (Snyder et al., 2000), and there is every reason to believe that the same may be true for children undergoing treatment (see McDermott & Snyder, 2000). As such, the CHS may serve as a predictor for successful treatment outcomes for children, and it may be sensitive enough to detect changes in children's hope as a function of treatment.

To date, the CHS has been used in six separate samples in our laboratories, with a total of 1,169 child research participants. Additionally, eight samples involving 744 children have been gathered by researchers in other laboratories. Thus, the research to date has sampled 1,913 children (roughly equal numbers of girls and boys) in 15 states across the United States. The age ranges of research participants have been from 7 through 16 years. Moreover, children without any identified problems have participated in the studies, as have children with psychological and physical problems. Furthermore, some initial attempts have been made to compare the Children's Hope Scale scores of children from differing racial backgrounds. For a scale that was published in 1997, this is a modest record—one that represents a start at having more researchers consider the CHS in their work. On this latter point, if hope is indeed our children's chance for a better future, then we adults would be wise to increase our efforts to understand it today.

Author's Note

This article is based, in part, on Snyder, Hoza, et al. (1997). For additional information about hope research, contact C. R. Snyder, 1415 Jayhawk Blvd., Department of Psychology, 340 Fraser Hall, University of Kansas, Lawrence, KS 66045 (crsnyder@ku.edu).

Appendix

Children's Hope Scale

---

1. I think I am doing pretty well.
2. I can think of many ways to get the things in life that are most important to me.
3. I am doing just as well as other kids my age.
4. When I have a problem, I can come up with lots of ways to solve it.
5. I think the things I have done in the past will help me in the future.
6. Even when others want to quit, I know that I can find ways to solve the problem.

Note: The total score is achieved by adding responses to the six items, where 1 = *none of the time*, 2 = *a little of the time*, 3 = *some of the time*, 4 = *a lot of the time*, 5 = *most of the time*, and 6 = *all of the time*. The three odd-numbered items tap agency, and the three even-numbered items tap pathways.

References

Asher, S. R., & Wheeler, V. A. (1985). Children's loneliness: A comparison of rejected and neglected peer status. *Journal of Consulting and Clinical Psychology, 53*, 500–505.

Barker, R., Dembo, T., & Lewin, K. (1941). Frustration and regression: An experiment with young children. *University of Iowa Studies in Child Welfare, 18*(1).

Barrera, M. E., & Maurer, D. (1981). The perception of facial expressions by the three-month-old. *Child Development, 52*, 203–206.

Bates, E., Camaioni, L., & Volterra, V. (1975). The acquisition of performances prior to speech. *Merrill Palmer Quarterly, 21*, 205–226.

Berger, K. E. (1991). *The developing person through childhood and adolescence.* New York: Worth.

Bretherton, I., & Beeghly, M. (1982). Talking about internal states: The acquisition of an explicit theory of mind. *Developmental Psychology, 18*, 906–921.

Callahan, B. M. (2000). *Ethnicity and hope in children*. Unpublished dissertation, University of Kansas, Lawrence.

Connell, J. P. (1985). A new multidimensional measure of children's perceptions of control. *Child Development, 56*, 1018–1041.

Corrigan, R. L. (1978). Language development as related to stage 6 object permanence development. *Journal of Child Language, 5*, 173–189.

Crandall, V. C., Crandall, V. J., & Katkovsky, W. (1965). A children's social desirability questionnaire. *Journal of Consulting and Clinical Psychology, 29*, 27–36.

Dodge, K. A. (1986). A social information processing model of social competence. In M. Perlmutter (Ed.), *Minnesota Symposium on Child Psychology: Vol. 18. Cognitive perspectives on children's social and behavioral development* (pp. 77–125). Hillsdale, NJ: Lawrence Erlbaum.

Gorsuch, R. L. (1983). *Factor analysis*. Hillsdale, NJ: Lawrence Erlbaum.

Harter, S. (1985). *Manual for the Self-Perception Profile for Children: Revision of the Perceived Competence Scale for Children*. Denver: University of Denver Press.

Hieronymous, A. N., & Hoover, H. D. (1985). *Iowa Test of Basic Skills*. Chicago: Riverside.

Hinton-Nelson, M. D., Roberts, M. C., & Snyder, C. R. (1996). Early adolescents exposed to violence: Hope and vulnerability to victimization. *American Journal of Orthopsychiatry, 66*, 346–353.

Hodgkins, N. M. (2001). The relationship of parental acceptance/rejection to hope and shame in adolescents. *Dissertation Abstracts International, 62*(1-B), 550.

Hoza, B., & Beery, S. H. (1993, March). *Assessing children's loneliness in the peer and family contexts*. Poster presented at the meeting of the Society for Research in Child Development, New Orleans, LA.

Kaplan, L. (1978). *Oneness and separateness*. New York: Simon & Schuster.

Kazdin, A. E., French, N. H., Unis, A. S., Esveldt-Dawson, K., & Sherick, R. B. (1983). Hopelessness, depression, and suicidal intent among psychiatrically disturbed children. *Journal of Consulting and Clinical Psychology, 51*, 504–510.

Kliewer, W., & Lewis, H. (1995). Family influences on coping processes in children with sickle cell disease. *Journal of Pediatric Psychology, 20*, 511–525.

Kopp, C. B. (1989). Regulation of distress and negative emotions: A developmental view. *Developmental Psychology, 25*, 343–354.

Kovacs, M. (1985). The Children's Depression Inventory (CDI). *Psychopharmacology Bulletin, 21*, 995–998.

Lane, S. (1992). Review of the Iowa Test of Basic Skills. In J. J. Kramer & J. C. Conoley (Eds.), *The eleventh mental measurement yearbook* (pp. 419–424). Lincoln: University of Nebraska, Buros Institute of Mental Measurements.

McDermott, D., & Snyder, C. R. (2000). *The great big book of hope: Help your children achieve their dreams*. Oakland, CA: New Harbinger Publications.

McNeal, R. E. (1998). Pre- and post-treatment hope in children and adolescents in residential treatment: A further analysis of the effects of the teaching family model. *Dissertation Abstracts International, 59*(5-B), 2425.

Menninger, K. (1959). The academic lecture on hope. *American Journal of Psychiatry, 116*, 481–491.

Nowicki, S., & Strickland, B. (1973). A locus of control scale for children. *Journal of Consulting and Clinical Psychology, 40*(1), 148–154.

Nunnally, J. C. (1978). *Psychometric theory* (2nd ed.). San Francisco: Jossey-Bass.

Pervin, L. A. (Ed.). (1989). *Goal concepts in personality and social psychology*. Hillsdale, NJ: Lawrence Erlbaum.

Roberts, M. C., Brown, K. J., Johnson, R. J., & Reinke, J. (2002). Positive psychology for children: Development, prevention, and promotion. In C. R. Snyder & S. J. Lopez (Eds.), *Handbook of positive psychology* (pp. 663–675). New York: Oxford University Press.

Schulman, M. (1991). *The passionate mind*. New York: Free Press.

Shorey, H. S., Snyder, C. R., Yang, X., & Lewin, M. R. (in press). The role of hope as a mediator in recollecting parenting, adult attachment, and mental health. *Journal of Social and Clinical Psychology*.

Skinner, E. A. (1992). Perceived control: Motivation, coping, and development. In R. Schwarzer (Ed.), *Thought control of action* (pp. 91–106). Washington, DC: Hemisphere.

Snyder, C. R. (1989). Reality negotiation: From excuses to hope and beyond. *Journal of Social and Clinical Psychology, 8,* 130–157.

Snyder, C. R. (1994). *The psychology of hope: You can get there from here.* New York: Free Press.

Snyder, C. R. (2002). Hope theory: Rainbows of the mind. *Psychological Inquiry, 13,* 249–275.

Snyder, C. R., Cheavens, J., & Sympson, S. (1997). Hope: An individual motive for social commerce. *Group Dynamics: Theory, Research, and Practice, 1,* 107–118.

Snyder, C. R., Harris, C., Anderson, J. R., Holleran, S. A., Irving, L. M., Sigmon, S., et al. (1991). The will and the ways: Development and validation of an individual-differences measure of hope. *Journal of Personality and Social Psychology, 60,* 570–585.

Snyder, C. R., Hoza, B., Pelham, W. E., Rapoff, M., Ware, L., Danovsky, M., et al. (1997). The development and validation of the Children's Hope Scale. *Journal of Pediatric Psychology, 22*(3), 399–421.

Snyder, C. R., Ilardi, S. S., Cheavens, J., Michael, S. T., Yamhure, L., & Sympson, S. (2000). The role of hope in cognitive behavior therapies. *Cognitive Therapy and Research, 24,* 747–762.

Snyder, C. R., & Lopez, S. J. (Eds.) (2002). *Handbook of positive psychology.* New York: Oxford University Press.

Snyder, C. R., Sympson, S. C., Ybasco, F. C., Borders, T. F., Babyak, M. A., & Higgins, R. L. (1996). Development and validation of the State Hope Scale. *Journal of Personality and Social Psychology, 70,* 321–335.

Stevenson, H. W., & Newman, R. S. (1986). Long-term prediction of achievement and attitudes in mathematics and reading. *Child Development, 57,* 646–659.

Stevenson, M. B., Ver Hoeve, J. N., Roach, M. A., & Leavitt, L. A. (1986). The beginning of conversation: Early patterns of mother-infant vocal responsiveness. *Infant Behavior and Development, 9,* 423–440.

Stotland, E. (1969). *The psychology of hope.* San Francisco: Jossey-Bass.

6 The Ethnic Identity Scale

Adriana J. Umaña-Taylor

University of Illinois at Urbana-Champaign

Identity formation is a critical developmental task that increases in salience during adolescence as individuals begin to grapple with the question "Who am I?" (Erikson, 1968). Given that the resolution of one's identity during this period is thought to serve as a guiding framework in adulthood (e.g., Swanson, Spencer, & Petersen, 1997), there is a growing interest in exploring adolescents' identity development. A component of global identity that has gained attention in recent years is adolescents' ethnic identity, particularly because as the United States becomes more diverse, ethnic identity may emerge as a particularly salient component.

Ethnic identity has been examined in relation to numerous outcome variables, such as self-esteem (see Umaña-Taylor, Diversi, & Fine, 2002), academic achievement (Arellano & Padilla, 1996), and individuals' ability to cope with discrimination (e.g., Phinney & Chavira, 1995). Findings tend to be mixed, with some studies providing evidence of significant associations between these constructs and other studies finding limited evidence regarding an association between ethnic identity and important outcome variables. A significant limitation of existing work is the lack of a theoretically grounded measurement tool that is appropriate for use with multiple ethnic and racial groups. In fact, scholars suggest that the divergent findings, which plague the literature on this topic, are in large part due to the variation in conceptualization and measurement of ethnic identity (see Umaña-Taylor et al., 2002, for a review). As such, there is a great need for a valid and reliable measure of ethnic identity that is applicable to a diverse group of individuals.

This chapter presents data from three studies, all of which provide preliminary evidence for the psychometric soundness of the Ethnic Identity Scale (EIS), which was designed to measure the multifaceted nature of ethnic identity (see Umaña-Taylor, Yazedjian, & Bámaca-Gómez, 2004).

Ethnic identity has been conceptualized using both Tajfel's (1981) social identity theory and Erikson's (1968) identity formation theory. Social identity theory posits that identity develops from both an individual's sense of belonging to a particular group and the affective component accompanying that sense of group membership. Furthermore, Tajfel suggests that individuals' self-esteem is derived from their sense of group belonging, and, consequently, those who maintain favorable definitions of group membership will also exhibit positive self-esteem (e.g., Phinney, Cantu, & Kurtz, 1997). However, if the social climate in which individuals' lives are embedded does not place value on the ethnic group and individuals experience discrimination or prejudice, they may display lower self-esteem than members of groups who do not have these experiences.

Alternatively, Erikson's (1968) identity formation theory posits that identity development occurs through a process of exploration and commitment to important identity domains of a broader self-concept. Yet, Erikson's postulations do not articulate that one's commitment to a component identity is necessarily always positive. Rather, Erikson indicates that individuals will, as a result of exploration, resolve their feelings about the role of a particular component identity (e.g., vocational, religious, sexual, political) within their broader social self. Furthermore, Erikson's theory suggests that the culmination of such a period of exploration will lead the individual to "reconcile his conception of himself and his community's recognition of him" (Erikson, 1959, p. 120). In other words, it is only through the process of exploration that individuals can come to a resolution regarding a particular identity. Thus, from an Eriksonian perspective, there are two critical components to the process of identity formation: exploration and commitment. Note that while social identity theory focuses more on the affective components of identity and how they are related to outcomes, Erikson's theory places greater emphasis on the process of identity development.

Marcia's (1980, 1994) operationalization of Erikson's theory of identity formation allows researchers to classify individuals, based on their degree of exploration and commitment, into one of four identity statuses: *diffuse, foreclosed, moratorium,* and *achieved*. According to this typology, individuals who have not explored or committed to an identity would be considered diffuse, and those who have explored but have not yet committed would be considered to be in moratorium. In contrast, individuals who have not explored, but have committed to a particular identity, would be considered foreclosed, whereas those who have both explored and committed would be considered achieved.

In terms of ethnic identity, Phinney (1989) drew on Tajfel's and Erikson's theories as well as Marcia's operationalization of Erikson's theory to develop a conceptualization of ethnic identity and eventually a measure that assessed ethnic identity. Phinney's (1992) Multigroup Ethnic Identity Measure (MEIM) includes 14 items that assess individuals' degree of exploration, commitment, participation in cultural activities, and affirmation and belonging regarding their ethnic group. Items are summed and a composite score is used to determine degree of ethnic identity achievement. Recent work (i.e., Roberts et al., 1999) suggests that a revised 12-item version of the MEIM should be utilized; however, the scoring remains the same: a sum score is created to determine individuals' degree of ethnic identity achievement.

Because the MEIM has been the most widely used measure of ethnic identity, past research has been conducted under the assumption that an *achieved* ethnic identity implies not only a greater amount of commitment and exploration but also a *positive identification* with the group. In such research, the process of ethnic identity (e.g., ways in which individuals have explored their identity and developed an understanding of how they feel about that group membership) has been examined but only in the context of one's positive response to one's ethnic group. Although Phinney's theoretical postulation does not assume a positive commitment to the group, the measurement tool based on that theoretical model does. Therefore, in using the MEIM, only individuals whose commitment to their ethnic identity is positive are characterized as having an achieved identity. Consequently, the measurement is incongruent with the theory, as one's commitment is confounded with one's affirmation of one's ethnic identity.

Furthermore, with current operationalizations of ethnic identity, it is difficult to understand the relationship between ethnic identity and various outcomes. For example, based on existing work with the MEIM, findings suggest that it may be unhealthy to have a low degree of identification with one's ethnic group (e.g., lower self-esteem). With the current operationalization of the construct, however, it is not possible to decipher which aspect of the ethnic identity formation process is associated with negative outcomes. With current methods, exploration, commitment, and affirmation toward one's ethnicity are examined jointly. The key to furthering our understanding of the aspects of ethnic identity formation that are associated with outcomes may lie in examining exploration, resolution, and affirmation as *distinct components* of ethnic identity as opposed to using a sum score of a measure that combines individuals' scores on the three constructs.

It is particularly important to address this issue given that current methods of assessing ethnic identity development are not entirely consistent with Erikson's original formulation of exploration and commitment. With current methods, identity resolution is examined along a continuum of exploration, commitment, and affirmation. Such a continuum precludes the possibility of creating *statuses* of ethnic identity by assuming a continuous process of identity negotiation that culminates in a positive assessment of ethnic group membership. Whereas Erikson's original conceptualization of commitment implied a resolution of how various component identities are related to the broader self, current definitions of commitment imply a positive assessment of the meaning of group membership.

As a result, the EIS was introduced (see Umaña-Taylor et al., 2004) as a measurement tool that could assess a typology for examining ethnic identity statuses that was consistent with Marcia's operationalization of Erikson's theory and Tajfel's social identity theory. This typology mirrors Marcia's, by examining whether individuals' degree of exploration and resolution regarding ethnicity is high or low. Consistent with Marcia's framework, the typology uses the statuses diffuse, foreclosed, moratorium, and achieved. Furthermore, the typology adds a third dimension that is in line with social identity theory. Based on individuals' scores on a measure of affirmation, a positive or negative label is assigned to their diffuse, foreclosed, moratorium, or achieved status. Thus, an individual who scores low on both exploration and commitment but high on affirmation would be categorized as diffuse positive, whereas an individual who scores low on all three components would be categorized as diffuse negative.

By developing a measure that independently assesses the three distinct components of ethnic identity formation and thereby allows for the classification of individuals into an ethnic identity typology, the framework through which ethnic identity is examined can be refined and can more clearly capture its variability. In other words, the proposed typology captures the experiences of individuals who feel that their ethnicity is an important component of their social selves, engage in a process of exploration, resolve their feelings, and choose to affirm the role that their ethnic identity plays in their lives. Additionally, it can capture the experiences of individuals who have explored their ethnicity and maintain a clear sense of what that group membership means to them, yet may not ascribe positive feelings toward their ethnic group.

Two studies were conducted to develop and explore the psychometric properties of the EIS (see Umaña-Taylor et al., 2004). This chapter provides a review of the findings from these two studies, in addition to providing additional information that was not presented in Umaña-Taylor et al., such as coefficient alphas of the subscales for each pan-ethnic/racial group in the sample. In addition, findings from a third study, a longitudinal study of Latino high school students, are explored and compared with findings from the initial two studies.

Method

Initially, two studies were conducted to examine the psychometric properties of the EIS. The first study used exploratory and confirmatory analyses to examine, refine, and confirm the factor structure of the EIS in a university sample. In addition, the psychometric properties of the refined measure were examined in the first study. The second study examined the methodological properties of the three subscales that were developed in Study 1 with a sample of high school students to determine whether the measure was valid and reliable with a younger adolescent population. Finally, a third study was conducted in which the psychometric properties of the EIS were further examined with a group of Latino 9th- and 10th-grade students.

In all three studies, adolescents completed a questionnaire that included the following measures: Umaña-Taylor et al.'s (2004) EIS, Rosenberg's (1979) Self-esteem Scale, and Umaña-Taylor's (2001) Familial Ethnic Socialization Measure. Questionnaires were self-administered and participation was voluntary. For high school students, written parental consent was obtained; active written consent was obtained from university students.

Measures

Ethnic Identity

The EIS includes 17 items, scored on a 4-point Likert scale, with responses ranging from *Does not describe me at all* (1) to *Describes me very well* (4). Items assessed the degree to which individuals (a) had engaged in exploring their ethnicity (e.g., I have read books, magazines, newspapers, or other materials that have taught me about my ethnicity), (b) had resolved issues related to their ethnicity (e.g., "I understand how I feel about my ethnicity"), and (c) felt positively about their ethnicity (e.g., "I dislike my ethnicity"). Negatively worded items were reverse scored such that higher scores indicated higher levels of exploration, resolution, and affirmation.

Race/Ethnicity

The following introduction and brief question preceded the EIS items in the questionnaire:

> The U.S. is made up of people of various ethnicities. Ethnicity refers to cultural traditions, beliefs, and behaviors that are passed down through generations. Some examples of the ethnicities that people may identify with are Mexican, Cuban, Nicaraguan, Chinese, Taiwanese, Filipino, Jamaican, African American, Haitian, Italian, Irish, and German. In addition, some people may identify with more than one ethnicity. When you are answering the following questions, we'd like you to think about what YOU consider your ethnicity to be. Please write what you consider to be your ethnicity here ___ and refer to this ethnicity as you answer the questions below.

The participant's response to this question was then used to create the variable *race/ethnicity*.

Self-esteem

Rosenberg's (1979) Self-esteem Scale was used to assess participants' global self-esteem. This measure comprises 10 items (e.g., "At times I think I am no good at all") with end points of *strongly disagree* (1) to *strongly agree* (4). Items were scored such that higher scores indicated higher self-esteem. This scale has been used with ethnically diverse populations (e.g., Mexican, Dominican, Puerto Rican, African American, and White adolescents) and has obtained moderate Cronbach's alphas (e.g., .79–85) with these samples (Der-Karabetian & Ruiz, 1997; Lorenzo-Hernandez & Quellette, 1998; Martinez & Dukes, 1997; Phinney et al., 1997). In the studies discussed in this chapter, the measure obtained alphas of .85 (Study 1), .88 (Study 2), and .87 (study 3).

Familial Ethnic Socialization

A revised version of the Familial Ethnic Socialization Measure (Umaña-Taylor, 2001) was used to assess the degree to which participants perceived that their families socialized them with respect to their ethnicity. The 12 items (e.g., "My family teaches me about our family's ethnic/cultural background" and "Our home is decorated with things that reflect my ethnic/cultural background") were rated on a 5-point Likert scale, with end points of *not at all* (1) and *very much* (5) and end points of *not at all* (1) and *very often* (5). Responses were coded so that higher scores indicated higher levels of familial ethnic socialization. The original version, consisting of 9 items, obtained a Cronbach's alpha of .82 with a sample of Mexican-origin adolescents (Umaña-Taylor, 2001). In the studies discussed in this chapter, the measure obtained alphas of .94 (Study 1), .92 (Study 2), and .94 (Study 3).

Reliability of the EIS

To examine the internal consistency of the EIS subscales, reliability coefficients were explored for each of the samples. For Studies 1 and 2, which were ethnically and racially diverse, alphas were examined across four major ethnic/racial groups (White, Latino, Black, and Asian). Because only Latino adolescents were sampled for Study 3, alphas were examined only for Latinos in that study. Reliability coefficients were moderately high for all samples, ranging from .72 to .93. Thus, the subscales demonstrated strong internal consistency across multiple ethnic and racial groups, as well as across age groups (i.e., high school vs. university).

Study 1

Data were gathered from 615 individuals who were attending either a 4-year university located in the Midwest ($n = 297$) or a 4-year university located on the West Coast ($n = 318$). The total sample included 164 males (27%) and 445 females (72%); six respondents did not provide this information. Participants ranged in age from 18 to 56 years ($M = 21.8, SD = 3.91$) and, in total, reported 193 different ethnic backgrounds (e.g., Polish, Mexican, Irish, and Eritrean). Respondents' self-reported ethnicity was used to classify participants into six major ethnic/racial groups: White ($n = 276, 45\%$), Latino ($n = 71, 12\%$), Asian ($n = 125, 20\%$), Black ($n = 49, 8\%$), multiethnic/-racial ($n = 41, 7\%$; e.g., Asian, Caucasian), and other ($n = 25, 4\%$; e.g., American). Twenty-eight participants (5%) did not report ethnic background.

Validity

Preliminary support for the measure's construct validity was provided by examining correlations among the three subscales (i.e., exploration, affirmation, and resolution), a measure of self-esteem, and a measure of familial ethnic socialization. Examination of the intercorrelations among the three subscales indicated that the exploration and resolution subscales were moderately correlated

Table 1. Correlations among EIS Subscales, Rosenberg Self-esteem Scale, and Umaña-Taylor Familial Ethnic Socialization Measure

	Study 1—university				Study 2—high school				Study 3—high school			
	1	2	3	4	1	2	3	4	1	2	3	4
1. Exploration												
2. Affirmation	.08				.17*				.13*			
	(292)				(212)				(325)			
3. Resolution	.65***	.11			.46***	.12			.57***	.12*		
	(298)	(292)			(214)	(217)			(325)	(325)		
4. Self-esteem	.16**	.10	.23***		.16*	.22**	.30***		.38***	.25***	.38***	
	(292)	(287)	(294)		(216)	(219)	(221)		(325)	(325)	(325)	
5. Familial ethnic socialization	.71***	−.01	.62***	.09	.66***	.05	.47***	.12	.60***	.10	.57***	.38***
	(294)	(289)	(296)	(294)	(213)	(217)	(218)	(220)	(323)	(323)	(323)	(323)

*p < .05. **p < .01. ***p < .001.

with one another (Table 1). Thus, individuals who reported high levels of exploration also reported high levels of resolution. Due to the correlational nature of the analyses, it is unclear whether exploration influences one's resolution or whether individuals who have resolved how they feel about their ethnicity are more apt to explore their ethnicity at greater lengths. It is possible that the relationship is bidirectional or that a third, unidentified, variable could be influencing both. Theoretically, one would expect that through exploration one can come to a resolution; however, it is possible that after one has resolved issues related to ethnicity, one will continue to explore and seek out activities that will expose one to one's ethnicity.

On the other hand, the affirmation subscale was not significantly related to either the exploration or the resolution subscales, suggesting that exploration and/or resolution regarding one's ethnicity is not necessarily related to the affect that one holds toward that ethnicity. According to Umaña-Taylor et al. (in press), these findings suggest that it is inaccurate to assume that individuals will feel positively about their ethnicity just because they have explored their ethnicity and/or feel that they have resolved how they feel about their ethnicity.

Because previous research has found significant positive relationships between ethnic identity and self-esteem (see Umaña-Taylor et al., 2002, for a review), as well as between ethnic identity and familial ethnic socialization (Umaña-Taylor & Fine, 2001), the construct validity of the EIS was examined by exploring the correlations among each subscale and measures of self-esteem and familial ethnic socialization. Results indicated that the exploration and resolution subscales were both positively associated with individuals' self-esteem and familial ethnic socialization. Thus, individuals who reported that their families had socialized them with regard to their ethnicity also tended to report higher levels of exploration and resolution regarding their ethnicity, which is consistent with previous research (i.e., Umaña-Taylor & Fine, 2001). Respondents' scores on the affirmation subscale, however, were not significantly correlated with their scores on self-esteem or familial ethnic socialization. Umaña-Taylor et al. (2004)

have argued that these findings may shed light on the modest relationship that has emerged between ethnic identity and self-esteem in previous studies. They argue that previous studies have combined individuals' scores on the three constructs (i.e., exploration, resolution, affirmation), and it is possible that the relationship that has emerged in previous work has been modest because the method of measuring ethnic identity introduced error by combining individuals' scores on affirmation with their scores on exploration and commitment.

Distribution of EIS Scale Scores

Because the EIS was developed with the intention of being able to categorize individuals into a typology, cutoff values for each of the subscales were identified, whereby individuals could be classified into eight groups based on their scores on each of the three subscales (i.e., all possible combinations of high/low affirmation, high/low exploration, high/low resolution). A variation of a K-means cluster analysis was used to determine cutoff values for each of the subscales (19.5, 20.5, and 9.5 for the exploration, affirmation, and resolution subscales). Respondents who scored above the cutoff value on a particular subscale were considered to score "high" on that subscale, and those who scored at or below the cutoff value were considered to score "low" on the subscale. The eight types were labeled diffuse negative, diffuse positive, foreclosed negative, foreclosed positive, moratorium negative, moratorium positive, resolved negative, and resolved positive. For example, the label *resolved positive* identifies individuals who scored above the cutoff value on all three subscales (i.e., *resolved* = high exploration and high commitment, *positive* = high affirmation). Using this categorization scheme, all individuals were classified into one of the eight types.

The distribution of scores indicated that only 10% of the sample reported low scores on the affirmation subscale (Table 2). Furthermore, the group with

Table 2. *Study 1 Means and Standard Deviations of Familial Ethnic Socialization and Self-esteem by EIS Type*

	N	%	\multicolumn{3}{c}{Familial ethnic socialization}			\multicolumn{3}{c}{Self-esteem}		
	N	%	n	M	SD	n	M	SD
Diffuse negative	11	3.8	11	32.82^c	12.06	11	31.55	6.67
Diffuse positive	88	30.3	86	29.09^{bdefgh}	10.90	86	31.42	4.38
Foreclosed negative	10	3.4	10	42.70^h	8.734	10	31.30	3.43
Foreclosed positive	51	17.6	51	37.67^{ad}	8.10	50	31.44	4.34
Moratorium negative	3	1.0	3	51.00^g	11.27	3	31.33	4.04
Moratorium positive	13	4.5	13	40.85^e	11.08	13	31.62	5.72
Resolved negative	5	2.0	3	49.67^f	8.39	4	28.75	2.75
Resolved positive	10	37.6	108	48.80^{abc}	8.28	106	33.17	4.50
F				32.23***			1.67	
				(7,277)			(7,275)	

Note: Values in same column with same superscript are significantly different from one another.

the largest number of people included those who had explored their ethnicity, had resolved issues about their ethnicity, and felt positively about their ethnicity (i.e., 38% of the sample). It is possible that the distribution of scores was driven, in part, by social desirability and individuals felt inclined to report positive affect toward their ethnicity (i.e., affirmation). Because previous research has not examined the distribution of individuals according to typology classifications, it is not possible to determine whether this is a typical distribution for this age group.

The next two largest groups were (1) those who had not explored or resolved, and felt positively about their ethnicity (i.e., 30%), and (2) those who had not explored but reported that they had resolved issues regarding their ethnicity and that they felt positively about it (i.e., 18%). This finding is critical because it demonstrates that it is possible to distinguish individuals who are diffuse or foreclosed. Thus, according to Umaña-Taylor et al. (2004), perhaps it is inaccurate to have a combined category of diffuse and foreclosed because they involve different processes.

The distribution of typology classifications was further explored with regard to ethnic minority/majority status. A majority of ethnic majority individuals (i.e., White) tended to fall into the diffuse positive category, which is associated with low exploration, low commitment, but positive feelings about one's ethnic group membership. On the other hand, the majority of Latino, Asian, and Black individuals tended to fall into the resolution positive category, indicating that they had explored, committed, and felt positively about their ethnic group membership. These patterns supported previous findings that suggested ethnic identity to be more salient for ethnic minority group members than for ethnic majority group members (e.g., Roberts et al., 1999).

Mean Differences between Types

In addition, Umaña-Taylor et al. (2004) conducted two analyses of variance (ANOVAs) to explore whether individuals' scores on familial ethnic socialization and self-esteem varied as a function of their typology classification. Individuals' scores on familial ethnic socialization varied significantly depending on EIS type, but individuals' self-esteem scores did not vary based on EIS type (Table 2).

Tukey's post hoc analyses indicated that (a) individuals who were classified as resolved positive reported significantly higher levels of familial ethnic socialization than individuals classified as foreclosed positive, diffuse positive, and diffuse negative ($p < .001$ for all), and (b) individuals classified as diffuse positive reported significantly lower levels of familial ethnic socialization than individuals classified as foreclosed negative, moratorium negative, moratorium positive, and resolved negative ($p < .01$ for all). Thus, adolescents who reported high levels of exploration, resolution, and affirmation (i.e., resolved positive) reported higher levels of familial ethnic socialization than those who reported feeling positively but not necessarily exploring (i.e., foreclosed positive) or resolving (i.e., diffuse positive).

Study 2

Data for Study 2 were drawn from a larger research project examining the influence of school context on ethnic identity (see Yazedjian, 2003). Data were gathered from adolescents attending a high school located in a large ethnically diverse city in the Midwest. The sample included 231 11th-grade high school students (45.5% males, 54.5% females). Age of participants ranged from 15 to 18 ($M = 16.6$, $SD = .59$). Participants reported 88 different ethnic backgrounds (e.g., Polish, Vietnamese, Mexican, Native American) from which racial classifications were created. Of all participants, 64 (28%) were White, 49 (21%) were Latino, 35 (11%) were Asian, 46 (20%) were Black, 3 (1%) were Native American, 18 (8%) were multiethnic/-racial, and 6 (3%) were classi- fied as other. A total of 10 participants (4%) did not report their ethnic/racial background.

Validity

In line with findings from Study 1, the exploration and resolution subscales were significantly positively correlated with one another (Table 1). With the high school sample, however, a significant positive relationship emerged be- tween adolescents' scores on the affirmation and exploration subscales. Thus, individuals who reported high levels of exploration regarding their ethnicity also tended to report high levels of resolution and affirmation toward their eth- nicity. Similar to Study 1, the affirmation subscale was not significantly related to the resolution subscale. These findings suggest that although adolescents who report exploring their ethnicity also tend to report feeling positively about their ethnicity, resolution regarding one's ethnicity is not necessarily related to the affect that one holds toward that ethnicity.

In addition, the intercorrelations among each subscale (i.e., exploration, af- firmation, and resolution), a measure of self-esteem, and a measure of familial ethnic socialization provided preliminary evidence for the construct validity of the EIS. The findings were similar to those obtained with the university sam- ple in Study 1: The exploration and resolution subscales were both positively correlated with adolescents' self-esteem and familial ethnic socialization, and adolescents' scores on the affirmation subscale were not related to their scores on familial ethnic socialization (Table 1). Contrary to findings in Study 1, ado- lescents' scores on the affirmation subscale were positively related to their self- esteem scores. Thus, as adolescents reported higher levels of affirmation (i.e., feeling positively about their ethnicity), they also tended to report higher levels of self-esteem.

Distribution of EIS Scale Scores

In line with Study 1, the distribution of scores for each classification of the typology was explored with the high school sample (Table 3). Because the means

Table 3. Study 2 Means and Standard Deviations of Familial Ethnic Socialization and Self-esteem by EIS Type

	N	%	Familial ethnic socialization			Self-esteem		
			n	M	SD	n	M	SD
Diffuse negative	6	2.9	6	37.33	8.55	6	23.33^{bdef}	4.03
Diffuse positive	45	21.6	43	28.93^{cde}	6.81	44	29.77^{ac}	5.53
Foreclosed negative	3	1.0	3	34.67	6.81	3	35.33	5.00
Foreclosed positive	55	26.4	54	35.31^{ad}	10.47	54	33.30^{cd}	4.71
Moratorium negative	2	1.0	2	37.00	7.07	2	23.50	.71
Moratorium positive	20	9.6	20	38.30^{be}	8.81	20	31.20^{e}	4.89
Resolved negative	3	1.0	3	42.33	10.60	3	30.00^{f}	5.03
Resolved positive	74	35.6	73	46.93^{abc}	9.71	73	32.99^{ab}	5.35
F				14.50***			5.57***	
				(7, 196)			(7, 197)	

Note: Values in same column with same superscript are significantly different from one another.

and standard deviations of high school students' scores on the three subscales were comparable to those of the university sample (data not shown), the cutoffs that were developed in Study 1 were applied to these data, and all individuals were classified into one of the eight types, as in Study 1.

The distribution of ethnic minority/majority individuals within each of the typology classifications did not appear to vary as much by minority/majority status as was the case with university students. Umaña-Taylor et al. (2004) suggest that one possibility is that differences in ethnic identity statuses between ethnic majority and ethnic minority individuals do not become evident until later developmental periods, and perhaps this trend is a result of less variability in levels of ethnic identity exploration and commitment during the high school years. This idea is in line with previous findings that suggest that exploration and commitment toward ethnicity show a developmental progression with age, with college students reporting significantly higher scores on ethnic identity achievement than high school students (Phinney, 1992).

In addition to exploring the distribution of scores, Umaña-Taylor et al. (2004) conducted ANOVAs to explore variations in self-esteem and familial ethnic socialization by typology classification. Results indicated that familial ethnic socialization and self-esteem both varied significantly depending on EIS type (Table 3). Tukey's post hoc analyses indicated that individuals classified as diffuse positive scored significantly lower on familial ethnic socialization than those classified as foreclosed positive ($p < .05$), moratorium positive ($p < .05$), and resolved positive ($p < .001$); individuals classified as foreclosed positive scored significantly lower on familial ethnic socialization than individuals classified as resolved positive ($p < .001$); and individuals classified as moratorium positive scored significantly lower on familial ethnic socialization than those classified as resolved positive ($p < .05$).

In terms of self-esteem, Tukey's post hoc analyses indicated that individuals classified as diffuse negative reported significantly lower self-esteem scores than those classified as foreclosed positive ($p < .001$), moratorium positive ($p < .05$), resolved negative ($p < .05$), and resolved positive ($p < .001$); individuals classified as diffuse positive reported significantly lower self-esteem scores than those classified as foreclosed positive and those classified as resolved positive ($p < .05$ for both).

These findings provide support for construct validity by demonstrating that individuals who scored low on exploration and/or resolution also scored low on familial ethnic socialization. Findings involving self-esteem also provide support for construct validity, in that those who had explored, resolved, and felt positively tended to have the highest self-esteem scores. In fact, those who had not explored or resolved issues seemed to have lowest levels of self-esteem, an idea that is consistent with social identity and Eriksonian perspectives (Umaña-Taylor et al., 2004). Umaña-Taylor and colleagues argue that perhaps the relationship that emerges between ethnic identity and self-esteem during this developmental period is due to adolescents' identities being less multifaceted than young adults' identities and, therefore, the weight that their ethnic identification bears on their overall feelings about themselves is stronger than it is in later developmental periods, when other aspects of one's identity may weigh in more heavily (e.g., occupational success, intimate relationships).

A second, more contextually driven, explanation is that a change in context (from an ethnically balanced high school to a more homogeneous university setting) could account for a lack of relationship between ethnic identity and self-esteem because in a university setting adolescents do not have the support for their culture that was evidenced in high school and, therefore, must derive their sense of self from other component identities. In fact, upon closer examination of exploration and resolution scores, when broken down by ethnic background, mean exploration scores increase significantly from high school to college for Latino and Black adolescents, whereas exploration scores decrease significantly for White adolescents. This increase in exploration for Latino and Black adolescents may occur because these adolescents are entering contexts where perhaps they must answer new questions (related to ethnicity) due to the ethnic homogeneity of a university setting. Additionally, the homogeneous setting may increase the salience of ethnicity and, as a result, prompt increased exploration. Furthermore, and theoretically consistent with the idea that increases in exploration may eventually lead to increased resolution, there is a parallel significant increase in resolution scores among Latino and Black adolescents in the university sample, thus suggesting that increases in exploration are associated with increased resolution.

Study 3

Data for Study 3 were drawn from a longitudinal study exploring ethnic identity development and academic success among Latino high school students. Data were gathered from five high schools in the Midwest. Ninth- and 10th-grade students who were self-identified as Latino or Hispanic in school records were invited to participate; in total, 325 students participated in the first wave of data collection (50.8% males, 49.2% females; M age = 15.3, SD = .75).

Validity

To further explore the validity of the EIS with a second sample of high school students, intercorrelations among the three subscales were examined. In line with findings from the previous two studies, the exploration and resolution subscales were significantly positively correlated with one another. In addition, similar to the high school sample from Study 2, a significant positive relationship emerged between adolescents' scores on the affirmation and exploration subscales. Unlike the previous two studies, adolescents' scores on affirmation were positively related to their scores on resolution. However, the effect size for this correlation (r = .12) was identical to the effect size for the sample in Study 2. Thus, it is likely that the significance that emerged in Study 3 was a result of the larger sample size.

Similar to the previous two studies, the intercorrelations among each subscale (i.e., exploration, affirmation, and resolution), a measure of self-esteem, and a measure of familial ethnic socialization provided evidence for the construct validity of the EIS. The findings were similar to those obtained in the previous studies: The exploration and resolution subscales were both positively correlated with adolescents' self-esteem and familial ethnic socialization, and adolescents' scores on the affirmation subscale were not related to their scores on familial ethnic socialization (Table 1). Contrary to findings in Study 1, but replicating findings in Study 2, adolescents' scores on the affirmation subscale were positively related to their self-esteem scores. Thus, as adolescents reported higher levels of affirmation (i.e., feeling positively about their ethnicity), they also tended to report higher levels of self-esteem.

Distribution of EIS Scale Scores

In line with the procedure followed in the previous two studies, the distribution of scores for each classification of the typology was explored in Study 3 (Table 4). In line with the previous two studies, the largest percentage of adolescents was classified as resolved positive. Furthermore, a small percentage of adolescents reported low affirmation scores. As previously mentioned, it is possible that adolescents do not feel comfortable reporting negative feelings toward their ethnicity, and, thus, an element of social desirability may be driving the results.

Additionally, one-way ANOVAs were conducted to explore whether individuals' scores on self-esteem and familial ethnic socialization varied as a function of their typology classification. As found in Study 2, results indicated that familial ethnic socialization and self-esteem both varied significantly depending on EIS type (Table 4). With regard to familial ethnic socialization, Tukey's post hoc analyses indicated that individuals classified as diffuse negative scored significantly lower on familial ethnic socialization than those classified as foreclosed

Table 4. Study 3 Means and Standard Deviations of Familial Ethnic Socialization and
Self-esteem by EIS Type

	N	%	Familial ethnic socialization			Self-esteem		
			n	M	SD	n	M	SD
Diffuse negative	11	3.4	11	29.00^{abc}	15.88	11	24.00^{ade}	6.48
Diffuse positive	23	7.1	23	31.04^{def}	11.00	23	26.35^{b}	4.26
Foreclosed negative	22	6.8	22	38.68^{gl}	8.29	22	25.91^{c}	4.24
Foreclosed positive	86	26.5	85	41.36^{adhk}	10.45	86	29.42^{e}	5.32
Moratorium negative	0	0.0	0	—	—	0	—	—
Moratorium positive	4	1.2	4	28.25^{ij}	11.53	4	26.00	3.56
Resolved negative	34	10.5	33	48.30^{beilk}	8.46	34	29.26^{d}	4.33
Resolved positive	145	44.6	145	49.85^{cfghj}	8.81	145	31.26^{abc}	5.23
F				24.97***			8.72***	
				(6, 316)			(6, 318)	

positive ($p < .01$), resolved negative ($p < .001$), and resolved positive ($p < .001$); individuals classified as diffuse positive scored significantly lower on familial ethnic socialization than those classified as foreclosed positive ($p < .001$), resolved negative ($p < .001$), and resolved positive ($p < .001$); individuals classified as foreclosed negative scored significantly lower on familial ethnic socialization than those classified as resolved negative ($p < .01$) and resolved positive ($p < .001$); individuals classified as foreclosed positive scored significantly lower on familial ethnic socialization than individuals classified as resolved negative ($p < .05$) and resolved positive ($p < .001$); finally, individuals classified as moratorium positive scored significantly lower on familial ethnic socialization than those classified as resolved negative ($p < .01$) and resolved positive ($p < .001$).

In terms of self-esteem, Tukey's post hoc analyses indicated that individuals classified as diffuse negative reported significantly lower self-esteem scores than those classified as foreclosed positive ($p < .05$), resolved negative ($p < .05$), and resolved positive ($p < .001$); individuals classified as diffuse positive reported significantly lower self-esteem scores than those classified as resolved positive ($p < .001$); and those classified as foreclosed negative reported significantly lower levels of self-esteem than those classified as resolved positive ($p < .001$).

Replicating findings from the previous two studies, findings from Study 3 provided support for construct validity by demonstrating that individuals who scored low on exploration and/or resolution also tended to score low on familial ethnic socialization. Furthermore, as in the previous studies, adolescents' scores on ethnic identity affirmation were not related to their scores on familial ethnic socialization. For self-esteem, findings also provided support for construct validity. Similar to findings in Study 2, those who had explored, resolved, and felt positively tended to have the highest self-esteem scores. In fact, those who had not explored or resolved seemed to have lowest levels of self-esteem, which, as previously mentioned, is consistent with social identity and Eriksonian perspectives. It is interesting to note that in both Studies 2 and 3, whose foci were high school students, a relationship between ethnic identity and self-esteem emerged.

However, this relationship did not emerge with the university sample. It will be important for future research to explore the idea previously introduced suggesting that adolescents' ethnic identity may be more influential on individuals' self-esteem during earlier developmental periods, when their identities are less multifaceted.

Conclusion

Previous methods of assessing ethnic identity have been based on continuous measures and do not provide information about the differential influence of each ethnic identity component on individual outcomes. Umaña-Taylor et al. (2004) developed and explored the validity and reliability of a measure (i.e., EIS) that would assess the three components of ethnic identity independently of one another (i.e., exploration, resolution, and affirmation) and would facilitate researchers' ability to classify individuals into an ethnic identity typology based on their scores on each component. In addition, the third study described in this chapter attempted to replicate the findings reported by Umaña-Taylor et al.

Taken together, the findings from the three studies provide preliminary evidence for the reliability and validity of the EIS among high school and university students. The three subscales obtained strong reliability coefficients, demonstrating good internal consistency. Moreover, support for the measure's construct validity emerged in all studies when the relationships among the subscales and measures of familial ethnic socialization and self-esteem were examined. Beyond providing evidence for the reliability and validity of the measure, these findings also highlight the importance of examining the three components of ethnic identity as individual factors, as opposed to using a sum score of the three scales. Both the intercorrelations among the subscales and the significant differences among the typology classification groups demonstrate the need to examine each component independently. Most important, the operationalization proposed in the current investigation allows the *method* of assessing ethnic identity to become congruent with both Erikson's and Tajfel's theoretical frameworks.

Although these findings provide new insights for understanding the multifaceted nature of ethnic identity formation, there are limitations to consider. Most important, before the measure can be used widely, it must be examined with other populations. For example, these samples represent only two geographical areas in the United States. Future studies should explore this measure with individuals living in other areas of the country. Although the United States is ethnically diverse, the ethnic composition of the population varies by locale. Salience of ethnic identity may also vary as a result of this contextual factor. Although an examination of the influence of context on ethnic identity formation was beyond the scope of this chapter, this is an area that warrants further study.

On a related note, future studies should examine a broader range of developmental periods. For example, Erikson (1968) argues that identity formation is a central task during adolescence. In line with this idea, researchers have found that exploration of one's ethnicity becomes increasingly evident during this developmental period. The current studies focused on individuals in high school and those enrolled in postsecondary education. However, because exploration regarding ethnicity has been noted as early as the seventh and eighth grades (Roberts et al., 1999), it will be important for future studies to examine the reliability and validity of this measure with younger populations.

Finally, although the studies discussed in this chapter included ethnically diverse populations, their purpose was to explore the psychometric properties of the EIS with a diverse sample, rather than to examine its validity across ethnic and racial groups. Thus, a critical next step is to explore the factorial invariance of the EIS by ethnic group. It will be important to explore whether the factor structure of the EIS varies by ethnic group due to varied experiences and meanings associated with ethnic identity across groups. Future studies should include large enough samples of a range of ethnic groups to enable an analysis of whether the factor structure is comparable across groups.

Despite these limitations, the combination of findings suggests that using a typology classification may be useful for understanding how different components of ethnic identity relate to outcomes such as self-esteem. Furthermore, the EIS appears to be reliable with multiple ethnic and racial groups, as well as with diverse age groups, and findings from the three studies provide preliminary support for the validity of the measure.

Author's Note

Address correspondence to Adriana J. Umaña-Taylor, Department of Human and Community Development, University of Illinois at Urbana-Champaign, Urbana, IL, 61801 (umana@uiuc.edu).

References

Arellano, A. R., & Padilla, A. M. (1996). Academic invulnerability among a select group of Latino university students. *Hispanic Journal of Behavioral Sciences, 18,* 485–507.

Der-Karabetian, A., & Ruiz, Y. (1997). Affective bicultural and global-human identity scales for Mexican-American adolescents. *Psychological Reports, 80,* 1027–1039.

Erikson, E. H. (1959). Identity and the life cycle. *Psychological Issues, 1* (Monograph No. 1). New York: International Universities Press.

Erikson, E. H. (1968). *Identity: Youth and crisis.* New York: W. W. Norton.

Lorenzo-Hernandez, J., & Quellette, S. C. (1998). Ethnic identity, self-esteem and values in Dominicans, Puerto Ricans, and African Americans. *Journal of Applied Social Psychology, 28,* 2007–2024.

Marcia, J. E. (1980). Identity in adolescence. In J. Adelson (Ed.), *Handbook of adolescent psychology* (pp. 159–187). New York: Wiley.

Marcia, J. E. (1994). The empirical study of ego identity. In H. A. Bosma, T. G. Graafsma, H. D. Grotevant, & D. J. de Levita (Eds.), *Identity and development: An interdisciplinary approach* (4th ed., pp. 281–321). Belmont, CA: Wadsworth.

Martinez, R. O., & Dukes, R. L. (1997). The effects of ethnic identity, ethnicity, and gender on adolescent well-being. *Journal of Youth and Adolescence, 26,* 503–516.

Phinney, J. S. (1989). Stages of ethnic identity development in minority group adolescents. *Journal of Early Adolescence, 9,* 34–49.

Phinney, J. S. (1992). The Multigroup Ethnic Identity Measure: A new scale for use with diverse groups. *Journal of Adolescent Research, 7,* 156–176.

Phinney, J. S., Cantu, C. L., & Kurtz, D. A. (1997). Ethnic and American identity as predictors of self-esteem among African American, Latino, and White adolescents. *Journal of Youth and Adolescence, 26*(2), 165–185.

Phinney, J. S., & Chavira, V. (1995). Parental ethnic socialization and adolescent coping with problems related to ethnicity. *Journal of Research on Adolescence, 5,* 31–53.

Roberts, R. E., Phinney, J. S., Masse, L. C., Chen, Y. R., Roberts, C. R., & Romero, A. (1999). The structure of ethnic identity of young adolescents from diverse ethnocultural groups. *Journal of Early Adolescence, 19,* 301–322.

Rosenberg, M. (1979). *Conceiving the self.* New York: Basic Books.

Swanson, D. P., Spencer, M. B., & Petersen, A. (1997). Identity formation in adolescence. In K. Borman & B. Schneider (Eds.), *The adolescent years: Social influences and educational challenges* (97th yearbook of the National Society for the Study of Education, pp. 18–41). Chicago: National Society for the Study of Education.

Tajfel, H. (1981). *Human groups and social categories.* Cambridge: Cambridge University Press.

Umaña-Taylor, A. J. (2001). *Ethnic identity development among Mexican-origin Latino adolescents living in the U.S.* Unpublished doctoral dissertation, University of Missouri, Columbia.

Umaña-Taylor, A. J., Diversi, M., & Fine, M. A. (2002). Ethnic identity and self-esteem among Latino adolescents: Distinctions among the Latino populations. *Journal of Adolescent Research, 17,* 303–327.

Umaña-Taylor, A. J., & Fine, M. A. (2001). Methodological implications of grouping Latino adolescents into one collective ethnic group. *Hispanic Journal of Behavioral Sciences, 23,* 347–362.

Umaña-Taylor, A. J., Yazedjian, A., & Bámaca-Gómez, M. Y. (2004). Developing the Ethnic Identity Scale using Eriksonian and social identity perspectives. *Identity: An International Journal of Theory and Research, 4,* 9–38.

Yazedjian, A. (2003). *Experiencing ethnicity: A case study of White, Black, Latino, and Asian adolescents in an urban high school.* Unpublished doctoral dissertation, University of Illinois at Urbana-Champaign.

II Healthy Habits, Positive Behaviors, and Time Use

7 Leisure Time Activities in Middle Childhood

Sandra L. Hofferth and Sally C. Curtin

University of Maryland, College Park

It is often assumed that how children spend their time affects their cognitive and social development. For example, parents complain that children spend too little time studying, reading, or helping around the house, and too much time watching television or hanging out with friends. A recent Centers for Disease Control health campaign ("VERB: It's What You Do") promotes physical activity. However, in spite of the use of language in which time is the measure of children's activities and behavior, time is rarely studied. In this chapter we take advantage of national data collected in 1997 to measure children's involvement in a variety of leisure time activities and whether variations in time use are associated with children's achievement and behavior.

The time that children spend in various activities can measure productive engagement and can also be indicative of their potential contributions to society as a whole. The benefits of certain activities, such as time spent in school and studying, are widely presumed. In economic terms, this time can be considered to reflect investments in "human capital" because the knowledge and learning skills gained can ultimately be used by the individual to earn money and also to contribute to the overall society.

The benefits of nonacademic uses of children's time, particularly leisure activities, are less obvious and the subject of this chapter. We use time diary data from the 1997 Child Development Supplement (CDS) of the Panel Study of Income Dynamics (PSID) to examine the amount of weekly time that children 6–12 years of age spend in various leisure activities—playing, studying, computer usage, watching television, art, hobbies, sports, reading, time outdoors, religious activities, housework, and shopping.

The Benefits of Leisure Time

There is wide variation around the world in the amount of leisure time available to children. In nonindustrial societies, the amount of leisure time children have is primarily dictated by necessity, such as climate and economic conditions (Larson & Verma, 1999). Even among postindustrial societies, there are differences in the leisure time available to children, but these are primarily attributable to the priorities and culture of the particular society. For example, children in North America have much more leisure time than children in East Asia owing to differences between countries in priorities for schoolwork versus other areas of personal and social development. East Asian children spend about 2–3 hours a week more in schoolwork than do North American children and have about the same amount less in leisure time. European children are intermediate between North American and East Asian children. Of this leisure time, however, North American and European children spend more time in structured activities, particularly sports, than East Asian children.

The benefits of leisure time depend on its use, with structured activities generally considered to be more beneficial than unstructured, and active more beneficial than passive. There has been extensive research on the potential effects of watching television (see below), but less on other, less frequent uses of leisure time. It is plausible that many uses of leisure time, both structured and unstructured, have the potential for positive outcomes for children. First, these activities can function as learning environments for mastering specific skills and techniques (Larson & Verma, 1999). A child participating in sports, for example, is learning the particular rules and becoming proficient at the skills required of the game chosen. A child participating in various arts and hobbies learns the specific techniques involved and can become more familiar with the culture surrounding the activity.

The other valuable aspect of these activities is that they can promote positive relationships with adults and with peers (Larson, 1994). An athletic team is coached by an adult, made up of peers, and supported by parents. Adults give lessons. Outdoor activities, hobbies, and arts activities often involve adults and peers. Such activities provide opportunities to work with adults other than parents in a variety of settings and roles. They also provide the opportunity to engage with peers in activities with common objectives and goals. Thus, many leisure activities can provide opportunities for learning and for positive behavioral and health outcomes, depending on the quality of the experience and the particular characteristics of the child.

Computer, Television, and Media Use

In the past decade, the use of electronic media has skyrocketed. The amount of time spent watching television is the largest of this category, averaging one quarter of children's free time, some 13–14 hours per week, 2 hours per day (Hofferth & Sandberg, 2001). However, the use of other media has risen. Today every school has computers, but so do most homes. Even in 1997, when our diary data were collected, the Internet had not penetrated into middle-class homes the way it has today. According to a 1998–1999 study, 69% of American homes had a computer and 45% had access to the Internet (Roberts, Foehr, Rideout, & Brodie, 1999). The same study estimated that children 8–13 years old spend 6.75 hours each day interacting with media, from television to games to CDs to computers (Roberts et al., 1999). While this may be an overestimate of time, it points to a high degree of media involvement. Here we examine computer and television viewing separately. In this study, watching videos refers to watching movies on video and not to playing video games. Future research also needs to include video games, which are heavily used by boys. Although television viewing may be individual in nature, parents often work on the computer with their children, and children often play video games together. Television viewing has been studied extensively; the nature of the programs viewed has been shown to be more important than total time (Anderson, Huston, Schmitt, & Linebarger, 2001). However, television may reduce achievement by displacing more positive activities.

Sports and Outdoor Activities

Between 1981 and 1997, there was a 35% increase in the amount of time 9- to 12-year-olds spent in sports activities (Hofferth & Sandberg, 2001). Consistent with the heightened emphasis on team activities, both boys and girls increased their participation. Although the passage of Title IX in the 1970s increased opportunities for girls, boys are more likely to participate in sports and spend about 50% more time at sports.

Previous research has shown a negative association between sports participation and delinquency; however, this appears to be due to the fact that delinquency reduces eligibility for sports participation rather than the other way around (Larson, 1994). Eccles found evidence that participation in team sports in high school can be associated with both better grades and increased alcohol use (Eccles & Barber, 1999).

Outdoor activities such as camping and walking comprise less than 30 minutes per week. Time spent actually declined for the 9- to 12-year age group (Hofferth & Sandberg, 2001).

Quiet Activities—Reading and Studying

The time children spend not only in school but also in school-related activities at home such as doing homework may boost their human capital and improve their cognitive achievement. Reading for pleasure is linked to higher verbal achievement (Hofferth & Sandberg, 2001). One would expect that studying would also be linked to development; however, causality may go the other direction such that children who are having problems in school may spend more time on homework.

Research shows that the weekly time U.S. children spent studying outside the school setting increased between 1981 and 1997 more for the younger than for the older children (Hofferth & Sandberg, 2001). Studying, of course, varies by age of child. In 1981, 3- to 5-year-olds were said to study about 25 minutes. In contrast, 6- to 8-year-olds spent 52 minutes studying, and 9- to 12-year-olds spent 3 hours 22 minutes studying. By 1997, children spent more time in school and day care at younger ages; the time spent on homework rose to 36 minutes a week for 3- to 5-year-olds (up 44%) in 1997, to 2 hours 8 minutes for 6- to 8-year-olds (up 144%), and to 3 hours 41 minutes (up 9%) for 9- to 12-year-olds.

Adolescents spend more time in homework than do younger children. Leone and Richards (1989) found children in grades 5–9 spend about 15 hours per week in class actually doing academic work and another 6.5 hours per week studying. By the time they get to age 16 or 17, teenagers in the United States report spending some 10 hours per week studying (Fuligni & Stevenson, 1995).

Hobbies and Art Activities

It is in activities developing specific skills that one would anticipate participation to have its greatest long-term benefits. Besides learning a skill, children learn about a specific craft or hobby that may sustain their interest until adulthood and beyond. Although overall time spent in them is quite small, the amount of time spent in hobbies and art activities more than doubled between 1981 and 1997 for school-age children (Hofferth & Sandberg, 2001). Girls spend more time than boys in art activities, which include dance and music lessons, gender-typed activities. Boys and girls spend about the same low amount of time in hobbies. Research shows that hobby participation in grades 9–10 is associated with less delinquency in grades 11–12 (Larson, 1994).

Household Work and Shopping

Household work would appear to combine skill building with needed family work. In preindustrial societies, children spend considerable time in the work of the family, estimated at 6.7 hours for 10- to 12-year-old girls in rural Bangladesh (Cain, 1980). Such children spend little time in school. While in preindustrial societies household work is not optional, in industrial societies household work time is considerably more variable and discretionary. Parents tend not to train children in gender-linked household tasks as much as in the rural past. In Western countries, children do not spend much time helping their parents with household chores. In 1997, two out of three 6- to 8-year-olds and three quarters of 9- to 12-years-olds spent some time doing chores around the house; 6- to 8-year-olds spent about 2 hours per week; and 9- to 12-year-olds spent 3.75 hours per week (about 30 minutes per day). The trends in household chores for children are similar to those of parents—a general decline in housework for women has been shown in numerous studies (Gershuny & Robinson, 1988). On the other side, more goods and services are purchased outside the home instead of being produced at home. The time children spent accompanying their parents shopping to purchase goods and services increased significantly over the same period. Weekly shopping time rose from 2 hours to almost 3 hours (Hofferth & Sandberg, 2001).

Play

Play and school are considered the "work" of children. Since there is so little discretion over time in school, which varies by community, we do not focus on it. Instead, we focus on play. Play as a category of time encompasses most of children's activities that are not formally organized, for example, board games and playing around the house. This informal play comprises about one quarter of children's free time. There was little change in time devoted to play between 1981 and 1997 (Hofferth & Sandberg, 2001).

Religious Activities

The last category of activities that we discuss is involvement in activities of religious organizations. This includes participation in classes and meetings, as well as attending religious services. Research has found evidence that family attendance at religious services is associated with positive behavior such as delayed entry into sexual activity (Udry & Billy, 1987). However, such attendance and related activities have been declining in the United States. Between 1981 and 1997, time spent in activities of religious organizations declined 22% for 6- to 8-year-olds and 44% for 9- to 12-year-olds (Hofferth & Sandberg, 2001).

Data and Methods

The 1997 Child Development Supplement

As mentioned earlier, data for this study on children's time use come from 24-hour time diaries used in the 1997 Child Development Supplement (CDS) of the Panel Study of Income Dynamics (PSID) (Hofferth, Davis-Kean, Davis, & Finkelstein, 1999). The PSID is a 30-year longitudinal survey of a representative sample of U.S. men, women, children, and the families in which they reside. In 1997, the PSID added a refresher sample of immigrants to the United States (since 1968) so that the sample represents the U.S. population in 1997. When weights are used, the PSID has been found to be representative of U.S. individuals and their families (Fitzgerald, Gottschalk, & Moffitt, 1998). Data were collected in 1997 on up to two randomly selected 0- to 12-year-old children of PSID respondents both from the primary caregivers and from the children themselves. Child interviews were completed with 2,380 households containing 3,563 children. The response rate was 90% for those families regularly interviewed in the core PSID and 84% for those contacted the first time this year for the immigrant refresher sample, yielding a combined response rate for both groups of 88%. Post-stratification weights based upon the 1997 Current Population Survey are used to make the data nationally representative. The individual-level child file used in this analysis is weighted by the product of the core PSID family weight, a post-stratification factor (by race and education of household head) based on comparison to the 1997 Current Population Survey, and a subselection weight that adjusts for the probability that a child in a given household was sampled and also for nonresponse of sampled children. This chapter focuses on 6- to 12-year-olds.

The CDS collected a complete time diary for 1 weekday and 1 weekend day for each sample child. The time diary, which was interviewer-administered to parent and child, asked several questions about the child's flow of activities over a 24-hour period beginning at midnight of the designated day. These questions ask the primary activity that was going on at that time, when it began and ended, and whether any other activity was taking place. In the coding process, children's activities are classified into 10 general activity categories (paid work, household activities, child care, obtaining goods and services, personal needs and care, education, organizational activities, entertainment/social activities, sports, hobbies, active leisure, passive leisure), and further subdivided into three-digit subcategories (such as parent reading to a child) that can be recombined in a variety of ways to characterize children's activities. Time spent traveling for the purposes of engaging in a specific activity is included in that category. Time spent doing secondary activities is not included here. For example, time spent doing housework with the television on where housework was the primary activity is not counted as time watching television. Thus, some activities that are often secondary may be underestimated. Given that many activities are occasional, we would not expect all children to engage in most of these on a daily basis. However, we want to abstract from this to describe the activities of American children in general. Since not all children do every activity each day, the total time children spend in an activity is a function of the proportion who engage in the activity and the time those participating spend in it. An estimate of weekly time is computed by multiplying weekday time (including those who do not participate and have 0 time) by 5 and weekend day time by 2, after removing children who do not have both a weekend and weekday diary.

Time use data are by their nature quite sensitive to errors resulting in extreme or unusually large values for a particular activity; an error in reporting has ramifications not only for estimates of time spent in that particular activity but in all other activities in the day as well. In addition, imputing daily values to a hypothetical week as we do here exacerbates these problems. The large sample size of the CDS diminishes the impact of these problems somewhat. Although care was taken during the data coding and cleaning stage to assure that all activities were temporally contiguous and that they summed to 24 hours for a given day, there are some outlying values in major activities that deserve special attention. Time use estimates were analyzed for extreme values, and where the authors deemed there to be a substantial probability of data error, that case was removed from the analyses completely. After selecting children 6–12 with two time diaries and excluding extreme values, the sample size was reduced to 1,461.

Robinson and Godbey (1997) distinguish among contracted time (work, school), committed time (household and child-care obligations), personal time (eating, sleeping, personal care), and free time (everything else). We generally use this model with some small changes because we are concerned with children, not adults. Since they have to be in school but don't have to work, we treat school rather than work as children's "contracted" time. Personal care refers to time spent eating, sleeping, and caring for their personal needs. Few children have "committed" time; we include household work and homework along with free time. The leisure time reported in this chapter is the time children have in a day when personal time (sleeping, eating, and personal care) and contracted time (time in school) are subtracted from the daily time. Free or discretionary time, therefore, consists of household work and shopping, studying, attendance at religious services, youth groups, visiting, sports, outdoors activities, hobbies, art activities (which includes dance and music lessons), playing, TV watching, reading, household conversations, and other passive leisure (which includes going to movies and sports events as a spectator). We discuss all of these except youth groups, visiting, household conversations, day care, and other passive leisure. The latter includes attending events, listening to CDs, and doing nothing. These activities comprise only a small fraction of children's time.

The Validity and Reliability of Time Diary Data

Substantial methodological work has established the validity and reliability of data collected in time diary form for adults (Juster & Stafford, 1985). For children, Hofferth (1999) compared maternal verbal reports of whether mothers read to their children every day with an estimate based upon two diary days, that is, whether a child was reported as read to either on a weekend day or a weekday in the time diary. The frequency from the stylized question was 47%, compared with 42% from the time diaries. While the report from the stylized question is higher than the time diary estimate, the correlation between the two measures is .34. As an additional test, Hofferth regressed verbal achievement on the stylized question and separately on the time diary question, in each case controlling for demographic factors. The coefficients were not significantly different. This suggests a high degree of validity of the time diary measures, compared with other existing measures. The same was done for television viewing, and again, the two different types of reports were quite similar. These are the only time measures asked in most surveys.

Measurement of the Demographic Control Variables

The demographic control variables used in these analyses include characteristics of the individual child, the head of the household, the family, and the
child's mother. Characteristics of the individual child include age and gender.
The age, gender, race/ethnicity, and education of the head of household are
also included. Characteristics of the family that are included in the multivariate
analysis are the number of children in the family, a combined family struc-
ture/working status of the parent(s) variable, and the ratio of family income to
needs, equivalent to the ratio of income to the poverty line. Finally, the mother's
score on the passage comprehension subtest of the Woodcock-Johnson Test of
Basic Achievement is also used a control variable (see below for more details).

Child Assessments and Analysis Plan

A child's cognitive development was assessed by using four subtests of the
Woodcock-Johnson Revised Test of Basic Achievement: letter–word identification (test of the children's ability to respond to letters and words), passage comprehension (test that measures vocabulary and comprehension skills), calculation (test of mathematical calculation performance), and applied problems (test
of skill in analyzing and solving practical numerical problems) (Woodcock &
Mather, 1989). A child's socioemotional development was measured by the
Behavior Problems Index, a 30-item scale that attempts to quantify the existence and severity of child behavior problems (Peterson & Zill, 1986). From this
scale, two subscales can be derived that measure two general types of behavior
problems: internalizing (distressed or withdrawn behavior) and externalizing
(aggressive behavior). We examine the effects of children's time use on cognitive
achievement and behavior, net of the demographic controls.

Results

Leisure Time

Table 1 shows the total amount of leisure time available to children by age
(6–8 years or 9–12 years) and gender of the child for a weekday and a weekend
day. On a given weekday, children 6–8 years old have about 331 minutes (5.5
hours) of leisure time compared with 353 minutes (5.8 hours) for children 9–
12 years old. While older children spend a little bit more time in school, they
sleep about a half hour less per day than younger children. This accounts for the
slightly higher leisure time for older children.

The amount of leisure time available to children on a weekend day is nearly
twice that of a weekday—646 minutes (10.7 hours) for children ages 6–8 and
663 minutes (11 hours) for children ages 9–12. The difference is the 6.5 hours
typically spent in school. Once again, the slightly higher amount of leisure time

Table 1. Average Minutes in Leisure and Nonleisure Time, by Age and Gender

	Weekday			Weekend day		
	Total	Male	Female	Total	Male	Female
			Children 6 to 8			
Nonleisure Time	1,109	1,104	1,116	794	781	809
Sleeping	592	584	602	638	628	650
Eating	63	66	60	85	85	86
Personal care	66	63	69	70	68	73
School time	387	390	385	—	—	—
Leisure Time	331	336	324	646	659	631
	($N = 596$)	($n = 307$)	($n = 289$)	($N = 596$)	($n = 307$)	($n = 289$)
			Children 9 to 12			
Nonleisure Time	1,087	1,097	1,079	777	763	788
Sleeping	561	566	556	629	624	633
Eating	58	58	57	78	79	77
Personal care	67	60	72	70	60	78
School time	402	412	394	—	—	—
Leisure Time	353	343	361	663	677	652
	($N = 865$)	($n = 427$)	($n = 438$)	($N = 865$)	($n = 427$)	($n = 438$)

available to the older children is primarily because they sleep less than younger children.

There are small differences in the amount of leisure time available to children by gender, with no consistent pattern. There is a 30-minute difference between groups at most. In general, girls tend to spend slightly more time in personal care and boys slightly more time at school, which affects the amount of leisure time available. There are no consistent patterns of gender differences in sleeping and eating time.

Participation in Leisure Activities

Table 2 lists the most common leisure activities, the proportion of children who engage in the activity in a typical week, and the average weekly hours engaged in the activity by age and gender of child. For children 6–8 years of age, watching television is the most universal use of leisure time, with 96% of children engaging in this activity. More than 9 out of 10 children of this age play, and about 8 in 10 participate in housework. Activities with the least frequent participation include hobbies (2%), using the computer (13%), and time spent in outdoor activities (excluding playing) (14%). Girls in this group are much more likely than boys to participate in art and shopping. Girls are slightly more likely than boys to read for pleasure, while boys are more likely to study.

Among children 9–12 years of age, television watching is also the most universal use of leisure time (94%), and more than 8 out of 10 children play and

Table 2. Proportion of Children Engaged in Various Leisure Activities and Average Weekly Hours Engaged in the Activities, by Age and Gender

	Proportion			Average weekly hours		
	Total	Male	Female	Total	Male	Female
		Children 6–8				
Leisure Activity				49.120	50.008	48.055
Playing	0.92	0.91	0.93	11.939	12.703	11.022
Studying	0.55	0.58	0.52	2.151	2.345	1.919
Using computer[a]	0.13	0.13	0.13	0.533	0.658	0.383
Watching TV	0.96	0.97	0.95	12.796	13.485	11.970
Art	0.23	0.15	0.34	0.729	0.398	1.125
Hobbies	0.02	0.02	0.02	0.068	0.032	0.111
Sports	0.76	0.76	0.75	5.295	6.159	4.257
Reading	0.43	0.40	0.46	1.157	1.161	1.152
Being outdoors	0.14	0.13	0.15	0.488	0.343	0.661
Religious activities	0.25	0.24	0.26	1.328	1.149	1.544
Housework	0.80	0.80	0.81	2.233	1.979	2.538
Shopping	0.48	0.40	0.56	2.476	2.228	2.773
Other[b]	NA	NA	NA	7.927	7.368	8.600
	(N = 596)	(n = 307)	(n = 289)	(N = 596)	(n = 307)	(n = 289)
		Children 9–12				
Leisure Activity				51.509	51.141	51.833
Playing	0.88	0.90	0.86	8.848	9.744	8.063
Studying	0.62	0.65	0.59	3.670	3.944	3.429
Using computer[a]	0.22	0.23	0.21	1.069	1.433	0.749
Watching TV	0.94	0.94	0.95	13.563	12.783	14.246
Art	0.22	0.14	0.28	0.929	0.446	1.352
Hobbies	0.04	0.03	0.04	0.146	0.112	0.175
Sports	0.76	0.83	0.69	6.452	8.711	4.471
Reading	0.35	0.29	0.40	1.250	0.981	1.486
Being outdoors	0.17	0.19	0.16	0.696	0.690	0.701
Religious activities	0.28	0.29	0.26	1.487	1.594	1.393
Housework	0.88	0.83	0.91	3.825	3.320	4.268
Shopping	0.46	0.39	0.53	2.300	1.737	2.793
Other[b]	NA	NA	NA	7.274	5.646	8.707
	(N = 865)	(n = 427)	(n = 438)	(N = 865)	(n = 427)	(n = 438)

Note: NA = not applicable.
[a] Also included under playing and studying.
[b] Total leisure time minus the listed activities except for time using computer.

participate in housework. Only 4% of these older children participate in art, and 17% participate in outdoor activities. Although computer usage was low in 1997 for all children, older children were almost twice as likely to use the computer (22%) as children 6–8 years of age (13%). As with the younger children, girls 9–12 years old are twice as likely as boys this age to participate in art and more than a third more likely to shop. The disparity between genders in reading is greater for older than younger children, with boys decreasing their participation with age more than girls. A higher proportion of older than younger children study, but boys are still more likely than girls to do so. Sports participation among older children reveals a gender disparity that is not evident for children 6–8 years of age. About 83% of boys 9–12 years of age participate in sports, compared with 69% of girls. This disparity develops because boys increase their participation in sports with age, while the reverse is true for girls.

The average weekly hours engaged in various leisure activities shown in Table 2 include both children who participate and those who do not, with the latter group contributing zero minutes. Children 6–8 years of age spend about 13 hours per week watching television and about 12 hours playing. These two activities occupy half their total weekly leisure time of 49 hours. These children spend a little over 2 hours per week studying and about 5 hours in sports. Children spend less than 1 hour of weekly leisure time using the computer or participating in art, hobbies, or outdoor activities. Religious activities and reading occupy only about 1 hour each of children's leisure time. The "other" category, which includes conversing, visiting, and passive leisure, amounts to about 8 hours per week. Boys spend more time playing, studying, watching television, and participating in sports, whereas girls spend more time doing housework and in other leisure activities.

Most of the same patterns that are evident for children 6–8 years old are also found for children 9–12 years old, except that older children spend more time studying and participating in sports than younger children, and less time playing. Gender differences persist except that whereas younger girls watch less television than boys, older girls watch more.

Day of Week Differences

In general, children's time use is similar on weekdays and similar on Saturday and Sunday, with small exceptions. On Fridays children spend much more time watching television compared with other weekdays (data not shown). Children spend more time in nearly all leisure activities on Saturday compared with Sunday, except for activities related to religious institutions. Organized religious activities occupy about 1 hour of children's leisure time on Sunday compared with less than 15 minutes on Saturday. Due to the similarity in time use among the weekdays and weekend days, with the exceptions mentioned above, we focus on a weekly estimate.

Cognitive Achievement

Table 3 shows the results of ordinary least squares regression of children's cognitive outcomes on their leisure time activities, controlling for demographic factors. Demographic factors such as parental education, number of children in the family, the child's gender, the mother's passage comprehension score, family structure/employment, and the ratio of income to needs significantly affect achievement. Even so, there are some significant effects of leisure activities.

Table 3. Regression of Child Outcomes on Children's Time Use and Control Variables

Variables	Woodcock-Johnson Test of Basic Achievement				Behavior Problems Index	
	Passage comprehension	Calculation	Letter-word	Applied problems	Internalizing	Externalizing
Playing (hr/week)	−0.08	−0.02	−0.05	−0.02	0.02+	0.03
Studying (hr/week)	−0.16	−0.23	0.00	−0.19	0.00	0.00
Time using computers (hr/week)	−0.05	0.26	−0.16	0.31+	−0.02	−0.02
Watching TV (hr/week)	−0.13**	−0.07	−0.08	−0.17***	0.01	0.03+
Art (hr/week)	0.19	−0.71**	0.14	−0.31	0.02	0.03
Hobbies (hr/week)	0.17	−0.42	0.49	0.03	0.06	0.06
Sports (hr/week)	0.09	0.13+	0.10	0.19**	−0.01	−0.01
Reading (hr/week)	0.33+	0.31	0.57**	0.38+	0.04	0.06
Outdoors (hr/week)	−0.09	−0.07	−0.27+	−0.25+	0.00	0.01
Religious activities (hr/week)	0.24+	0.29+	0.23	0.03	0.04	0.05
Housework (hr/week)	−0.46***	−0.45***	−0.67***	−0.33**	0.12***	0.13***
Shopping (hr/week)	0.29+	0.06	0.36+	−0.02	0.00	−0.03
Child is African American	−1.52	0.95	−1.46	−5.96***	−1.34***	−1.20+
Child is Hispanic	−6.68+	−2.93	−5.86+	−13.52***	−1.88**	−0.62
Child is other race (White omitted)	1.34	−0.33	10.24+	0.04	0.16	−1.03
Parent's education—high school	4.23**	5.28**	2.63	6.23***	−0.35	−1.34**
Parent's education—some college	7.28***	8.37***	6.50**	7.95***	−0.34	−1.70**
Parent's education—college Age of child	8.70***	11.15***	8.37***	11.78***	−0.49	−2.05***
	0.00	0.02	0.08***	0.02	0.01+	0.00
Age of family head	0.00	−0.03	−0.11	0.08	0.01	−0.01
Number of children in family	−2.12***	−0.31	−2.25***	−0.94	−0.23+	−0.12
Child is male	−3.14***	−0.48	−4.13***	2.03+	0.36+	1.58***
Mother's passage score	0.86***	0.62***	0.98***	0.68***	0.20	0.11
Two parents—both work	−1.39	0.25	−3.40+	−0.79	2.18***	1.92+
Two parents—neither works/wife works	−5.30+	−9.32***	−7.23**	−6.45**	1.26***	1.22+
Female head—works	−1.11	−2.02	−2.17	−0.15	2.11***	1.45+
Female head—does not work	−2.62	0.35	−5.21+	1.77	1.88**	1.85+
Male head	−1.53	−0.17	−0.19	−1.44	−0.05	−0.14+
Ratio of income to needs	0.37+	0.86***	0.71***	0.54**	−0.13	−0.36**
R-square	0.28	0.22	0.26	0.30	0.10	0.09
N	1,132	1,125	1,138	1,135	1,325	1,325

***$p < .001$. **$p < .01$. *$p < .05 + p < .10$ two-tailed test.

Positive Indicators

Time spent reading is positively associated with scores on the passage comprehension, letter–word, and applied problems tests. Time spent participating in sports is associated with positive scores on the calculation and applied problems tests. Other positive associations include time participating in religious activities for the passage comprehension and calculation test scores and shopping for the passage comprehension and letter–word scores. The literature discussed earlier consistently shows reading and sports to be positive indicators for high achievement and church involvement to be positive for children's development. Thus these findings are not surprising. The strong positive association for shopping is unexpected. More research needs to be conducted on the activities involved in shopping. If this involves parent–child talking and decision making, shopping could be helpful to developing verbal skills. Time spent shopping is not associated with the calculation score, which would be expected if it were linked to math skills.

Negative Indicators

As many people would predict, the time spent watching television is negatively associated with scores on the passage comprehension and applied problems tests. This is probably because it reduces the amount of time spent in positive activities, such as reading. Time spent in art activities is negatively associated with the calculation test score, and time in outdoor activities is negatively associated with letter–word and applied problems scores. These negative results may reflect selectivity. Children who are less interested in schoolwork and academics may be the most likely to participate in art activities and to spend time in outdoor activities. The strongest and most consistent finding is a negative association between the time that children spend doing housework and all of the achievement test scores. While this is surprising, it may reflect something about the families in which children spend more time in household work. It doesn't reflect family size and family income, since they are both controlled. Too-heavy home responsibilities may interfere with achievement.

Behavior Problems

Many demographic variables, particularly parental education and family structure/work and maternal warmth (Table 3), have strong associations with behavioral problems, but few of children's leisure time activities are associated with such problems. Time spent watching television is associated with more externalizing behavior problems, but the coefficient is quite small and the significance is marginal. Time spent playing is marginally associated with internalizing problems, but again the coefficient is quite small. The amount of time children spend doing housework is positively associated with both types of behavior problems, and this coefficient is reasonably large. Given its negative association with achievement and positive association with behavior problems, more research needs to be done on the meaning of household work for children and the circumstances in which they do more or less of it.

Summary and Conclusions

In general, the amount of leisure time available on a typical weekday to children 6–12 years, by age or gender, averages 5.5 to 6 hours. Virtually all groups had twice the leisure time on a weekend day (about 10.5 to 11.25 hours) compared with a weekday because they spent no time in school. Friday was the weekday with the most leisure time available, averaging over 1 hour more than Thursday, the day with the least amount of leisure time. Nearly all of this difference was accounted for by the difference in time spent in school. Children had about 1 hour more leisure time on Saturday than Sunday because they slept more on Sunday.

The vast majority of children were likely to use some of their leisure time watching television, playing, and doing housework, and about half of children's leisure time was spent watching television and playing. This was true on weekends, as well as weekdays. Only a very small proportion of children used leisure time to engage in hobbies and participate in outdoor activities, and very little time was spent in these activities. Girls were more likely than boys to participate in art, reading, and shopping, whereas boys were slightly more likely to study. At older ages, boys participated in sports more than girls, and at all ages they spent more time at it.

Three activities can be considered as measures of positive behavior in middle childhood: reading for pleasure, religious activities, and participation in sports. Considerable previous research focused on reading as positive behavior. Our research based upon actual time spent supports reading for pleasure as a positive indicator of children's leisure time. Reading is consistently associated with higher cognitive test scores. Participation in sports activities has been studied among adolescents. It is, for children in middle childhood, consistently associated with higher achievement test scores. Thus it qualifies as an indicator of positive behavior for them as well. Time spent at religious services and in activities of religious organizations is not as frequently measured. Time spent in religious activities is consistently positively related to achievement and could be used as a measure of positive behavior.

At the time this survey was conducted, the use of computers at home was experiencing rapid growth. Even with the relatively small amount of time spent by children in our study and with their young age, we found a positive association with applied problem scores. More research needs to be conducted as to what type of, and under what circumstances, computer use benefits children before considering it as a positive indicator of behavior. Some of the other activities expected to be positively associated with cognitive achievement and lower behavior problems simply occurred too infrequently to obtain in a diary. The shortcoming of the time diary methodology is that it more accurately reflects regular than occasional activities.

Finally, this study separated shopping from housework. We know that time spent in household work has been declining for women and children, whereas time spent shopping has been increasing. There is a presumption that time spent helping out around the house is a positive use of children's time. However, we found no evidence to support this. In fact, more time spent in household work is negatively associated with achievement and positively associated with behavior problems. We do not yet know how to interpret the positive association between shopping and achievement. More research needs to be conducted before including shopping as an indicator of positive behavior.

A number of leisure time activities were found to have negative associations with achievement and, therefore, are not positive behavior indicators. This includes art and outdoor activities. Television watching can be viewed as a negative measure since more time spent watching TV was associated with lower achievement and having more behavior problems. One indicator that was unexpectedly negative is studying. While never statistically significant, the coefficient was uniformly negatively associated with achievement, suggesting that studying follows poor performance rather than leading to good performance.

In sum, this study has identified several activities that could be included as positive indicators (reading, religious activities, and sports), and several for which more research needs to be conducted (computer use and shopping).

Authors' Note

Funding from the National Institute of Child Health and Human Development (NICHD) supported data collection for the Child Development Supplement to the Panel Study of Income Dynamics in 1997. Funding from the NICHD Family and Child Well-Being Research Network (VO1HD-37563) supported the preparation of this chapter. Address correspondence to Sandra L. Hofferth, University of Maryland, Department of Family Studies, Marie Mount Hall, College Park, Maryland 20742-7500 (Hofferth@umd.edu).

References

Anderson, D. R., Huston, A. C., Schmitt, K. L., Linebarger, D. L., & Wright, J. (2001). *Monographs of the Society for Research in Child Development. Vol. 66: Early Childhood Television Viewing and Adolescent Behavior* (W. Overton, Ed.). Boston: Blackwell.

Cain, M. (1980). The economic activities in a village in Bangladesh. In R. Evenson, C. Florencio, & F. White (Eds.), *Rural household studies in Asia* (pp. 188–217). Kent Ridge, Singapore: Singapore University Press.

Eccles, J., & Barber, B. (1999). Student council, volunteering, basketball, or marching band: What kind of extracurricular involvement matters? *Journal of Adolescent Research, 14,* 10–43.

Fitzgerald, J., Gottschalk, P., & Moffitt, R. (1998). An analysis of sample attrition in panel data: The Michigan Panel Study of Income Dynamics. *Journal of Human Resources, 33*(2), 251–299.

Fuligni, A. J., & Stevenson, H. W. (1995). Time use and mathematics achievement among American, Chinese, and Japanese high school students. *Child Development, 66,* 830–842.

Gershuny, J., & Robinson, J. P. (1988). Historical changes in the household division of labor. *Demography, 25*(4), 537–552.

Hofferth, S. (1999, May 27–28). *Family reading to young children: Social desirability and cultural biases in reporting.* Paper presented at the Workshop on Measurement of and Research on Time Use, Committee on National Statistics, Washington, DC: National Research Council.

Hofferth, S., Davis-Kean, P., Davis, J., & Finkelstein, J. (1999). *1997 User Guide: The Child Development Supplement to the Panel Study of Income Dynamics.* Ann Arbor: University of Michigan, Institute for Social Research.

Hofferth, S., & Sandberg, J. (2001). Changes in American children's time, 1981–1997. In S. Hofferth & T. Owens (Eds.), *Children at the millennium: Where have we come from, where are we going?* (pp. 193–229). New York: Elsevier Science.

Juster, F., & Stafford, F. P. (1985). *Time, goods, and well-being.* Ann Arbor: University of Michigan, Institute for Social Research.

Larson, R. (1994). Youth organizations, hobbies, and sports as developmental contexts. In R. Silbereisen & E. Todt (Eds.), *Adolescence in context: The interplay of family, school, peers, and work in adjustment* (pp. 46–65). New York: Springer-Verlag.

Larson, R., & Verma, S. (1999). How children and adolescents spend time across the world: Work, play, and developmental opportunities. *Psychological Bulletin, 125*(6), 701–736.

Leone, C., & Richards, M. (1989). Classwork and homework in early adolescence: The ecology of achievement. *Journal of Youth and Adolescence, 18,* 531–548.

Peterson, J. L., & Zill, N. (1986). Marital disruption and behavior problems in children. *Journal of Marriage and the Family, 48,* 295–307.

Roberts, D. F., Foehr, U. G., Rideout, V. J., & Brodie, M. (1999). *Kids & media @ the new millennium.* Menlo Park, CA: Henry J. Kaiser Family Foundation.

Robinson, J. P., & Godbey, G. (1997). *Time for life: The surprising ways Americans use their time.* University Park: Pennsylvania State University Press.

Udry, J. R., & Billy, J. (1987). Initiation of coitus in early adolescence. *American Sociological Review, 52,* 841–855.

Woodcock, R., & Mather, N. (1989). *W-J-R Tests of Achievement: Examiner's manual.* Allen, TX: DLM Teaching Resources.

8 Healthy Habits among Adolescents: Sleep, Exercise, Diet, and Body Image

Kathleen Mullan Harris

University of North Carolina and
The Carolina Population Center

Rosalind Berkowitz King

National Institute for Child Health and Human Development

Penny Gordon-Larsen

University of North Carolina and
The Carolina Population Center

Healthy habits among children lay the groundwork for positive youth de-velopment (Danner, 2000; Ge, Elder, Regnerus, & Cox, 2001; Siegel, Yancey, Aneshensel, & Schuler, 1999; U.S. Department of Health and Human Services [USDHHS], 1996). Most fundamental to the developing child are health habits involving sleep, diet, and exercise. This chapter reviews the literature on physi-cal activity, diet, and sleep among adolescents, and explores available indicators of these health habits using data from the National Longitudinal Study of Ado-lescent Health (Add Health).

We focus on adolescents because this is the life stage when youth begin to exercise their independence from parental control and monitoring and when parents begin to grant children more autonomy to make their own decisions and judgments about what they eat, how long they sleep, and in what forms and level of intensity they engage in physical activity. Adolescence also marks the stage of rapid physical development when notions of an ideal body image become especially salient in young people's lives as they develop self-conceptions of their own body image. With unique data from Add Health, we explore body image indicators which can be both a consequence and a cause of healthy habits involving diet and exercise during adolescence. Finally, adolescence is the life stage when individuals begin to formulate their healthy habits, setting patterns that continue into adulthood (Andrade, Benedito-Silva, Domenice, Arnhold, & Menna-Barreto, 1993; Must, Jacques, Dalal, Bajema, & Dietz, 1992; Serdula et al., 1993).

Attention to healthy habits in adolescence has heightened as obesity has become a serious public health problem affecting nearly 25% of all U.S. children (USDHHS, 1996). Concern over adolescent obesity has mounted owing to its rapid increase in prevalence, its persistence into adulthood, and its associated health consequences, including morbidity and mortality (Must et al., 1992; National Institutes of Health [NIH], 1995; Serdula et al., 1993). For example, there has been a dramatic increase in the incidence of Type II diabetes ("adult-onset") in adolescents in parallel with the national increase in prevalence of obesity (Pinhas-Hamiel & Zeitler, 1996). Adolescent obesity is a major antecedent of adult obesity, CHD risk, increased morbidity and mortality (Bao et al., 1997; Must et al., 1992; NIH, 1995), and even increased risk of breast cancer (Hulka, Liu, & Lininger, 1994). Moreover, the consequences of adolescent obesity extend beyond its health effects to impacts on SES status and reduced chances for marriage (Averett and Korenman, 1999).

Literature Review

Exercise and Diet

Physical activity has been associated with a wide range of beneficial health outcomes in adults, including bone and cardiovascular health and a reduction in selected cancers (NIH, 1987). Physical activity during childhood and adolescence may have a positive impact on growth and development and psychological and emotional outcomes that may continue into adulthood (Ross & Hayes, 1988; USDHHS, 1996). Inactivity, in particular TV viewing, has been associated with obesity in cross-sectional studies of children, adolescents, and adults (Gortmaker, Sobal, Peterson, Colditz, & Dietz, 1996). Physical activity habits, and specifically inactivity, track significantly from adolescence to young adulthood (Raitakari et al., 1994). Minority adolescents have consistently high levels of inactivity and low levels of activity, and these trends are exaggerated for females (Andersen, Crespo, Bartlett, Cheskin, & Pratt, 1998; Gordon-Larsen, McMurray, & Popkin, 1999; Sallis, Zakarian, Hovell, & Hofstetter, 1996; Wolf et al., 1993).

Body composition is ultimately affected by total energy expenditure relative to energy intake. Physical activity accounts for 15%–40% of total energy expenditure, more for children than for adults (Bouchard, Shepard, & Stephens, 1993). Resting metabolic rate and the thermic effect of food are relatively invariant to most voluntary behaviors. In contrast, level of physical activity is voluntary, more easily modified, and is the component of total energy expenditure most linked with child obesity (Johnson, Burke, & Mayer, 1956, were among the first to show this).

Adolescent physical activity includes work at school or home, travel-related activity, activity during work for those with jobs, participation in individual and team sports, and leisure activities (play). Adolescent inactivity typically includes sedentary pastimes associated with energy expenditure near or only marginally above the resting metabolic rate (e.g., television viewing, reading). The intervention and epidemiology literature generally differentiates physical activity and inactivity when studying their relationship to obesity, and there is evidence that reducing inactivity is more important than increasing more vigorous activity (Epstein, Saelens, & O'Brien, 1995). While activity and inactivity are obviously related (particularly at the extremes given the allocation of a finite amount of time during a day), there are sufficient grounds to study them separately.

Methods for measuring physical activity/inactivity include questionnaires, heart rate monitors, and accelerometers (Janz, 1994; Mathews & Freedson, 1995; Pereira et al., 1997). Each has strengths and weaknesses. Questionnaires typically collect information on only one or two activities that take up a great deal of time (e.g., viewing television), while a few use more detailed recall or historical measures of multiple activities (Matsudo, 1996). Despite these weaknesses, questionnaires remain the most feasible method for large samples and have been validated with more precise measures of physical activity/inactivity (Pereira et al., 1997). While they do not measure physical activity with enough accuracy to quantify total energy expended in activity, questionnaires are nonetheless useful for ranking individuals by activity level with reasonable reliability and validity.

Diet, especially energy and fat intake, is theoretically a key determinant of energy balance and, consequently, obesity. There is great difficulty measuring diet and relating it to adolescent obesity in the United States because of the difficulties with measurement of diet in large population studies in general and because of differential misreporting related to obesity. While human clinical studies support a diet–obesity relationship (Obarzanek et al., 1994), there is a surprisingly meager population literature to confirm these findings. Shah and Jequier (1991) reviewed 11 studies on food intake in youth and noted that only 3 reported a positive relationship of food intake and obesity. Furthermore, no study in the United States or Europe has been able to adequately measure and then study how diet affects the onset of overweight and/or changes in the level of body fatness. The Add Health data cannot add much, as they are inadequate to provide meaningful measures of total energy, energy density, or proportion of energy from fat, the latter being viewed as a key determinant of total energy intake (Bray and Popkin, 1998). In this chapter, however, we do explore healthy and unhealthy food intake as part of adolescents' diet.

Body Image

One of the defining features of adolescence is rapid physical development brought on by puberty. Puberty typically involves rising levels of estrogen and testosterone, the hormones related to reproductive capability. In addition to triggering changes directly related to that capability, such as menarche, rising hormonal levels trigger the development of secondary sex characteristics such as breast development in girls and facial hair in boys. Both boys and girls also experience a height spurt and weight gain. However, the nature of the weight gain tends to differ: For boys, the increase is typically in the form of increased muscle mass, whereas girls see an increasing portion of their body composition shift toward fat (Petersen & Taylor, 1980).

These physiological changes take place within a socially defined structure of norms and expectations about the meanings of womanliness and manhood (Martin, 1996). For boys, increasing muscle mass fits with the high value currently placed on a powerful muscular male body type (Bordo, 1999). In contrast, girls whose bodies are adding fat encounter an ideal female image that emphasizes thinness and angularity (Brumberg, 1997). The majority of past research has focused on documenting this ideal among middle-class White girls; recent explorations among other groups, such as African American girls, has shown this ideal to be less pervasive but gaining influence (Duke, 2002; Story, French, Resnick, & Blum, 1995). Some studies have suggested that mass media may play a role in influencing the development of weight concerns and weight control practices among preadolescents and adolescents (Field et al., 2001; Milkie, 1999).

Not living up to these ideals is linked to detrimental outcomes for both boys and girls. Adolescents who are dissatisfied with their body image are at increased risk for physical and emotional problems such as excessive dieting and depression (Ge et al., 2001; Siegel et al., 1999). Girls, especially White girls, are at greatest risk of developing eating disorders (Lovejoy, 2001).

A preference for thinness is prevalent in middle- and upper-SES White American culture (Rand & Kuldau, 1990), and this preference may affect behaviors such as eating habits, dieting, and activity patterns. The cultural obsession with thinness may be less pervasive among Blacks, Asians, or Hispanics compared to non-Hispanic Whites. In general, perceptions of overweight and weight reduction activities are less common in Black than White women (Felts, Tavasso, Chenier, & Dunn, 1992).

The relationship between body image, diet, and exercise is a reciprocal one. Adolescents' body weight and stature are a function of biological factors and eating and exercise behavior; in turn, diet and physical activity have direct effects on body weight and risks of obesity. Body image, however, incorporates the individuals' interpretation of their own body weight and stature compared to cultural norms and messages about the ideal weight and stature. This added component of self-perception can therefore affect eating and physical activity behavior independent of actual body weight. We therefore explore indicators of body image with important implications for understanding adolescent behaviors involving diet and exercise.

Sleep Habits

While the relationship between exercise, diet, and body image is widely studied, the relationship between sleep and other healthy habits has not received much attention. Research on sleep is mainly focused on changing patterns across age and by gender, predictors of changing patterns of sleep, especially as they relate to sleep problems, and the relationship between sleep problems and other outcomes. Much of the research on youth sleep habits focuses on sleep problems and sleep deprivation (e.g., Guilleminault, 1987; Morrison, McGee, & Stanton, 1992). The development of good sleep habits in adolescence is critical, as many adult insomniacs report that their problem began in adolescence (Hauri, Percy, Olmstead, & Sateia, 1980). A few studies have examined how sleep deprivation is related to school performance and daytime functioning in adolescence, documenting negative effects on mental and physical health (Danner, 2000; Wolfson & Carskadon, 1998). Clearly, it is impossible to sort out the direction of influence here, but concern over chronic sleep deprivation among adolescents in particular has targeted school start times as one important cause of sleep deprivation and an avenue for policy intervention (Danner, Hutchins, & Hooks, 2001; Manber et al., 1995).

Sleep patterns of adolescents have been investigated by means of electro-physiological recordings (Coble, Kupfer, Taska, & Kane, 1984) and questionnaire-based surveys, mainly self-reports (Lee, Blair, & Jackson, 1999; Wolfson & Carskadon, 1998). During childhood, the sleep schedule on school days and weekends is generally constant, wake times in particular (Petta, Carskadon, & Dement, 1984). When children enter adolescence, major changes in sleep patterns occur, mainly characterized by a delay in the sleep period. Adolescents tend to stay up later at night and to sleep later in the morning than do pre-pubescent children (Dahl & Carskadon, 1995). This delay in the sleep period is especially pronounced on weekends.

While age is the key determinant of changing sleep patterns, gender and puberty status are also associated with the timing of sleep, especially on weekends (Laberge et al., 2001). In prepubertal children there is generally no gender difference in sleep patterns (Wolfson, 1996). However, numerous studies based on self-reports have noted significant gender differences in adolescent sleep patterns, with girls reporting longer sleep hours and sleeping later on weekends (Lee et al. 1999; Wolfson & Carskadon, 1998). There is evidence that puberty status, and the fact that girls start puberty earlier than boys, may explain the longer sleep patterns of girls (Laberge et al., 2001). Surprisingly, most sleep research has been done on White samples, or where there is racial and ethnic diversity in the sample, racial differences have not been investigated (e.g., Danner, 2000). Our exploratory work on sleep habit indicators will examine both age and race/ethnicity differentials.

Data

Our data come from the National Longitudinal Study of Adolescent Health (Add Health). Add Health is a nationally representative study of adolescents in grades 7 through 12 in the United States in 1995. As detailed in Harris et al. (1997), Add Health was designed to help explain the causes of adolescent health and health behavior with special emphasis on the effects of multiple contexts of adolescent life. The study used a school-based design to select a stratified sample of 80 high schools with selection probability proportional to size. For each high school, a feeder school was also selected with probability proportional to its student contribution to the high school. The school-based sample therefore has a pair of schools in each of 80 communities. An in-school questionnaire was administered to every student who attended each selected school on a particular day during the period of September 1994 to April 1995 and was completed by more than 90,000 adolescents.

In a second level of sampling, adolescents and parents were selected for in-home interviews. From the school rosters, a random sample of some 200 students from each high school–feeder school pair was selected, irrespective of school size, to produce the core in-home sample of about 12,000 adolescents. A number of special oversamples were also selected for in-home interviews, including ethnic samples, physically disabled adolescents, and a genetic sample. The in-home interviews were conducted between April and December 1995, yielding "Wave I data." The core plus the special samples produced a total sample size of 20,745 adolescents in Wave I. A parent, generally the mother, was also interviewed in Wave I. All adolescents in grades 7 through 11 in Wave I (plus 12th graders who were part of the genetic sample) were targeted roughly 1 year later for the Wave II in-home interview. The content of the Wave II interview was similar to that of the Wave I interview.

We limit our sample to adolescents aged 12 through 19 at Wave I to capture the typical school ages of 7th through 12th graders, eliminating the handful of 11-, 20-, and 21-year-olds in these grades. In our analysis of physical activity indicators we eliminate disabled youth (adolescents who use a walking aid). We use Wave I data to maximize our sample size for our indicator analysis with the exception of diet (questions only available at Wave II) and body image when we must use Wave II data, when measured height and weight were taken (as opposed to self-reported height and weight in Wave I). Sampling weights that adjust for the differential sampling probabilities of adolescents responding to the two in-home interviews have been developed and are used throughout our analysis. Sample sizes for Wave I data with valid sample weights are over 18,000 adolescents; Wave II sample size with valid weights for the body image analysis is about 13,000.

Measurement

Measures of healthy habits in adolescence do not lend themselves to the development of constructs or scales of "healthy habits," because the measures are so specific to the particular health habit, and it would be difficult to decide how or whether to weight each habit or cluster of behaviors representing the habit. We therefore do not attempt to develop such constructs (using factor analysis, for example); although we note in the discussion that an index of "healthy habits" might be possible, where points are assigned for engagement in "good habits" in each realm of diet, physical activity, sleep, and body image.

Sleep habits are measured by responses to three questions in the Wave I Add Health survey. Sleep hours are reported in response to the question, "How many hours of sleep do you usually get?" We examine both the continuous measure of sleep hours and a categorical measure with four categories: < 7 hours; 7–8 hours; 9 hours; and 10+ hours. We measure bedtime hour by responses to the question, "What time do you usually go to bed on week nights?" We categorize bedtime hour into four categories: < 10 : 00 p.m.; 10:00–10:59 p.m.; 11:00–11:59 p.m.; and < 12 : 00 a.m. A final question, "Do you usually get enough sleep?" (with a yes or no response), we use to validate our bedtime and sleep hours indicators.

Physical activity is measured by a standard physical activity behavior recall in Add Health that is similar, although not identical, to self-report questionnaires used and validated in other large-scale epidemiological studies (e.g., Andersen et al., 1998). A series of questions, listed below, asks about participation in moderate to vigorous physical activity (5–8 metabolic equivalents), in units of times per week. One metabolic equivalent represents the resting metabolic rate, or 3.5 ml O_2/kg body weight/minute.

Moderate–Vigorous

1. During the past week, how many times did you go rollerblading, roller-skating, skateboarding, or bicycling?
2. During the past week, how many times did you play an active sport, such as baseball, softball, basketball, soccer, swimming, or football?
3. During the past week, how many times did you do exercise, such as jogging, walking, karate, jumping rope, gymnastics, or dancing?

Respondents indicated the number of times in which they engaged in moderate to vigorous physical activity for each set of activities according to the following four categories: 0; 1–2; 3–4; and 5+ times per week. We create a dichotomous variable indicating a 1 for respondents who engage in any moderate to vigorous physical activity 5+ times per week in line with the Surgeon General's physical activity recommendations.

Inactivity can be measured by TV viewing, video viewing, and computer or video game use, which are reported by the adolescent as hours/week over the past week (i.e., "How many hours a week do you watch television?"). Quantifying inactivity has received far less attention than physical activity (Dietz, 1996), and little, if anything, is published in the literature regarding the reliability and validity of inactivity data. We use the hours of TV viewing per week to measure inactivity. Similar patterns are obtained using the video viewing and computer use, but we decided not to combine these with TV viewing because they may also represent educational activities.

Diet measures attempt to capture healthy and unhealthy food choices by adolescents. Unhealthy choices are measured by the number of times the adolescent eats fast food in a week. We create two categories: seldom (0 or 1 time) and often (2+ times). Healthy food choices are measured by the number of servings of fruits and vegetables the adolescent eats in a week. Again, we create two categories: few (0 or 1 serving each of fruit and vegetables) and moderate (2+ servings each of fruit and vegetables/week).

Actual weight status is based on adolescents' body mass index (BMI). Interviewers measured and weighed adolescents in Wave II to obtain their height and weight. Measurements were in feet and inches and pounds, with the BMI equaling (weight in kilograms/height in meters^2). We express actual weight relative to height as a categorical variable by comparing adolescents' BMIs to the appropriate percentiles for age (in months) and gender from the most recent reference curves published by the Centers for Disease Control (2002) and the National Center for Health Statistics (Kuczmarksi et al., 2000). We categorized those below the 5th percentile as "underweight" and those at or above the 85th percentile as "at risk for overweight" (abbreviated as "overweight" hereafter). Adolescents in the middle percentile range (at or above 5% and below 85%) were classified as "normal weight."

Perceived weight is measured in response to the question, "How do you think of yourself in terms of weight?" Response categories included very underweight, slightly underweight, about the right weight, slightly overweight, very overweight. We grouped together the two underweight and two overweight responses to create a three-category measure that is parallel to actual weight: underweight, average weight, and overweight.

Weight concordance is based on the comparison of actual and perceived weight measures. Respondents were categorized as having a perception that is **heavier** than their actual weight ("thinks heavier"), **accurate** for their actual weight ("thinks same"), and **lighter** than their actual weight ("thinks lighter"; see Table 6). For example, a female adolescent who is underweight but perceives herself as average weight would fall into the "thinks heavier" category (i.e., thinks she is heavier than she really is), whereas a male adolescent who is overweight but perceives himself as average weight would fall into the "thinks lighter" category (i.e., thinks he is lighter than his actual weight indicates).

Dieting behavior is based on the question, "Are you trying to lose weight, gain weight, or stay the same weight?" Responses include (1) lose weight; (2) gain weight; (3) stay the same weight; and (4) not trying to do anything about weight. Because so few girls respond that they are trying to gain weight and so few boys respond that they are trying to lose weight, we analyzed the "lose weight" response (relative to everything else) only for girls and the "gain weight" response (relative to everything else) only for boys.

Gender is based on the respondent's report from the in-school survey.

Race/ethnicity is measured by responses to a racial identification question and a Hispanic origin question. We combined the information on race and Hispanic ethnicity to create one variable that has four categories: non-Hispanic White, non-Hispanic Black, Hispanic, and Asian. For simplicity in presentation and owing to small sample sizes, we eliminated adolescents of "other" race (largely Native American and "other" [unknown] race).

Age is calculated as the elapsed years between the month, day, and year of birth and the month, day, and year of interview. For presentation purposes we categorize age into two groups: pre- and early adolescence, ages 12–15; and older adolescents, those 16–19.

Analyses

Our exploratory analyses involve arraying descriptive data on each of the four domains of healthy habits (sleep, physical activity and inactivity, diet, and body image) separately for females and males by race/ethnicity and age. Where we have multiple measures of healthy habits in a domain, we attempt to validate the central measure of interest.

Sleep Habits

The average number of hours that adolescents in grades 7–12 in 1995 usually sleep is 7.84 ($N = 18,864$).

Table 1 shows the distribution of adolescents according to our categories of sleep hours by race/ethnicity and age. Sleep deprivation is defined as less than 6 hours of sleep a night (Danner, 2000), and we have shown that less than 7 hours is about 1 hour or more below the overall mean, so the < 7

Table 1. Distribution of Female and Male Sleep Hours by Race/Ethnicity and Age

Category	Sleep Hours			
	< 7	7–8	9	10+
By race/ethnicity ($N = 18,277$)				
Female				
Non-Hispanic White	14.87	60.03	15.56	9.54
Non-Hispanic Black	24.82	53.41	11.26	10.51
Hispanic	13.25	59.29	18.59	8.87
Asian	22.94	55.51	14.15	7.41
Male				
Non-Hispanic White	12.19	58.88	18.04	10.89
Non-Hispanic Black	19.53	58.29	11.59	10.59
Hispanic	14.76	56.08	17.35	11.81
Asian	18.08	63.97	12.39	5.57
By age ($N = 18,786$)				
Female				
12–15	10.34	57.97	19.79	11.90
16–19	23.56	59.46	10.00	6.97
Male				
12–15	6.77	55.05	23.25	14.93
16–19	20.81	62.24	10.34	6.62

category identifies adolescents who are not getting sufficient sleep at night. The modal category is 7–8 hours, and certainly the category of 9 hours represents healthy sleep habits for adolescents. The category of 10 hours or more cannot necessarily be defined as "unhealthy," but it is fairly far above the mean and therefore is nonnormative (and as the table indicates is more common for younger adolescents). Table 1 helps identify which race and ethnic groups, and which age groups of adolescents fall into these various patterns of sleep.

Among females, non-Hispanic Black and Asian youth are more likely to get insufficient sleep at night (< 7 hours) and less likely to fall within the healthy sleep habit range of 7–9 hours. Differences within the 10+ sleep hours category are minor, with the exception that Asian girls are the least likely to sleep 10 hours or more a night. The race and ethnicity patterns are the same for males, with somewhat smaller differences. In general, non-Hispanic White boys tend to get the most sleep, and Asian boys the least sleep at night. Note, however, that the majority of boys and girls across all race and ethnic groups fall within the healthy range of 7–9 hours a night.

The age patterns in Table 1 show that more than 20% of the older girls and boys usually get fewer than 7 hours of sleep a night, compared to 10% of the younger girls and 7% of the younger boys. Moreover, the younger girls and boys are much more likely than the older adolescents to get 9 or 10+ hours of sleep a night.

We also explored the related sleep habit of adolescents' weekday bedtime hour by race/ethnicity and age (not shown). Bedtime hour is categorized into four bedtimes, with < 10 : 00 p.m. a fairly early bedtime for adolescents and after midnight a rather late bedtime on a weekday. The majority (about 60%) of girls and boys go to bed between 10:00 p.m. and midnight. Over 20% of girls and a little less than 20% of boys go to bed before 10:00 p.m. on the weekdays, and more boys go to bed after midnight than girls. We find Black females to have the least healthy bedtime hour, as they are least likely to go to bed before 10:00 p.m. and most likely to go to bed after midnight, consistent with their lower sleep hours in Table 1. Age patterns confirm that girls and boys in pre- and early adolescence have earlier bedtimes than older adolescents. Bedtime hour does a better job of validating sleep hours as an indicator of healthy sleep habits by age than by race and ethnicity because wake-up times vary by age (Danner et al., 2001; Manber et al., 1995), but are likely to vary *within* race and ethnic groups (owing to a number of factors in addition to age).

We further validate the sleep hours indicator by exploring the relationship between sleep hours and whether the adolescent reports that he or she gets enough sleep by race/ethnicity and age (not shown). Among those girls and boys who report that they do not sleep enough, a larger percentage report less than 7 hours of sleep a night, and this is especially the case for Black and Asian girls and boys. Moreover, a very small percentage (3%–12%) of Black and Asian girls and boys get more than 8 hours of sleep (9 and 10+ categories). In contrast, adolescents who perceive that they sleep enough are much less likely to report less than 7 hours as their usual sleep hours a night, and more likely to fall within the healthy range of 7–9 hours a night. However, the race and ethnicity pattern is still evident. Even among Black and Asian girls and boys who report that they get enough sleep, their likelihood of getting less than 7 hours a night is higher than it is among White and Hispanic girls and boys who report getting enough sleep.

We find a similar relationship between sleep hours and whether adolescents perceive that they get enough sleep by age (not shown), with the pattern most dramatic for older adolescents. For example, among older adolescent girls who do not sleep enough, 42% report less than 7 hours of sleep a night compared to only 13% with less than 7 hours among those who report that they get enough sleep. Overall, sleep hours appears to be a valid measure for healthy sleep habits.

Physical Activity and Inactivity

Turning to physical activity and exercise, in Table 2 we show the percentage distribution of engaging in physical activity according to the categories of 0, 1–2, 3–4, and 5+ moderate to vigorous physical activities a week, where 5+ times per week represents the Surgeon General's physical activity recommendations. We find that boys are more likely to be physically active than girls, but even so, less than 50% of boys meet the healthy habit recommendations of 5+ activities a week and a little more than one quarter of girls engage in 5+ activities a week. The

Table 2. *Percentage of Female and Male Adolescents Engaging in Physical Activity, by Race/Ethnicity and Age*

Category	Moderate to Vigorous Physical Activity Bouts/Week			
	0	1–2	3–4	5+
By race/ethnicity ($N = 18{,}471$)				
Female				
Non-Hispanic White	5.68	32.59	34.13	27.60
Non-Hispanic Black	9.80	36.85	34.30	19.05
Hispanic	4.72	32.75	35.96	26.57
Asian	5.63	21.78	41.14	31.44
Male				
Non-Hispanic White	4.89	21.66	30.27	43.19
Non-Hispanic Black	4.41	20.47	34.67	40.45
Hispanic	4.35	17.50	31.28	46.87
Asian	1.74	21.87	34.42	41.97
By age ($N = 18{,}819$)				
Female				
12–15	3.41	25.92	36.34	34.33
16–19	9.64	40.83	32.48	17.05
Male				
12–15	1.98	14.77	30.85	52.40
16–19	7.30	27.61	31.35	33.73

good news is that a small percentage of girls (6%) and boys (4%) get absolutely no exercise on a weekly basis. Modal categories are 1–4 activities a week for girls and 5+ for boys.

Race and ethnicity differences are consistent with prior research (Andersen et al., 1998; Wolf et al., 1993). Non-Hispanic Black girls are the most likely to get no exercise (9.8%) and the least likely to engage in 5+ physical activities (19%) per week. Asian girls are among the most physically active. In contrast, race and ethnicity differences among boys are relatively minor, with Hispanic boys the most active and Black boys the least.

Age differences show an overrepresentation of younger adolescents in the high exercise category of 5+ activities a week and less representation in the less active categories of 0 or 1–2 activities a week relative to older adolescents for both girls and boys. Among older girls, almost 10% get no weekly exercise and only 17% engage in the recommended 5 or more moderate to vigorous physical activities a week. Although the level of exercise is higher for older male adolescents, the pattern is the same, with 7% getting no exercise and only one third engaging in 5 or more physical activities a week. With the exception of pre- and early-adolescent boys, the majority of adolescents exercise less than what is recommended to maintain health in adolescence. The distributions in Table 2 suggest that a simple indicator of healthy habits involving exercise would be the yes–no dichotomy of engaging in 5+ moderate to vigorous physical activities a week.

Table 3 displays our indicator of inactivity, average hours of TV viewing per week for girls and boys by race/ethnicity and age. On average, boys tend to watch about 2 more hours of TV than girls. Consistent with previous research, non-Hispanic Black girls and boys spend the most time watching TV (Gordon-Larsen et al., 1999; Sallis et al., 1996). The differential is especially prominent for girls, where Blacks watch an average of 20 hours a week, compared to Asian girls, who watch 15.8 hours, Hispanic girls, who watch 13.8 hours, and White girls, who watch about 13 hours. Among boys, Blacks and Asians watch the most TV, followed by White and Hispanic boys, who watch an average of 5 less hours per week.

Table 3. Average Hours of TV Viewing per Week among Female and Male Adolescents, by Race/Ethnicity and Age

Category	Female	Male
By race/ethnicity ($N = 18,407$)		
Non-Hispanic White	13.28	15.55
Non-Hispanic Black	20.44	21.22
Hispanic	13.81	14.74
Asian	15.82	19.83
By age ($N = 18,754$)		
12–15	15.72	18.47
16–19	13.28	14.74

Table 4. Diet Choices of Adolescents by Race/Ethnicity and Age

A. Percentage of Female and Male Adolescents Who Have Fast Food Two or More Times per Week by Race/Ethnicity and Age

Category	Female	Male
By race/ethnicity ($N = 13,301$)		
Non-Hispanic White	54.39	60.16
Non-Hispanic Black	58.70	59.47
Hispanic	53.36	53.76
Asian	53.57	61.79
By age ($N = 13,536$)		
12–15	51.67	54.14
16–19	60.52	67.27

B. Percentage of Female and Male Adolescents Who Have Two or More Servings Each of Fruits and Vegetables per Week by Race/Ethnicity and Age

Category	Female	Male
By race/ethnicity ($N = 13,301$)		
Non-Hispanic White	36.90	38.50
Non-Hispanic Black	31.67	32.94
Hispanic	50.74	46.77
Asian	41.91	38.68
By age ($N = 13,536$)		
12–15	39.46	40.16
16–19	32.49	35.11

Inactivity is the one indicator in which younger adolescents do not demonstrate healthier habits than older adolescents. On average, younger girls watch 2.5 hours more TV than older adolescent girls, and younger boys watch about 3 hours more TV than older adolescent boys. Although this measure of inactivity is well accepted in the field, further work to validate this measure in Add Health is needed.

Diet

Table 4, section A, shows the frequency with which adolescents make the unhealthy diet choice of fast food, and section B the frequency of the healthy diet choice of fruits and vegetables by race/ethnicity and age. Boys eat fast food more frequently than girls as almost 60% of boys eat fast food two times or more a week compared to about 54% of girls. Among girls, non-Hispanic Blacks make the less healthy choice of fast food more often than the other racial and ethnic groups, who all have about equal percentages of eating fast food two or more times a week. Among boys, Hispanics choose fast food less often than Whites, Blacks, and Asians.

Age differences show that older adolescents eat fast food more frequently than younger adolescents. If we acknowledge that adolescents aged 16–19 typically have more independence and autonomy to make their own diet decisions, it appears that this independence is associated with less healthy choices.

Panel B of Table 4 shows the distributions on eating two or more servings of fruit and two or more servings of vegetables a week by race/ethnicity and age. Differences between girls and boys are minor on this diet indicator, perhaps because fruits and vegetables are less subject to adolescent choice and more under the influence of family eating behaviors. About 38% of both girls and boys have two or more servings each of fruits and vegetables. Race and ethnicity differences are evident, however. Hispanic youth eat fruits and vegetables most frequently, as 51% of girls and 47% of boys have two or more servings of fruits and two or more servings of vegetables a week. Asian youth eat fruits and vegetables less frequently than Hispanics, but more frequently than Whites and Blacks. Blacks have the lowest frequency of eating fruits and vegetables. This pattern suggests that perhaps the immigrant diet more often includes fruits and vegetables, even with acculturation of eating behaviors over generations (Gordon-Larsen, Harris, Ward, and Popkin, 2003).

Age patterns indicate that younger adolescents eat fruits and vegetables more frequently than older adolescents, again suggesting that as adolescents gain more independence from family eating norms, their diets tend to be less healthy.

Body Image

Our final domain of healthy habits addresses adolescents' self-perceptions about their body weight, or what we refer to as body image. This indicator represents the degree to which adolescents have a healthy view of their body weight. We begin by first presenting the distributions on actual weight status based on BMI (body mass index). In Table 5 we show the percentages of female and male adolescents who fall into the three categories of underweight, normal weight, and overweight by race/ethnicity and age. Consistent with findings from the obesity research, Black girls are more likely to be overweight, followed by Hispanic girls, White girls, and then Asian girls, who are the least likely to be overweight and the most likely to be underweight (Popkin & Udry, 1998). More than two thirds of White and Asian girls fall within the normal weight range, while over 30% of Black and Hispanic girls fall within the overweight range. Among boys, Blacks do not stand out as being overweight, but they are less likely than the other groups to be underweight. Age patterns show decreasing prevalence of overweight status and slightly increasing prevalence of underweight status as girls and boys age into late adolescence.

When we examine perceived weight of adolescent girls and boys by race/ethnicity (not shown), we find that race and ethnic differences in perceptions of overweight status are *dissimilar* to the race and ethnic differences in actual weight for girls indicated in Table 5. In particular, a similar percentage of Hispanic girls (44%), Black girls (40%), and White girls (39%) perceive themselves to be overweight, indicating that Black girls have more accurate

Table 5. Distribution of Female and Male Adolescents' Actual Weight Based on BMI Categories, by Race/Ethnicity and Age (N = 12,966)

Category	% Underweight	% Normal	% Overweight
By race/ethnicity			
Female			
Non-Hispanic White	7.14	70.35	22.51
Non-Hispanic Black	5.10	55.77	39.14
Hispanic	7.68	61.54	30.78
Asian	18.20	70.00	11.80
Male			
Non-Hispanic White	9.10	64.20	26.70
Non-Hispanic Black	5.14	68.61	26.25
Hispanic	9.36	61.78	28.86
Asian	10.42	67.33	22.24
By age			
Female			
12–15	6.36	66.08	27.56
16–19	8.73	68.34	22.94
Male			
12–15	7.38	64.59	28.04
16–19	10.23	64.92	24.86

perceptions of their overweight status than the other groups, who all overestimate their overweight status, especially Whites and Asians. Perceptions of underweight status are also overestimated by all race and ethnic groups. Among Whites, Asians, and Hispanics, almost a third of the girls who have BMIs in the normal range perceive that their weight is not normal.

Among boys, a larger percentage perceive themselves to be underweight than is actually the case, and this is especially true for Black boys. Such results confirm previous research on body image showing that girls tend to aspire to the cultural ideal of thinness as they are especially likely to perceive that they are overweight, with the exception of Black girls, who seem to be less sensitive to this ideal (Dawson, 1988; Duke 2002; Felts et al., 1992). Boys, on the other hand, aspire to muscular body images and tend, therefore, to perceive their weight to be too low more often than it actually is. In contrast, girls' and boys' perceptions of weight do not vary as much by age (not shown).

We also find that girls' tendencies to perceive their weight to be heavier than it is are more pronounced among older adolescents, suggesting that the cultural ideal of thinness increases in later adolescence for girls (not shown). The pattern for boys is relatively the same across age categories.

Table 6 shows the distribution of actual and perceived weight concordance for girls and boys by race/ethnicity and age. White, Hispanic, and Asian girls are more likely to think they are heavier than they are compared to Black girls, who are more likely to think they are lighter than they are. Asian girls express the lowest concordance, with especially high percentages thinking they are either heavier or lighter than they actually are. Boys generally think they are lighter than they are, especially Black boys. Similar to earlier age patterns, we see lower

Table 6. Distribution of Female and Male Adolescents' Concordance Between Actual and Perceived Weight, by Race/Ethnicity and Age (N = 12,966)

Category	% Thinks Lighter	% Thinks Same	% Thinks Heavier
By race/ethnicity			
Female			
Non-Hispanic White	8.47	69.21	22.32
Non-Hispanic Black	16.46	70.25	13.29
Hispanic	11.91	67.98	20.10
Asian	16.57	51.38	32.05
Male			
Non-Hispanic White	23.30	67.82	8.88
Non-Hispanic Black	29.70	65.23	5.08
Hispanic	24.91	64.35	10.75
Asian	23.87	66.50	9.62
By age			
Female			
12–15	11.44	70.49	18.07
16–19	8.93	65.57	25.50
Male			
12–15	23.99	68.03	7.98
16–19	25.18	65.51	9.31

concordance as adolescents age, with older girls more likely to think they are heavier than they are and older boys more likely to think they are lighter than they are. As an indicator of healthy body image, these concordance measures in Table 6 are probably the most illustrative and parsimonious.

We validate these healthy body image indicators by exploring their associations with dieting behavior for girls and with attempts to gain weight for boys (not shown). A strong linear relationship is observed for all race and ethnic groups and across adolescent age groups such that girls who think they are lighter than they are, are less likely to try to lose weight and girls who think they are heavier than they are, are more likely to try to lose weight than girls who perceive their weight correctly. Given that our earlier results show that girls tend to perceive themselves to be heavier than they actually are, such dieting behavior is not healthy. A linear relationship also emerges across race/ethnicity and age such that boys who think they are lighter than they are, are more likely to be trying to gain weight and boys who think they are heavier than they are, are less likely to be trying to gain weight compared to boys who perceive their weight correctly. The age pattern indicates that a muscular body image becomes more salient in later adolescence for boys.

Relationships among Healthy Habits Indicators

A final step in this exploratory work is an assessment of the extent to which these indicators are related to one another and are capturing an underlying

Table 7. Regression Coefficients Relating Each Healthy Habits Indicator in the Columns with Each Healthy Habits Indicator in the Rows (equations adjust for age and sex)

	Independent Variable			
Dependent Variable	5+ bouts of phy activ/week	2+ fruits and veggies/week	Fast food 2+ times/week	Hours of TV viewing/week
BMI (weight for height)	−.393**	−.23	−.48**	.024**
Hours of sleep	.02**	.01**	−.02**	.003
Sleep enough	.28**	.23**	−.13*	−.001
TV hours	−.86**	−2.80**	.86**	
Fruits and vegetables	.46**		−.15*	
Fast food	−.04	−.15*		
Unhealthy body image (thinks heavier than are)				
Females	−.09	−.08	−.13	
Males	−.32**	−.25	−.06	

Note: BMI and TV hours are estimated with linear regression; hours of sleep are estimated with poisson regression; sleep enough, fruit and vegetables, and fast food are estimated with logistic regression; body image is estimated with logistic regression on the sample of adolescents who think they are either heavier than their actual weight or the same as their actual weight, $N = 10,944$ boys and $N = 10,937$ girls (we drop those who think they are thinner than they actually are). Because some of our measures are only available at Wave II, we use the Wave II sample for all other regressions with an average N of 13,000.

concept of "healthy habits." If adolescents adopt healthy habits in general, then they should engage in healthy habits across the array of indicators that we have examined here, and adoption of one healthy habit should be correlated with adoption of other healthy habits. In Table 7 we show the degree and direction of the statistical association between the various healthy habits indicators we have employed in our analysis. We present results from a number of regression equations in which we regress the various healthy habits indicators on each other, adjusting for age and sex (with the exception of body image, in which we run separate male and female models). We display the regression coefficient for each equation as a measure of the degree of relatedness between the two habits. The size of the coefficients cannot be compared because the measurement scales of both the independent and dependent variables vary across indicators as do the estimation procedures. Because some of the indicators are only available at Wave II, we use the Wave II sample.

The results are reassuring as they show fairly consistent and significant associations among our healthy habits indicators in the expected directions. For example, results in the first row indicate that BMI is highly correlated with activity and inactivity. Adolescents who engage in 5 or more moderate to vigorous bouts of physical activity a week have a lower BMI. Similarly, inactive adolescents who watch more hours of TV tend to have higher BMIs than adolescents who watch less TV. Diets that frequently include fast food are related with lower BMIs, an unexpected result; but perhaps this reflects highly active adolescents with little time to eat. Healthy sleep habits (hours and reports that adolescents sleep enough) are associated with greater physical activity and healthy diets that include more fruits and vegetables and less fast food. In addition, adolescents who are physically active and have healthy diets tend to watch fewer hours of TV, and physically active adolescents eat more fruits and vegetables. For reasons that are unclear, having an unhealthy body image by perceiving one's weight to be heavier than it actually is, is correlated only with less exercise among boys (bottom two rows of Table 7).

Across the array of 19 associations among the healthy habits of exercise, diet, and sleep that we examine, 16 are statistically significant and in all but one (fast food and BMI), the relationship is in the expected direction. That is, engagement in a healthy habit in one domain is correlated with engagement in a healthy habit in another domain. Thus, we conclude that the indicators of healthy habits that we have developed here are highly interrelated and capture the same underlying concept of "healthy habits."

Discussion and Conclusions

These analyses of healthy habits suggest several effective and practical measures of healthy habits as indicators of positive youth development. Sleep hours as an indicator of sufficient sleep or sleepiness and sleep deprivation can be used to represent healthy sleep habits. Whether adolescents engage in the Surgeon General's recommended level of physical activity of 5 or more moderate to vigorous physical activities a week is our choice for a healthy exercise indicator. Hours of TV viewing is an effective proxy for inactivity among youth. Add Health does not really have the data to develop a healthy diet indicator, but the two we examined were clearly related to other healthy habits (Table 7) and therefore serve as useful proxies for healthy diet choices, with the frequency of consuming fruits and vegetables a better barometer of healthy habits than consumption of fast food. Finally, body image represents a unique healthy habits indicator that captures the various dimensions of healthy habits, including exercise, weight, and eating and dieting behavior, and blends in the psychological component of self-perception and self-image. The body image indicator we recommend is our measure of concordance between actual and perceived weight.

Our exploratory analysis and validation of indicators provided evidence in support of previous research on differentials in healthy habits by race/ethnicity and age. In particular, we find that Black adolescents, and especially Black girls, are particularly disadvantaged in their healthy habits. Blacks tend to sleep fewer hours a night (Black girls have the latest bedtime hour), have lower levels of physical activity, higher levels of inactivity watching TV, less healthy diets, especially Black girls, and tend to be more likely to be overweight. The one exception is that Blacks, and Black girls in particular, tend to have a healthier body image, which puts them at lower risk of eating disorders and depression.

Although we only use cross-sectional data, the age cohort trends seem to suggest that adolescent developmental trajectories in healthy habits are discouraging. As adolescents age they get less sleep, less exercise, make less healthy food choices, and tend to have less healthy body images. Maintaining the healthy habits that younger adolescents display remains an ambitious goal for parents and health policy workers alike, as adolescents carry these habits with them into the early formative educational and career years of young adulthood.

Our analysis indicated that our sleep, diet, and physical activity indicators are valid measures of the concept of healthy habits, and although we argue that an index of "healthy habits" does not make conceptual sense, these indicators are interrelated and capture an underlying dimension of healthy habits in adolescence. Future work needs to examine the statistical relationships between our healthy habits indicators and developmental outcomes for youth, analysis that is beyond the scope of the work presented here. It is possible that different healthy habits may be associated with different developmental outcomes.

Authors' Note

We are grateful to the National Institute of Child Health and Human Development for their support through grant P01 HD31921 as part of the Add Health project, a program project designed by J. Richard Udry (PI) and Peter Bearman, and funded by NICHD to the Carolina Population Center, University of North Carolina at Chapel Hill, with cooperative funding participation of 17 other federal agencies.

We also acknowledge support to Harris through the Family and Child Well-being Research Network, grant U01 HD37558, of the National Institute of Child Health and Human Development.

We thank Annie Latta for her assistance with the tables and Shannon Cavanagh for her thoughtful contributions on the background and analyses of body image.

References

Andersen, R. E., Crespo, C. H., Bartlett, S. J., Cheskin, L. J., & Pratt, M. (1998). Relationship of physical activity and television watching with body weight and level of fatness among children: Results from the Third National Health and Nutrition Examination Survey. *Journal of the American Medical Association, 279*, 938–942.

Andrade, M. M. M., Benedito-Silva, A. A., Domenice, E. E., Arnhold, I. J., & Menna-Barreto, L. (1993). Sleep characteristics of adolescents: A longitudinal study. *Journal of Adolescent Health, 14*, 401–406.

Averett, S., & Korenman, S. (1999). Black-white differences in social and economic consequences of obesity. *International Journal of Obesity and Related Metabolic Disorders, 23*(2), 166–173.

Bao, W., Srinivisan, S. R., Valdez, R., Greenlund, K. J., Wattigney, W. A., & Berenson, G. S. (1997). Longitudinal changes in cardiovascular risk from childhood to young adulthood in offspring of parents with coronary artery disease. *Journal of the American Medical Association, 278*, 1749–1754.

Bordo, Susan. (1999). *The male body: A new look at men in public and in private.* New York: Farrar, Straus & Giroux.

Bouchard, C. A., Shephard, R. J., & Stephens, T. (Eds.). (1993). *Physical activity, fitness, and health consensus statement* (27–29). Champaign, IL: Human Kinetics.

Bray, G. A., & Popkin, B. M. (1998). Dietary fat intake does affect obesity! *American Journal of Clinical Nutrition, 68*, 1157–1173.

Brumberg, J. J. (1997). *The Body Project: An intimate history of American girls*. New York: Random House.

Centers for Disease Control. (2002). BMI: Body mass index. BMI for children and teens. National Center for Chronic Disease Prevention and Health Promotion. Document available online at http://www.cdc.gov/nccdphp/dnpa/bmi/bmi-for-age.htm

Coble, P. A., Kupfer, D. J., Taska, L. S., & Kane, J. (1984). EEG sleep of normal healthy children. Part I. Findings using standard measurement methods. *Sleep, 7*, 289–303.

Dahl, R. E., & Carskadon, M. A. (1995). Sleep and its disorders in adolescence. In R. Ferber & M. Kryger (Eds.), *Principles and practice of sleep medicine in the child* (pp. 19–27). Philadelphia: Saunders.

Danner, F. (2000). Sleep deprivation and school performance. *Sleep, 23*, 255–256.

Danner, F., Hutchins, G., & Hooks, K. (2001). Adolescent sleep and school start times. *Sleep, 24*, A11.

Dawson, D. A. (1988). Ethnic differences in female overweight: Data from the 1985 National Health Interview Survey. *American Journal of Public Health, 78*, 1326–1329.

Dietz, W. H. (1996). The role of lifestyle in health: The epidemiology and consequences of inactivity. *Proceedings of the Nutrition Society, 55*, 829–840.

Duke, L. (2002). Get real! Cultural relevance and resistance to the mediated feminine ideal. *Psychology & Marketing, 19*, 211–233.

Epstein, L. H., Saelens, B. E., & O'Brien, J. G. (1995). Effects of reinforcing increases in active versus decreases in sedentary behavior in obese children. *International Journal of Behavioral Medicine, 2*, 41–50.

Felts, M., Tavasso, D., Chenier, T., & Dunn, P. (1992). Adolescents' perceptions of relative weight and self-reported weight loss activities. *Journal of School Health, 62*, 372–376.

Field, A. E., Camargo, C. A., Jr., Taylor, C. B., Berkey, C. S., Roberts, S. B., & Colditz, G. A. (2001). Peer, parent, and media influences on the development of weigh concerns and frequent dieting among preadolescent and adolescent girls and boys. *Pediatrics, 107*, 56–60.

Ge, Xiaojia, Elder, G. H., Jr., Regnerus, M., & Cox, C. (2001). Pubertal transitions, perceptions of being overweight, and adolescent psychological maladjustment: Gender and ethnic differences. *Social Psychology Quarterly, 64*, 363–375.

Gordon-Larsen, P., Harris, K. M., Ward, D. S., & Popkin, B. M. (2003). Exploring increasing overweight and its determinants among Hispanic and Asian immigrants to the US: The National Longitudinal Study of Adolescent Health. *Social Science and Medicine, 57*, 2023–2034.

Gordon-Larsen, P., McMurray, R. G., & Popkin, B. M. (1999). Adolescent physical activity and inactivity vary by ethnicity: The National Longitudinal Study of Adolescent Health. *Journal of Pediatrics, 135*, 301–306.

Gortmaker, S. L., Sobal, A. M., Peterson, K., Colditz, C. A., & Dietz, W. H. (1996). Television viewing as a cause of increasing obesity among children in the United States. *Archives of Pediatric and Adolescent Medicine, 150*, 536–562.

Guilleminault, C. (Ed.). (1987). *Sleep and its disorders in children*. New York: Raven Press.

Harris, K. M., Florey, F., Tabor, J. W., Bearman, P. S., Jones, J., & Udry, J. R. (2003). The National Longitudinal Study of Adolescent Health: Research Design (http://www.cpc.unc.edu/projects/addhealth/design.html).

Hauri, P., Percy, L., Olmstead, E., & Sateia, M. (1980). Childhood onset insomnia. *Sleep Research, 9*, 201.

Hulka, B. S., Liu, E. T., & Lininger, R. A. (1994). Steroid hormones and risk of breast cancer. *Cancer, 74*(Suppl. 3), 1111–1124.

Janz, K. F. (1994). Validation of the CSA accelerometer for assessing children's physical activity. *Medicine and Science in Sports and Exercise, 26*, 369–375.

Johnson, M. L., Burke, B. S., & Mayer, J. (1956). Relative importance of inactivity and overeating in the energy balance of obese high school girls. *American Journal of Clinical Nutrition, 4*, 37.

Kuczmarksi, R. J., Ogden, C. L., Guo, S. S., Grummer-Strawn, L. M., Flegal, K. M., Mei, Z., et al. (2000). *CDC growth charts: United States*. Advance data from vital and health statistics; no. 314. Retrieved October 15, 2001, from National Center for Health Statistics. Web site: http://www.cdc.gov/nchs/data/series/sr_11/sr11_246.pdf

Laberge, L., Petit, D., Simard, C., Vitaro, F., Tremblay, R. E., & Montplaisir, J. (2001). Development of sleep patterns in early adolescence. *Journal of Sleep Research, 10,* 59–67.

Lee, C., Blair, S., & Jackson, A. (1999). Cardiorespiratory fitness, body composition, and all-cause and cardiovascular disease mortality in men. *American Journal of Clinical Nutrition, 69,* 373–380.

Lovejoy, M. (2001). Disturbances in the social body: Differences in body image and eating problems among African American and White women. *Gender & Society, 15,* 239–261.

Manber, R., Pardee, R., Bootzin, R., Kuo, T., Rider, A., Rider, S., et al. (1995). Changing sleep patterns in adolescence. *Sleep Research, 24,* 106.

Martin, K. (1996). *Puberty, sexuality, and the self: Boys and girls at adolescence.* New York: Routledge.

Mathews, J. E., & Freedson, P. S. (1995). Field trial of a three-dimensional activity monitor: Comparison with self report. *Medicine and Science in Sports and Exercise, 27,* 1071–1078.

Matsudo, V. K. R. (1996). Measuring nutrition status, physical activity, and fitness, with special emphasis on populations at nutritional risk. *Nutrition Reviews, 54,* S79–S96.

Milkie, M. A. (1999). Social comparisons, reflected appraisals, and mass media: The impact of pervasive beauty images on Black and White girls' self-concepts. *Social Psychology Quarterly, 62,* 190–210.

Morrison, D., McGee, R., & Stanton, W. R. (1992). Sleep problems in adolescence. *Journal of the American Academy of Child and Adolescent Psychiatry, 31,* 94–99.

Must, A., Jacques, P. F., Dallal, G. E., Bajema, C. J., Dietz, W. H. (1992). Long-term morbidity and mortality of overweight adolescents: A follow-up of the Harvard Growth Study of 1922 to 1935. *New England Journal of Medicine, 327,* 1350–1355.

National Institutes of Health. (1987). Consensus Development Conference on Diet and Exercise in Non-Insulin-Dependent Diabetes Mellitus. *Diabetes Care, 10,* 639–644.

National Institutes of Health. (1995). Physical activity and cardiovascular health. NIH Consensus Statement Online, December 18–20, 1–33.

Obarzanek, E., Schreiber, G. B., Crawford, P.B., Goldman, S.R., Barrier, P.M., & Frederick, M.M. (1994). Energy intake and physical activity in relation to indexes of body fat: The National Heart, Lung, and Blood Institute Growth and Health Study. *American Journal of Clinical Nutrition, 60,* 15–22.

Pereira, M. A., FitzGerald, S. J., Gregg, E. W., Joswiak, M. L., Ryan, W. J., Suminski, R. R., et al. (1997). A collection of physical activity questionnaires for health-related research. *Medicine and Science in Sports and Exercise, 29,* S1–S205.

Petersen, A., Taylor, B. (1980). The biological approach to adolescence. In J. Adelson (Ed.), *Handbook of Adolescent Psychology* (pp. 117–158). New York: Wiley and Sons.

Petta, D., Carskadon, M., & Dement, W. (1984). Sleep habits in children aged 7–13 years. *Sleep Research, 13,* 86.

Pinhas-Hamiel, O., & Zeitler, P. (1996). Insulin resistance, obesity, and related disorders among black adolescents. *Journal of Pediatrics, 129,* 319–321.

Popkin, B. M., & Udry, J. R. (1998). Adolescent obesity increases significantly in second and third generation U.S. immigrants: The National Longitudinal Study of Adolescent Health. *Journal of Nutrition, 128,* 701–706.

Raitakari, O. T., Porkka, K. V. K., Taimela, S., Telama, R., Rasanen, L., & Viikari, J. S. A. (1994). Effects of persistent physical activity and inactivity on coronary risk factors in children and young adults: The Cardiovascular Risk in Young Finns Study. *American Journal of Epidemiology, 140,* 195–205.

Rand, C. S. W., & Kuldau, J. M. (1990). The epidemiology of obesity and self-defined weight problem in the general population: Gender, race, age, and social class. *International Journal of Eating Disorders, 9,* 329–343.

Ross, C. E., & Hayes, D. E. (1988). Exercise and psychologic well-being in the community. *American Journal of Epidemiology, 127,* 762–771.

Sallis, J. F., Zakarian, J. M., Hovell, M. F., & Hofstetter, C. R. (1996). Ethnic, socioeconomic, and sex differences in physical activity among adolescents. *Journal of Clinical Epidemiology, 49,* 125–134.

Serdula, M. K., Ivery, D., Coates, J. R., Freedman, D. S., Williamson, D. F., & Byers, T. (1993). Do obese children become obese adults? A review of the literature. *Preventive Medicine, 22,* 167–177.

Shah, M., & Jequier, R.W. (1991). Is obesity due to overeating and inactivity, or to a defective metabolic rate? A review. *Annals of Behavioral Medicine, 13,* 73–81.

Siegel, J. M., Yancey, A. K., Aneshensel, C. S., & Schuler, R. (1999). Body image, pubertal timing, and adolescent mental health. *Journal of Adolescent Health, 25,* 155–165.

Siervogel, R. M., Roche, A. F., Guo, S. M., Mukherjee, D., & Chumlea, W. C. (1991). Patterns of change in weight/stature from 2 to 18 years: Findings from long-term serial data for children in the Fels Longitudinal Growth Study. *International Journal of Obesity, 15,* 479–485.

Story, M., French, S. A., Resnick, M. D., & Blum, R. W. (1995). Ethnic/racial and socioeconomic differences in dieting behaviors and body image perceptions in adolescents. *International Journal of Eating Disorders, 18,* 173–179.

U.S. Department of Health and Human Services. (1996). *Physical activity and health: A report of the Surgeon General.* Atlanta, GA: U.S. Department of Health and Human Services, Centers for Disease Control and Prevention, National Center for Chronic Disease Prevention and Health Promotion.

Wolf, A. M., Gortmaker, S. L., Cheung, L., Gray, H. M., Herzog, D. B., & Colditz, C. A. (1993). Activity, inactivity, and obesity: Racial, ethnic, and age differences among schoolgirls. *American Journal of Public Health, 83,* 1625–1627.

Wolfson, A. R. (1996). Sleeping patterns of children and adolescents. *Child and Adolescent Psychiatric Clinics of North America, 5,* 549–568.

Wolfson, A., & Carskadon, M. (1998). Sleep schedules and daytime functioning in adolescents. *Child Development, 69,* 875–887.

9 Adolescent Participation in Organized Activities

Bonnie L. Barber and Margaret R. Stone

University of Arizona

Jacquelynne S. Eccles

University of Michigan

There is good evidence that participating in school and community-based activities is associated with both short- and long-term indicators of positive development (e.g., Barber, Eccles, & Stone, 2001; Eccles & Gootman, 2002; Eccles & Templeton, in press; Larson, 2000; Mahoney & Cairns, 1997; Roth, Brooks-Gunn, Murray, & Foster, 1998; Youniss & Yates, 1997). Sociological research has documented a link between adolescents' extracurricular activities and adult educational attainment, occupation, and income (Otto, 1975, 1976; Otto & Alwin, 1977). Participation in organized activities is also positively related to achievement, educational aspirations, self-esteem, ability to overcome adversity, active participation in the political process and volunteer activities, leadership qualities, and physical health (e.g., Barber et al., 2001; Holland & Andre, 1987; Marsh & Kleitman, 2002; Scales, Benson, Leffert, & Blyth, 2000; Youniss, Yates, & Su, 1997).

There has been far less developmental research on constructive leisure activities than on other contexts such as family and school (Kleiber, 1999), but some progress has been made in understanding the mechanisms whereby constructive organized activities facilitate healthy development. First, they provide a developmental forum for initiative and engagement in challenging tasks, and allow participants to express their talents, passion, and creativity (Csikszentmihalyi, 1991; Klieber, 1999; Larson, 2000). Second, organized activities help adolescents meet their need for social relatedness, providing a broad range of opportunities for social development (Fletcher & Shaw, 2000; Youniss et al., 1997). Third, participation may also promote the development of assets such as social, physical, and intellectual skills, meaningful roles and empowerment, positive identity, constructive peer networks, and clear expectations and boundaries (e.g., Eccles & Barber, 1999; Marsh & Kleitman, 2002, 2003; Perkins, Borden, & Villarruel, 2001).

Activity Participation, Social Identity, and Peer Group

To explain the connection between activities and positive development, we have proposed a synergistic system connecting activity involvement with peer group composition and identity exploration (Barber, Stone, Hunt, & Eccles, in press; Eccles & Barber, 1999). Specifically, we believe that enhanced outcomes result for adolescents who experience a confluence of activity participation, activity-based identity adoption, and a benign peer context. Previous research, including our own, has demonstrated the pervasive connections between each of these three factors and numerous outcomes.

The activities adolescents choose can reflect core aspects of their self-beliefs. Therefore, voluntary participation in discretionary extracurricular activities provides an opportunity for adolescents to be personally expressive and to communicate to both themselves and others that "this is who I am" or "this is what I believe I am meant to do." In addition, extracurricular activity settings provide the opportunity to enhance identification with the values and goals of the school (Barber et al., in press; Marsh, 1992; Marsh & Kleitman, 2003).

Activities also help structure one's peer group: Adolescents in extracurricular activities have more academic friends and fewer friends who skip school and use drugs than adolescents who do not participate in activities (Eccles & Barber, 1999). In turn, having more academic and less risky friends predicts other positive outcomes for adolescents. Conversely, being part of a peer network that includes a high proportion of youth who engage in, and encourage, risky behaviors predicts increased involvement in risky behaviors and decreased odds of completing high school and going on to college. Some activities facilitate membership in positive peer networks; others facilitate membership in more problematic peer networks (Dishion, Poulin, & Burraston, 2001). The critical mediating role of peer affiliations in the link between extracurricular activities and youth outcomes has also been documented by Eder and Parker (1987), Kinney (1993), and Youniss, McLellan, Su, and Yates (1999).

Measures of Activity Involvement

Participation in school and community activities can be measured in a number of ways. Mahoney (Mahoney, 2000; Mahoney & Cairns, 1997) has used the approach of coding participation from school yearbook information available for the participants in his local area study. He uses the photographs of participants in extracurricular activities, and a record of student names and positions of status within the activity. Yearbook activity photos overlapped closely with lists provided by school personnel. Mahoney has categorized activities into nine domains (academics, athletics, fine arts, student government, service, press activities, school assistants, vocational activities, and royalty activities). In his analyses, rather than focus on type of activity, Mahoney generally uses information about number of activities, or a categorical variable reflecting any activity involvement contrasted with no involvement (Mahoney, 2000; Mahoney & Cairns, 1997). Although this method seems useful, noninvasive, and valid, it is restricted to local area studies that have access to yearbooks and administrators.

Marsh and colleagues have used large national samples (e.g., the National Education Longitudinal Study) to test several models of the function of extracurricular activities (Marsh, 1992; Marsh & Kleitman, 2002, 2003). In one study (see Marsh & Kleitman, 2002), three measures were employed to reflect the number of school-based activities undertaken and the time spent overall on such participation in 10th and 12th grade, and two to represent the level of participation in structured and unstructured activities outside of school. Summary indices were also created to reflect overall involvement.

In this chapter we report on our use of survey questions to assess activity participation in a local study. We also report information on concurrent and predictive validity of the measure.

Study Design and Sample

The measures of constructive organized activity involvement come from the Michigan Study of Adolescent Life Transitions (MSALT). This is a longitudinal study that began with a cohort of 6th graders drawn from 10 school districts in southeastern Michigan in 1983. The majority of the sample is White and comes from working- and middle-class families living in primarily middle-class communities based in small industrial cities around Detroit. We have followed approximately 1,800 of these youth through nine waves of data collection: two while they were in the 6th grade (1983–1984); two while they were in the 7th grade (1984–85); one while they were in the 10th grade (spring 1988); one while they were in the 12th grade (spring 1990); one in 1992–1993, when most were 21–22 years old; one in 1996–1997, when most were 25–26; and one in 2000–2002, when most were 29–30. The validity analyses presented here include 1,425 respondents (759 females and 666 males) who participated in the 10th-grade survey.

Approximately 88% of the participants were European American; 8%, African American; 1%, Asian American; 1%, Latino; 1%, Native American; and 1%, other, including mixed-race individuals. We included mother's report of her education as one measure of family socioeconomic status using a 4-point ordinal scale with 1 = *less than high school diploma* (11%), 2 = *high school diploma* (43%), 3 = *some college* (27%), and 4 = *bachelor's degree or more* (19%).

Approximately 6% of participants came from families with incomes of less than $10,000 in 1983; 12% with $10,000 to $20,000; 44% between $20,000 and $40,000; and 38%, $40,000 and more. Approximately 71% of participants lived with two biological parents, 13% with a parent and stepparent, and 16% with a single biological parent. Nearly 10% of participants (49 females and 76 males) had been rated by their teachers in sixth grade as suffering from a limiting physical, mental, or emotional condition.

Survey and school record data from approximately 900 MSALT participants were used for longitudinal analyses discussed in this report. Activity data were collected at 10th grade (Wave 5) when participants were approximately 16 years old. Prospective outcomes are discussed for 12th grade (Wave 6), and 2 years (Wave 7), 6 years (Wave 8), and 10 years (Wave 9) after high school graduation. Some of these results have been previously reported (Barber et al., 2001; Barber et al., in press; Eccles & Barber; 1999).

Measures of Activity Participation

Activity Involvement

At 10th grade, adolescents were provided with a list of 16 sports and 30 school and community clubs and organizations and asked to check all activities in which they participated (see the Appendix). To measure sports participation, we asked: "Do you compete in any of the following school teams (varsity, junior varsity, or other organized school program) *outside of PE*?" Cheerleading, though listed in both the sports section of the measure and the activities section, is coded as a "School Involvement" activity and not as a sport. To measure participation in nonsport activities, we asked: "Do you participate in any of the following activities or clubs at school?" We also asked about a range of activities outside of school: "Do you participate in any of the following clubs or activities outside of school?" This measure was created for the survey by the research team based on their previous research in schools. It was refined through pilot testing with local high school students.

Analyses of the Measure

Distribution of Responses

The Appendix summarizes the distribution of participation in school and community activities by gender. We computed a total number of activities by summing all the in-school and out-of-school clubs and activities that were checked. On average, these adolescents participated in between one and two activities and/or clubs. Girls participated at higher rates than boys, and 31% of the sample did not participate in any activities or clubs. Because sports were so common, we aggregated them separately by summing the different teams checked. Not surprisingly, boys participated on more different teams than girls. However, 45% of the sample had not competed on any school athletic team. Finally, we calculated the breadth of the adolescents' participation by summing the number of different types of activities (art, performing art, religious, leadership, sports, academic, service) for each adolescent (participation in several different sports [or several different performing arts] only counted as one type of activity). Girls also participated in a wider range of activities than boys (Eccles & Barber, 1999).

Missing Data and Subgroup Usage

Data regarding individual activities items were missing for approximately 10% of the sample. We attribute the missing data largely to the length of time allowed by schools for the completion of the survey and to differential reading ability. The items regarding activities were on pages 34–36 of a 51-page survey. Those who completed the survey did not differ from those who did in terms of sex, family income, family structure, and maternal education. However, there was a higher rate of missing data for disabled participants. Specifically, individuals with mental and emotional disabilities, as rated by teachers in junior high school, were less likely to provide data regarding activities than were those not so identified by teachers. Individuals with physical disabilities, on the other hand, provided data at the same rate as those not identified by teachers as having a physical disability.

Shortened Version

In Grade 12, sports participation was assessed by asking participants, "Do you compete in any school teams (varsity, junior varsity, or other organized school program) *outside of PE*?" Nonsport extracurricular involvement was assessed with the question, "Do you participate in any activities or clubs at school or outside of school?" Responses to these questions were coded using the number of teams or clubs listed by the participant, and the types (team vs. individual, male-typed vs. female-typed) of sports and activities. The 1,008 responses for sports were as follows: 567 did not compete in any sports; 245 listed one; 146 listed two; 42 listed three; 4 listed four; 3 listed five; and 1 listed six sports. For the 999 who responded to the activities question, 509 were not involved; 231 listed one; 146 listed two; 40 listed three; 44 listed four; 14 listed five; and 15 listed six or more activities. The difficulty with this format is coding the data after the open-ended responses are collected. Important information can be lost if too much collapsing is done during coding, and handwriting can be difficult to understand, particularly for less common types of clubs.

In the area of sports participation, we have done some comparisons with time use data that suggest we need both types of information. Students were asked, "About how many hours do you usually spend each week taking part in an organized sport?" Responses ranged from 0 = *none* to 7 = *21 or more hours per week*. Although the cross-tabulations for this variable and the sports question listed in the previous paragraph are distributed generally in ways one would have predicted (athletes spend more time taking part in organized sport each week), there are some cells that are interesting. For example, 16% of those who report no time spent on sports say they are on at least one sports team at school. We see this not as a validity problem but rather as important information: Those who play on fall teams may not spend time in the spring playing organized sports. Therefore, although time use may be an important indicator in some ways, we argue that the membership on a team may have impact even in the absence of current time spent practicing (through connection to adults at school, peer group, identity, and attachment to school).

Having used both checklists stipulating each sport and activity and general questions about sports and activities, with a follow-up question requiring students to list their activities, we prefer the former. Coding is simplified in this strategy, and there is less risk for students to give information only about the activities in which they *currently* participate. We believe, for instance, that students may miss reporting on football if they fill out the survey in spring.

Data Reduction

In order to understand patterns related to participation in various types of activities, we grouped the extracurricular activities into five categories: *prosocial activities*—church attendance and/or participation in volunteer and community service activities; *team sports*—participation on one or more school teams; *performing arts*—participation in school band, drama, and/or dance; *school involvement*—participation in student government, pep club, and/or cheerleading; and *academic clubs*—participation in debate, foreign language, math, or chess clubs, science fair, or tutoring in academic subjects.

Participants were coded as participating if they had checked off at least one activity or club within the broad category. The distribution of females and males in these activity types is included in the Appendix, as are the activities coded in each category. Consistent with results reported above, the males were more likely to engage in at least one sport activity than females. In contrast, females were significantly more likely to be involved in prosocial, performing arts, and school involvement activities (see Table 1).

We also assessed whether mother's education was related to participation in any of these five general categories. Both academic club participation and

Table 1. Participation in General Activity Types, by Gender

Type	Examples	% Females	% Males
Performing arts	School band, drama, dance	43	21
Team sports	School sport teams, except cheerleading	46	67
Academic clubs	Debate, foreign language, math, and chess clubs, science fair, tutoring in academic subjects	16	11
School involvement	Student government, pep club, cheerleading	23	8
Prosocial activities	Church attendance, volunteer and community service	27	16

prosocial activity involvement were significantly related to maternal education: Adolescents with mothers having a college degree or higher were more than twice as likely to be involved in academic clubs and prosocial activities as adolescents with mother having a high school degree or less. Similar trends were evident for both team sports and performing arts. These differences in maternal education, and the expected links of maternal education with many of the variables used to examine validity, lead us to include maternal education as a covariate in our analyses.

Construct Validity of the Measure

Our measure of activities correlates well with our measures of identity, characteristics of peer groups, and relevant measures of values and abilities.

Identity Categories

The Breakfast Club (Hughes, 1985) was a prominent film when our study participants were in the 10th grade. We asked the participants to indicate which of five characters (the Princess, the Jock, the Brain, the Basketcase, or the Criminal) was most like them. Twenty-eight percent selected the Jock identity, 40% the Princess, 12% the Brain, 11% the Basketcase, and 9% the Criminal.

We examined the extent to which adolescents in each particular activity identified one as a member of a social identity category. For this question, we analyzed the proportion of students in each sport or organization that claimed each social identity. A series of chi-squared analyses revealed that social identities were differentially distributed across sports and activities (Barber et al., in press). Not all athletes saw themselves as Jocks, especially among female athletes. The highest proportion of female athletes who considered themselves to be Jocks played basketball, softball, soccer, volleyball, and track. However, female athletes also often self-identified as Princesses (especially gymnasts and swimmers) rather than Jocks. The vast majority of cheerleaders saw themselves as Princesses rather than Jocks, lending support to our decision to exclude cheerleading from the sports composite. Overall, 22% of female athletes considered themselves to be Jocks, which is substantially higher than in the general female population (13%).

Sixty-nine percent of the male athletes self-identified as Jocks; this was especially true for those who played basketball, football, baseball, ice hockey, and wrestling. These five sports also had the fewest participants who self-identified as Brains. Overall, male athletes were unlikely to label themselves as Brains (14% of athletes compared to 20% of all males).

Although the distribution of the five identity groups across the nonsport activities was less extreme, the patterns were what one would expect (Barber et al., in press). Among the females, the Princesses were overrepresented in pep club and dance; the Brains were overrepresented in the band and orchestra and underrepresented in dance. Among the males, the Brains were overrepresented in foreign language clubs, math and science clubs, and band or orchestra; the Basketcases and Princesses were overrepresented in drama. Although few males self-identified as Princesses, the male Princesses were also overrepresented in dance, foreign language club, and band.

We think these data indicate important variability across activities and sports. Not all extracurricular involvement is equal. In fact, even within the category of sports, the teams seem to vary considerably from each other in the types of students who participate and in the meanings attached to team membership. These differences are reflected in the identities of participants. Therefore, we should expect differences in the benefits and risks that may accompany different activities. It is because of this variability that we recommend collecting very specific data about activities, not just counts of the total number of activities or general time use. Our question can certainly be collapsed into subcategories, but if the details are not collected, the more precise information will be unavailable.

Concurrent Prediction to Peer Group

Activity settings provide a peer group as well as a set of tasks. To the extent that one spends a lot of time in these activity settings with the other participants, it is likely that one's friends will be drawn from among the other participants. We have examined characteristics of the peer group for those who participated in the different types of activities (Eccles & Barber, 1999). At 10th grade, the peer group characteristics were consistent with the kinds of associates we expected in the different activity types. The peer groups for participants were generally characterized by a higher proportion of friends who planned to attend college and were doing well in school than were peer groups for nonparticipants. Adolescents involved in prosocial activities had fewer friends who used alcohol and drugs than their peers; they also had few friends who skipped school. Finally, consistent with the association of sports participation with increased drinking (Eccles & Barber, 1999), adolescents who participated in team sports had a higher proportion of friends who drank than those who did not participate in team sports.

Concurrent Prediction to Self-Concept and Task Value

Participation in team sports, as one would expect, was associated with higher levels of both self-concept of sports ability and task value for sports, after controlling for gender and ethnicity. Those who participated in team sports had a significantly higher self-concept of sports ability than nonparticipants, $F(1, 1248) = 306.84$, $p < .001$, Ms = 5.1 and 3.8, respectively. Athletes valued sports more highly as well, $F(1, 1248) = 409.83$, $p < .001$, Ms = 5.8 and 4.0, respectively. Interestingly, participants in school involvement activities also valued sports more highly than nonparticipants, $F(1, 1238) = 12.292$, $p < .001$, Ms = 5.4 and 4.9, respectively, and had a higher self-concept of sports ability, $F(1, 1238) = 7.330$, $p < .01$, Ms = 4.8 and 4.5, respectively. Follow-up analysis indicated that this effect held for boys but not girls. No other activity type predicted to higher self-concept or valuing of sports. However, performing arts participation predicted to a *lower* self-concept of sports ability, $F(1, 1246) = 7.417$, $p < .01$, Ms $= 4.4$ and 4.6, respectively, and lower valuing of sports, $F(1, 1246) = 8.669$, $p < .01$, Ms $= 4.8$ and 5.1, respectively. Follow-up analysis indicated that this effect also held only for boys. Clearly, achievement-related beliefs differ among activity types, suggesting the importance of maintaining distinctions.

Predictive Validity: High School Outcomes

In this section, we report on our previously published findings on the relation between 10th-grade extracurricular activity involvement and later psychological and behavioral outcomes (from Eccles & Barber, 1999). We examine whether specific types of extracurricular activities are more beneficial or risky than others.

Prosocial Activity Involvement

Adolescents involved in prosocial activities in 10th grade reported less alcohol and drug use; this difference was especially marked at grade 12, 2 years after the activity data were collected. Regression analyses indicated that the students who were involved in activities like attending religious services and doing volunteer work showed less of an increase in these risky behaviors over the high school years than their noninvolved peers, indicating that prosocial involvement can be a protective factor with regard to the usual age-related increases in these risky behaviors. Involvement in prosocial activities at grade 10 was also positively related to both liking school in the 10th grade and a higher GPA at the 12th grade.

Team Sports

Involvement in team sports at grade 10 predicted higher rates of drinking alcohol at grade 12. Involvement in team sports also served as a protective condition for academic outcomes. Sport participants liked school more in the 10th and 12th grades, and had higher 12th-grade GPAs than nonparticipants.

Performing Arts

Those adolescents who were involved in performing arts at grade 10 were less frequently engaged in risky behaviors at both grade 10 and 12 than those who were not. This was particularly true for alcohol-related behaviors. However, when we controlled for prior levels of drinking in longitudinal regression analyses, we found no evidence that 10th-grade involvement in performing arts affected the direction or magnitude of change in drinking behavior over the high school years. Participation in performing arts was also related to greater liking of school at both 10th and 12th grades and to higher 12th-grade GPA.

School-Involvement Activities

Participation in school-spirit and student government related clubs was not related consistently to engagement in risky behaviors. In contrast, it was positively related to liking school at grade 10 and to 12th-grade GPA.

Academic Clubs

Participation in academic clubs was primarily related to academic outcomes. Adolescents who participated in academic clubs had higher than expected high school GPAs than those who did not, even after controlling for aptitude and maternal education.

Longitudinal Analyses: Prediction to Outcomes in Young Adulthood

Our measure of activities relates to numerous positive long-term outcomes. For these analyses, some of which have been previously reported in Barber et al. (2001), we have also used the five activity type categories rather than specific individual activities. We examined the association between grade 10 activity involvement and subsequent (Wave 8 and/or Wave 9) young adult educational and occupational attainment, civic engagement, and psychological well-being. Analyses of covariance (ANCOVAs) were used with activity involvement and gender as predictors, and with mother's education (and high school math and verbal aptitude when applicable) as covariates.

Educational Attainment

Participation in all five of the activity types was positively related to completing more *years of education*; however, participation in prosocial activities was not a significant predictor once maternal education and aptitude score covariates were added. Logistic regressions examining the effects of participation net of gender, ethnicity, maternal education, and academic ability, indicated that *college graduation* (by age 25) was significantly related to participation in sports (Wald $\chi^2 = 6.655$, $p < .05$), school involvement activities (Wald $\chi^2 = 5.059$, $p < .05$), and academic clubs (Wald $\chi^2 = 8.251$, $p < .01$). Rates for college completion were consistently higher for participants than for nonparticipants: for team sports, 39% versus 30%; for school involvement, 47% versus 32%; and for academic clubs, 56% versus 31%.

Occupational Outcomes

Sports participation was positively related to reporting having more job autonomy at age 24 (after controlling for gender, ethnicity, and maternal education). Similarly, sports predicted greater likelihood of having a job with a future, rather than a short-term job, at age 24 (Barber et al., 2001). Having jobs with higher Socioeconomic Index (SEI) scores (after controlling for gender, ethnicity, maternal education, and academic ability) was predicted by 10th-grade school involvement activity participation 12 years later at Wave 9, $F(1, 335) = 4.704$, $p < .05$; $Ms = 62.55$ for participants and 57.61 for nonparticipants. Having participated in a sport was also related at the trend level, $F(1, 337) = 3.656$, $p < .06$; $Ms = 60.40$ for sports participants and 56.74 for nonparticipants.

Civic Engagement

After controlling for gender, maternal education, and ethnicity, 10th-grade prosocial activity participation predicted to increased involvement in volunteer work, $F(1, 645) = 22.00$, $p < .001$; $Ms = 1.7$ for participants and 1.2 for nonparticipants, and civic organizations, $F(1, 644) = 4.14$, $p < .05$; $Ms = 1.6$ for participants and 1.4 for nonparticipants, at age 25–26. At age 29–30, 10th-grade prosocial activity participation continued to predict increased involvement in volunteer work, $F(1, 489) = 3.58$, $p < .06$; $Ms = 1.5$ for prosocial activity participants and 1.3 for nonparticipants.

Psychological Adjustment

Repeated measures MANOVA's with a four-level time component (Waves 5, 6, 7, and 8) nested within person were run for psychological well-being and are reported in detail elsewhere (Barber et al., 2001). Two main effects emerged for activities: athletes reported lower isolation ($M = 3.0$) than nonathletes ($M = 3.2$); and participants in prosocial activities reported higher self-esteem ($M = 5.0$) than did nonparticipants ($M = 4.8$). Suicide attempts at Wave 8 were associated with participation in performing arts ($\chi^2 = 3.89$, $p < .05$): 11% for participants, 6% for nonparticipants. Performing arts participants were also significantly more likely to report having visited a psychologist ($\chi^2 = 15.16$, $p < .001$): 22% for participants versus 11% for nonparticipants.

Recommendations

We have found that our measure of activity participation at grade 10 is related to identity, peer group composition, and to achievement-related values. It is also an important predictor of alcohol use, GPA, educational and occupational attainment, civic engagement, and psychological adjustment. Based on our work with these items, we suggest it is best to have a checklist of sports and activities, because the detailed information on specific activities is differentially predictive of a broad set of outcomes.

Collapsing into such activity types as prosocial, sports, and academic clubs illustrates one fruitful use of these types of questions. We have also tried other combinations of these items. The *total number of clubs and activities* predicted greater attachment to school, higher 11th-grade GPA, increased likelihood of college attendance, lower rates of getting drunk in 12th grade, and less frequent use of marijuana in 12th grade (regressions controlling for verbal and math ability, maternal education and gender; Barber & Eccles, 1997). The last two regressions also controlled for the 10th-grade level of the risk behavior, and thus indicated that participation in more activities predicted a smaller increase than average in substance use from 10th to 12th grade. What is important to note is that being in more than one activity is related to better outcomes than being in only one (which is better than being in none), so that a simple question about activity involvement that did not tap the total number would miss such a connection. The *number of sports teams* also predicted increased likelihood of college attendance and 11th-grade GPA. This is consistent with Marsh and Kleitman's (2003) evidence that increasing levels of athletic participation are associated with increasing benefits.

Another way to use these items is to construct an index of breadth, or eclectic participation. We found that the extent of participation across a *broad range* of activity domains (number of different types of activities) such as music, art, sports, leadership, and community service predicted greater school attachment, higher GPA, and greater likelihood of college attendance, even after controlling for academic aptitude (Barber & Eccles, 1997). Greater breadth, or eclectic participation, was better than participation in only one domain, which in turn was better than none.

Finally, given the interesting relation we find between sports and drinking, we think it is important to keep sports separate from other activities. In fact, in some of our current work we are finding that among sports, there is also variability in links to academic outcomes and substance use (Eccles, Barber, Stone, & Hunt, 2003), so it is advantageous to know which sport the adolescent plays. Our bottom line is that detailed information about participation is desirable, and in checklist format it does not take prohibitively long to collect.

Appendix

MSALT Questions on Participation in School Sport, Organization, and Club Activities (Participation rates for females and males are in parentheses.)

Answer the following questions about the current school year.

Do you (did you) compete in any of the following *school teams* (varsity, junior varsity, or other organized school program) outside of physical education? (Check all that apply)

___ Baseball (46%, 67%)   ___ Soccer (4%, 8%)
___ Basketball (11%, 25%)   ___ Softball (17%, 3%)
___ Cheerleading (12%, 0%)   ___ Swimming/Diving (12%, 13%)
___ Field hockey (1%, 2%)   ___ Tennis (9%, 8%)
___ Football (3%, 32%)   ___ Track/Cross country (12%, 16%)
___ Golf (1%, 9%)   ___ Volleyball (17%, 5%)
___ Gymnastics (5%, 1%)   ___ Wrestling (1%, 16%)
___ Ice hockey (1%, 9%)
___ Other (Please Specify)_____

Which of the following activities or clubs *at school* do you (did you) do in this school year? (Check all that apply)

___ Art (9%, 8%)

___ Band or orchestra (19%, 14%)

___ Career-related club (3%, 2%)

___ Chess club (0%, 1%)

___ Computer club (1%, 2%)

___ Dance (14%, 5%)

___ Pep club/Cheerleading/Boosters (12%, 3%)

___ ROTC (0%, 3%)

___ S.A.D.D. (10%, 3%)

___ Science fair (11%, 5%)

___ Service clubs (3%, 2%)

___ Other (Please Specify) _____

___ Debate club/Forensics (1%, 1%)

___ Drama (13%, 6%)

___ Foreign language club (13%, 5%)

___ Gaming club (D&D) (0%, 3%)

___ Math club (0%, 1%)

___ Peer counseling (4%, 1%)

___ Sports clubs (13%, 26%)

___ Student government (11%, 5%)

___ Tutoring in math, science, or computers (2%, 2%)

___ Tutoring in other academic subjects (1%, 1%)

Do you (Did you) participate in any of the following clubs or activities *outside of school*? (Check all that apply)

___ Athletic/recreational club (16%, 28%)

___ Scouts/Girls, Boys Clubs/Ys (2%, 5%)

___ Junior Achievement (1%, 2%)

___ Church groups (18%, 11%)

Other (Please Specify)_____

___ Pop or rock band (6%, 9%)

___ 4-H (4%, 2%)

___ Political campaign (0%, 1%)

___ Volunteer/service work (14%, 5%)

References

Barber, B. L., & Eccles, J. S. (1997, April). *Student council, volunteering, basketball, or marching band: What kind of extracurricular involvement matters?* Paper presented at the biennial meeting of the Society for Research on Child Development, Washington, DC.

Barber, B. L., Eccles, J. S., & Stone, M. R. (2001). Whatever happened to the Jock, the Brain, and the Princess? Young adult pathways linked to adolescent activity involvement and social identity. *Journal of Adolescent Research, 16*, 429–455.

Barber, B. L., Stone, M. R., Hunt, J., & Eccles, J. S. (in press). Benefits of activity participation: The roles of identity affirmation and peer group norm sharing. In J. L. Mahoney, R. W. Larson, & J. S. Eccles (Eds.), *Organized activities as contexts of development: Extracurricular activities, after-school and community programs.* Mahwah, NJ: Lawrence Erlbaum.

Csikszentmihalyi, M. (1991). "An investment theory of creativity and its development": Commentary. *Human Development, 34*(1), 32–34.

Dishion, T. J., Poulin, F., & Burraston, B. (2001). Peer group dynamics associated with iatrogenic effects in group interventions with high-risk young adolescents. In D. W. Nangle & C. A. Erdley (Eds.), *The role of friendship in psychological adjustment* (pp. 79–92), San Francisco: Jossey-Bass/Pfeiffer.

Eccles, J. S., & Barber, B. L. (1999). Student council, volunteering, basketball, or marching band: What kind of extracurricular involvement matters? *Journal of Adolescent Research, 14*, 10–43.

Eccles, J. S., Barber, B. L., Stone, M. R., & Hunt, J. (2003). Extracurricular activities and adolescent development. *Journal of Social Issues, 59*, 865–889.

Eccles, J. S., & Gootman, J. A. (Eds.). (2002). *Community programs to promote youth development.* Washington, DC: National Academy Press.

Eccles, J. S., & Templeton, J. (in press). Extracurricular and other after-school activities for youth. *Review of Research in Education.*

Eder, D., & Parker, S. (1987). The cultural production and reproduction of gender: The effect of extracurricular activities on peer-group culture. *Sociology of Education, 60*(3), 200–213.

Fletcher, A. C. & Shaw, R. A. (2000). Sex differences in associations between parental behaviors and characteristics and adolescent social integration. *Social Development, 9*(2), 133–148.

Holland, A., & Andre, T. (1987). Participation in extracurricular activities in secondary school: What is known, what needs to be known? *Review of Educational Research, 57*, 437–466.

Hughes, J. (Director). (1985). *The Breakfast Club* [Motion picture]. United States: Universal Studios.

Kinney, D. A. (1993). From nerds to normals: The recovery of identity among adolescents from middle school to high school. *Sociology of Education, 66*(1), 21–40.

Kleiber, D. (1999). *Leisure experience and human development: A dialectical approach.* New York: Basic Books.

Larson, R. W. (2000). Toward a psychology of positive youth development. *American Psychologist, 55*, 170–183.

Mahoney, J. L. (2000). School extracurricular activity participation as a moderator in the development of antisocial patterns. *Child Development, 71*(2), 502–516.

Mahoney, J. L., & Cairns, R. B. (1997). Do extracurricular activities protect against early school dropout? *Developmental Psychology, 33*, 241–253.

Marsh, H. W. (1992). Extracurricular activities: Beneficial extension of the traditional curriculum or subversion of academic goals? *Journal of Educational Psychology, 84*, 553–562.

Marsh, H., & Kleitman, S. (2002). Extracurricular school activities: The good, the bad, and the nonlinear. *Harvard Educational Review, 72*(4), 464–514.

Marsh, H. W., & Kleitman, S. (2003). School athletic participation: Mostly gain with little pain. *Journal of Sport and Exercise Psychology, 25*, 205–228.

Otto, L. B. (1975). Extracurricular activities in the educational attainment process. *Rural Sociology, 40*, 162–176.

Otto, L. B. (1976). Extracurricular activities and aspirations in the status attainment process. *Rural Sociology, 41*, 217–233.

Otto, L. B., & Alwin, D. F. (1977). Athletics, aspirations, and attainments. *Sociology of Education, 50*(2), 102–113.

Perkins, D. F., Borden, L. M., & Villarruel, F. A. (2001). Community youth development: A partnership in action. *School Community Journal, 11*(2), 39–56.

Roth, J., Brooks-Gunn, J., Murray, L., & Foster, W. (1998). Promoting healthy adolescents: Synthesis of youth development program evaluations. *Journal of Research on Adolescence, 8*, 423–459.

Scales, P. C., Benson, P. L., Leffert, N., & Blyth, D. A. (2000). Contribution of developmental assets to the prediction of thriving among adolescents. *Applied Developmental Science, 4*, 27–46.

Youniss, J., McLellan, J. A., Su, Y., & Yates, M. (1999). The role of community service in identity development: Normative, unconventional, and deviant orientations. *Journal of Adolescent Research 14*(2), 248–261.

Youniss, J., & Yates, M. (1997). *Community service and social responsibility in youth.* Chicago: University of Chicago Press.

Youniss, J., Yates, M., & Su, Y. (1997). Social integration: Community Service and marijuana use in high school seniors. *Journal of Adolescent Research Special Issue: Adolescent Socialization in Context: Connection, Regulation, and Autonomy in Multiple Contexts, 12*(2), 245–262.

10 Positive Interpersonal and Intrapersonal Functioning: An Assessment of Measures among Adolescents

Brian K. Barber

University of Tennessee

The welcome shift in focus from negative to positive aspects of adolescents currently being pursued by many social science and public health researchers (e.g., Arnett, 1999; Barber & Erickson, 2001; Halpern-Felsher, Millstein, & Irwin, 2002; Larson, 2000; Yates & Youniss, 1999) brings with it the important challenge of identifying, revising, and/or developing adequate measurement instruments. Efficient progress in understanding adolescent competence rests largely on this key task of solidifying reliable and valid measures that can be used in the substantial research that is sure to follow this trend in attention to the positive aspects of adolescent functioning. Accordingly, the study presented in this chapter thoroughly assesses the psychometric properties of several indices of positive adolescent functioning to determine their adequacy for use in future research.

Not unlike measuring maladaptive behavior, assessing competence or positive functioning is complex, given the intricate nature of adolescent experience. However, unlike the traditional approach to studying adolescent problem behaviors that has organized inquiry by type or severity of specific problems (e.g., internalized and externalized problem syndromes and their many subcategories, as in Achenbach & Edelbrock, 1987), assessing positive adolescent functioning might better be organized according to the developmental tasks that face children in the second decade of life. Developmental theory suggests that adolescence is characterized by at least two fundamental domains of adolescent functioning: the intrapersonal and the interpersonal. Competent functioning in both of these domains is used as a marker of successful development

147

and preparation for advancement to the challenges yet to come in the adult years.

Competent intrapersonal functioning emerges with the development of two interrelated components of identity formation: the consolidation of self and the self's increasing awareness of others. Both are central to many theoretical approaches to adolescence. Indeed, according to Erikson (1968), a basic task of adolescence is the establishment of an autonomous self-concept that recognizes a self in the past, present, and future. Further, with increased cognitive and emotional capacities coincident with adolescence, youth develop the capacity to recognize others, understand their differences, and assume their perspectives during social interaction. These skills or attributes are critical to successful navigation of the many interactions adolescents will encounter in the educational, occupational, romantic, and family realms of life. Therefore, one way to examine positive adolescent functioning is to assess adolescent feelings or satisfaction with self and the degree to which adolescents are able to focus outside of self on others. In the present analyses, intrapersonal functioning is assessed specifically by measures of *self-esteem*, *perspective taking*, and *empathy*.

Theory on adolescents also gives key importance to social competence, or interpersonal functioning. Thus, beyond development of the self–other dynamic described above, adolescents face increasing opportunities and requirements to interact with peers and adults in various contexts. This opportunity arises because of longer hours spent away from the home—either at school or in the labor force. Such opportunity is augmented by required or desired interaction with peers, dating partners, teachers, and other adults in the community (coaches, religious leaders, employers, community leaders, etc.). Particularly—and contrary to earlier theoretical interpretations that dismissed the continued value of the parent-adolescent relationship—research has documented well the enduring need and desire of youth to maintain and enhance relationships with parents or other significant adult caregivers (e.g., Baumrind, 1991; Steinberg, 1990). Thus, in the current study, interpersonal functioning is assessed specifically with indexes of *social initiative*, *peer connection*, *communication with mother*, and *communication with father*.

While theory is clear on the importance to adolescents of developing and exercising intra- and interpersonal competencies, empirical documentation of these competencies, the extent to which they are relevant to population subgroups, how they develop, and how they enhance later functioning lags behind. The first step in addressing these issues is the establishment of reliable assessment tools for research. This chapter contributes to that effort by thoroughly testing the reliability of seven measures of positive adolescent functioning, all but one of which are established scales but have not been thoroughly assessed for psychometric adequacy. The resulting foundational information will be used in future research to document the conceptual organization of these dimensions of adolescent experience, patterns of change in them over time, and the predictive validity of the seven measures.

Measures of Positive Interpersonal and Intrapersonal Functioning

Data to evaluate these measures of positive adolescent functioning come from the Ogden Youth and Family Project (OYFP), a longitudinal study of families with adolescents in Ogden, Utah, that was funded by the National Institute of Mental Health. Although the OYFP sought information on adolescent mental and social problems (e.g., Barber, 1996, 2002; Barber & Erikson, 2001), it was also designed to assess the positive dimensions of adolescent experience. To that end, the project included seven scales of positive adolescent functioning, drawn from a variety of sources (see Appendix). The present study is the initial step in the analyses of the OYFP data for these scales.

Our first general goal in this study was to analyze the seven measures as thoroughly as possible to maximize confidence in their reliability. Thus, we assessed adolescent reports on these measures over five consecutive annual assessments. For each of the five waves of data, analyses were also conducted separately on eight relevant demographic subgroups: males and females, poor and not poor, Whites and non-Whites, Mormons and non-Mormons. In other words, for every scale, each psychometric statistic (kurtosis, skewness, and Cronbach's alpha) was calculated 45 separate times—for eight groups and the entire sample in each of 5 years (when the scale was available for all years). Our intent was to ensure that conclusions about the reliability of these scales were credible, in that they held as adolescents developed over time and they applied to youth of varying demographic statuses over time.

Our second general goal was to determine if reduced versions of these scales also met reliability requirements. This was important because self-reported measures like these are frequently used in large national surveys that have restrictions on space. To this end, both five-item and three-item versions of every scale were assessed as described above.

Our third goal was to provide evidence regarding the validity of the scales, drawing both on the published literature and cross-sectional analyses of data from the first wave of the Ogden Youth and Family Project.

Reliability

To evaluate reliability, all scales were assessed for kurtosis, skewness, and Cronbach's alpha, as well as mean and standard deviation. Kurtosis is a measure of the relative peakedness or flatness of a distribution. Skewness refers to the extent to which the desirable normal distribution has been shifted to the left or the right, resulting in a longer tail of the distribution in the direction of the skew. Both kurtosis and skew are centered on zero, and the closer to zero the coefficients are, the better. Cutoffs for acceptability are somewhat arbitrary. The standard set for this study was plus or minus 2.0, which is a fairly stringent level. Alpha is a common measure of interitem consistency. The maximum alpha value is 1.0, and higher values indicate higher reliability. The standard for acceptability used in this study was .70, a minimum level often invoked in studies of this type. To ensure that estimates of these parameters were not unduly influenced by item nonresponse, scale scores for all measures were calculated with the requirement that either 80% (for the five-item scales) or 67% (for the three-item scales) of the items in every scale had a response. Cases not meeting this requirement were dropped from the sample for these analyses.

The baseline sample of the OYFP was a random sample of fifth- and eighth-grade classrooms in the Ogden City School District in 1994, with an oversampling of Hispanic families to match the proportion of this, the largest ethnic minority group in the city. The overall sample consisted of 933 families with adolescent children. The sample was split about equally by sex and grade. Seventy-one percent of the students were White (including 16% Hispanic), 84% were from middle-income families, and 46% were Mormon. In the first year, an extensive self-report survey of family interaction, personality, youth behavior, and peer, school, and neighborhood experiences was administered to the students in classrooms. Later waves of the survey were done by multiple mailings to the students' homes.

Both fifth- and eighth-grade cohorts were followed for 4 years, until 1997. The younger cohort was surveyed an additional time in 1998. The participation rate in the first year (in-class assessment) was over 90%. No follow-up of absentees was done. Multiple mailings following standard mail survey methodology (Dillman, 1978) were employed to maximize response rates in the subsequent years of data collection. Response rates were 84% (780) in 1995, 78% (725) in 1996, 80% (749) in 1997, and 71% in 1998 (352; younger cohort only). Tests revealed that respondents differed from nonrespondents only in a higher percentage of Mormons represented among the respondents.

Data from the younger cohort were used in the current analyses because the five data points for that cohort span the transitions to both middle and high school, as well as the years during which the bulk of pubertal development is achieved. Thus, in addition to the across-time and across-group parameters of the analysis, it was also possible to assess whether the reliability of these scales endures through the two major normative changes associated with adolescent development: pubertal and school transitions.

In a first round of analyses, we used exploratory factor analysis with oblimin rotation in conjunction with consideration of item face validity to reduce each of the seven scales to a five- and a three-item version (see Appendix). In a second round, we computed the mean, standard deviation, kurtosis, skew, and alpha for both versions of each scale (except the empathy scale, which has only a three-item version) for the entire sample, as well as for the eight major demographic subgroups described previously. As an example, computations of all statistics for the self-esteem scale are presented in Table 1.[1]

In evaluating the 45 separate coefficients for each type of statistic for each of the five- and three-item scales, the following standard was used to judge the

---

[1] Results for the other six scales are available from the author.

Table 1. Psychometric Findings for Self-Esteem, by Year and Demographic Subgroup

		5-Item scale						3-Item scale				
	N	Mean	SD	Kurtosis	Skew	Alpha	N	Mean	SD	Kurtosis	Skew	Alpha
Full sample												
1994	436	3.85	0.81	0.61	−0.67	0.77	470	3.81	0.90	0.20	−0.68	0.72
1995	372	4.13	0.69	0.39	−0.66	0.81	370	4.10	0.76	0.05	−0.63	0.73
1996	344	4.02	0.72	0.61	−0.71	0.83	343	4.02	0.81	0.46	−0.77	0.81
1997	357	4.00	0.84	1.57	−1.10	0.86	357	3.98	0.93	1.24	−1.11	0.86
1998	322	3.86	0.89	0.14	−0.70	0.88	322	3.84	0.99	−0.01	−0.73	0.86
Males												
1994	247	3.84	0.87	0.14	0.59	0.79	246	3.79	0.98	−0.12	−0.62	0.73
1995	204	4.18	0.69	−0.04	−0.61	0.81	203	4.16	0.72	−0.01	−0.61	0.67
1996	181	4.12	0.66	−0.56	−0.38	0.79	181	4.13	0.72	−0.34	−0.53	0.75
1997	193	4.02	0.89	1.34	−1.13	0.88	193	4.04	0.98	1.44	−1.27	0.88
1998	177	3.87	0.89	0.65	−0.83	0.88	177	3.89	0.96	0.48	−0.85	0.85
Females												
1994	225	3.86	0.73	1.37	−0.77	0.73	224	3.84	0.82	0.64	−0.76	0.69
1995	168	4.08	0.68	0.94	−0.74	0.81	167	4.16	0.80	0.00	−0.62	0.78
1996	163	3.92	0.77	0.89	−0.86	0.85	162	3.86	0.88	0.42	−0.81	0.84
1997	164	3.98	0.78	1.98	−1.07	0.84	164	3.91	0.87	1.11	−0.93	0.83
1998	145	3.84	0.90	−0.40	−0.56	0.88	145	3.79	1.02	−0.45	−0.61	0.88
Not poor												
1994	390	3.89	0.79	0.92	−0.76	0.76	388	3.86	0.87	0.32	−0.72	0.70
1995	308	4.17	0.68	0.58	−0.71	0.81	306	4.14	0.74	0.17	−0.66	0.71
1996	288	4.05	0.70	1.02	−0.78	0.82	287	4.04	0.77	0.59	−0.76	0.78
1997	299	4.04	0.81	1.58	−1.08	0.86	299	4.01	0.91	1.23	−1.09	0.85
1998	273	3.88	0.86	0.33	−0.72	0.87	273	3.87	0.94	0.14	−0.73	0.85
Poor												
1994	75	3.65	0.87	0.15	−0.34	0.82	75	3.63	0.95	−0.26	−0.36	0.72
1995	59	3.92	0.73	−0.18	−0.46	0.82	59	3.89	0.85	−0.46	−0.46	0.78
1996	51	3.89	0.84	−0.62	−0.31	0.86	51	3.87	0.95	−0.25	−0.63	0.86
1997	55	3.84	0.96	1.32	−1.14	0.89	55	3.85	1.04	1.25	−1.18	0.91
1998	46	3.63	1.07	−0.73	−0.43	0.91	46	3.62	1.22	−0.90	−0.49	0.91
White												
1994	305	3.91	0.81	0.66	−0.74	0.81	303	3.90	0.89	0.43	−0.78	0.74
1995	240	4.23	0.63	0.20	−0.70	0.78	238	4.21	0.70	0.20	−0.75	0.69
1996	217	4.11	0.72	1.41	−0.98	0.83	217	4.12	0.77	0.98	−0.93	0.80
1997	242	4.07	0.82	1.66	−1.12	0.86	242	4.06	0.91	1.46	−1.15	0.87
1998	219	3.87	0.89	0.41	−0.77	0.88	219	3.85	0.99	0.22	−0.79	0.85
Non-White												
1994	167	3.73	0.79	0.75	−0.58	0.70	167	3.66	0.92	0.00	−0.54	0.67
1995	132	3.98	0.75	0.38	−0.47	0.84	132	3.91	0.82	−0.13	−0.37	0.76
1996	127	3.88	0.70	−0.13	−0.31	0.80	126	3.83	0.83	0.14	−0.55	0.79
1997	115	3.87	0.87	1.48	−1.09	0.86	115	3.82	0.97	0.94	−1.07	0.84
1998	103	3.83	0.89	−0.36	−0.58	0.86	103	3.84	0.98	−0.49	−0.62	0.88
Non-Mormon												
1994	272	3.81	0.82	0.40	−0.61	0.77	270	3.77	0.91	−0.03	−0.58	0.70
1995	200	4.08	0.72	0.38	−0.64	0.80	200	4.02	0.81	−0.11	−0.57	0.71
1996	179	3.93	0.74	1.08	−0.76	0.82	178	3.90	0.83	0.81	−0.77	0.77
1997	163	3.92	0.87	1.29	−1.02	0.86	194	3.91	0.97	0.77	−1.01	0.86
1998	161	3.84	0.88	0.26	−0.64	0.87	161	3.82	0.99	−0.11	−0.68	0.87

(*continued*)

Table 1. (Continued)

	5-Item scale					3-Item scale				
	N	Mean	SD	Kurtosis	Skew	Alpha	N	Mean	SD	Kurtosis	Skew	Alpha

	N	Mean	SD	Kurtosis	Skew	Alpha	N	Mean	SD	Kurtosis	Skew	Alpha
Mormon												
1994	200	3.90	0.78	1.03	−0.76	0.78	200	3.87	0.89	0.64	−0.84	0.74
1995	172	4.20	0.65	0.31	−0.64	0.83	170	1.20	0.69	0.22	−0.62	0.76
1996	165	4.13	0.69	−0.19	−0.62	0.83	165	4.14	0.77	−0.09	−0.77	0.83
1997	194	4.10	0.80	2.11	−1.22	0.87	163	4.07	0.89	2.07	−1.26	0.86
1998	161	3.87	0.90	0.09	−0.77	0.89	161	3.86	0.98	0.13	−0.80	0.86

Note: N = number in sample; SD = standard deviation; alpha = Cronbach's alpha.

psychometric adequacy of the scales:

1. The alpha value for the full sample averaged over the years of assessment must reach or exceed .70.
2. A minimum of 75% of the tests of alpha across sample subgroups and years must reach or exceed .70.
3. The kurtosis value and the skew value for the full sample averaged over the years of assessment must not exceed ± 2.00.
4. A minimum of 75% of the tests of kurtosis and skewness across sample subgroups and years must not exceed ± 2.00.

The overall results of these evaluations indicate that with only two exceptions (the three-item empathy scale and the five-item communication-with-mother scale), both the five- and three-item versions of all seven measures of positive adolescent functioning have acceptable psychometric properties (Table 2). Given the demanding standard for acceptability used in this study, these results indicate strong support for the reliability of these positive adolescent functioning scales, whether formed as five- or three-item versions.

Inspection of the relatively few instances where the psychometric properties fell below the standard revealed the following trends: (a) Problems with kurtosis occurred only for the five-item communication-with-mother scale. (b) For poor youth, alphas dipped below the minimum standard of .70 (but never below .60) in at least 1 of the 5 years for all scales except self-esteem and communication with father. And (c) for non-White youth, alphas dipped below the minimum standard of .70 (but never below .62) in at least 1 of the 5 years for all scales except peer connection, communication with mother, and communication with father. Thus, there is some evidence that poor and non-White youth (which are not mutually exclusive groups) perceived less consistency among the items making up several of the scales studied here than did the other sample subgroups. However, this may in part be an artifact, since the samples sizes for both of these groups were relatively much smaller than for the other groups, which may have impacted the strength of the reliability estimates (see, for example, the sample sizes [N] in Table 1).

Table 2. Psychometric Properties of Scales of Positive Youth Functioning Across 5 Years and Eight Demographic Subgroups

Scale	Number of subgroup tests	Average alpha for full sample	Percentage of subgroup tests where alpha >= .7	Average kurtosis for full sample	Percentage of subgroup tests where kurtosis <= ±2	Average skew for full sample	Percentage of subgroup tests where skew =< ±2	Psychometrically adequate
				Intrapersonal Functioning				
Self-esteem	40							
5 items		.83	100	.66	98	.77	100	Yes
3 items		.80	90	.39	98	.78	100	Yes
Perspective Taking	32[a]							
5 items		.85	100	.36	100	.10	100	Yes
3 items		.78	88	.36	100	.78	100	Yes
Empathy	32[a]							
3 items		.72	63	.37	100	.78	100	No
				Interpersonal Functioning				
Social Initiative	32[b]							
5 items		.81	100	.17	100	.42	100	Yes
3 items		.72	75	.35	100	.48	100	Yes
Peer Connection	24[a,b]							
5 items		.77	100	.30	100	.67	100	Yes
3 items		.75	88	.07	100	.65	100	Yes
Communication with Mother	24[c]							
5 items		.90	100	1.71	**58**	1.12	100	No
3 items		.86	96	1.47	79	1.25	100	Yes
Communication with Father	24[c]							
5 items		.70	100	1.71	100	1.12	100	Yes
3 items		.70	100	.66	100	.83	100	Yes

Note: Years = 1994–1998; subgroups = males/females, poor/not poor, Whites/non-Whites, and Mormons/non-Mormons. Alpha = Cronbach's alpha. Boldface percentages indicate that the value does not meet the standard of psychometric adequacy for this study.
[a] Scale was not available in 1995.
[b] Scale was not available in 1994.
[c] Scale was not available in 1997 and 1998.

Validity

Tests of predictive validity are also necessary to provide evidence that these scales do indeed tap competent functioning. Again, given that we used established scales in this report, there is already published evidence of predictive validity for such scales in that they have, typically independently, been correlated with relevant elements of the adolescents' social and personal world. As examples: Self-esteem has been linked to family structure (Mandara & Murray, 2000), parenting (Bush, Peterson, Cobas, & Supple, 2002), participation in school sports (Erkut & Tracy, 2002), and psychological functioning (Barber, Ball, & Armistead, 2003); social initiative has been linked to parenting, peer relations, and adolescent problem behaviors (Barber & Erickson, 2001); empathy and perspective taking have been linked to adolescent dating and peer aggression (McCloskey & Lichter, 2003) and adult romantic relationships (Long et al., 1999; Rowan, Compton, & Rust, 1995); and parent–adolescent communication has been linked to family structure (Baer, 1999), adolescent moral thought (White, 2000), problem behaviors (Hartos & Power, 1997), and risk factors for violence among adolescents (Beyers, Loeber, Wilkstroem, & Stouthamer-Loeber, 2001).

For preliminary analyses of validity in the data used in the present study, we selected the 1996 data set because all measures were available in that year, and we calculated correlations using the entire sample. First, as to demographic variables, gender of adolescent was significantly associated with self-esteem (3-item version −.17 and 5-item version −.15; females higher), communication with father (3-item version −.18 and 5-item version −.19; females higher), and peer connection (5-item version .19; males higher). Age of adolescent was significantly associated with perspective taking (both 3- and 5-item versions .15; higher with age) and peer connection (5-item version .11; higher with age). Family structure (single vs. dual-parent families) was significantly associated with self-esteem (3- and 5-item versions −.12; adolescents from dual-parent families higher) and communication with father (3-item version −.13 and 5-item version −.15; adolescents from dual-parent families higher).

We also correlated the measures of positive adolescent functioning with four aspects of the adolescents' personal and social world available in the data set that should be related significantly with positive functioning: academic achievement, parental psychological control, antisocial behavior, and depression. All measures of positive adolescent functioning (with the exception of peer connection) were significantly correlated with academic achievement (a single, self-reported variable on grade performance), with correlations ranging from .11 (perspective taking, 3-item version) to .39 (social initiative, 5-item version). Again with the exception of peer connection, all measures of positive adolescent functioning were significantly associated with parental psychological control (8-item Psychological Control Scale–Youth Self-Report; Barber, 1996) with coefficients ranging from −.16 (social initiative, 5-item version) to −.43 (communication with mother, 3-item version). Again with the exception of the peer connection scales, all measures of positive adolescent functioning were associated with antisocial behavior (13-item subscale of the Child Behavior Checklist–Youth Self-Report;

Achenback & Edelbrock, 1987), with correlations ranging from −.28 (perspective taking, 3-item version) to −.42 (communication with father, 5-item version). All measures of positive adolescent functioning were significantly associated with depression (Children's Depression Inventory; Kovacs, 1992), with coefficients ranging from −.13 (peer connection, 3- and 5-item versions) to −.52 (self-esteem, 5-item version).

There is, therefore, ample evidence of the validity of these measures of positive adolescent functioning, both from past studies and in the data set analyzed for the present study. This, together with the reliability and psychometric evidence presented earlier, recommends their use (either the 3- or 5-item versions) in future studies. The one exception to this is the peer connection measure, which, although psychometrically sound, was not associated with the standard and basic measures of an adolescent's personal and social worlds that were predictive of all of the other scales. This scale is a relatively new and untested measure, and it is clear that it does not tap the type of positive functioning illustrated by the other measures tested here and elsewhere. This is likely due to the fact that adolescents can bond effectively with peers, regardless of the relative pro- or antisocial nature of the other aspects of their lives.

As was suggested above for construct validity, future work could contribute meaningfully to understanding positive adolescent functioning by moving beyond the univariate assessment of its validity to testing more complex models of development and socialization. What will be particularly informative will be an assessment of the measurement framework—itself embedded in a conceptual framework that will result from the analyses described above—in elaborated models of the social experience of adolescents. One such framework that we will pursue in this regard is the socialization framework of connection with significant others, regulation of behavior, and respect for psychological autonomy that has proved useful in discriminating among other elements of adolescent functioning (e.g., Barber & Olsen, 1997).

Summary and Next Steps

In an effort to contribute to the growing research that is attending to competence in adolescence, we analyzed the reliability and validity of seven existing self-report measures of positive adolescent functioning. In so doing, we can now provide evidence of the psychometric adequacy of theoretically relevant variables that might be used in future studies.

The main strength of our study is its methodology. First, we analyzed measures that tap two major aspects of adolescent development: the self–other dynamic, whereby adolescents simultaneously recognize self and other; and social competence, whereby adolescents establish healthy relationships with key others in their lives, that is, intrapersonal and interpersonal functioning. Second, these measures were tested in 5 consecutive years of self-reports from the same sample of adolescents. Beyond the basic value of this longevity of assessment, the particular span of years—fifth through ninth grade—included the two major normative transitions of adolescence (puberty and school transitions), allowing for the detection of any change in scale adequacy during these physical and social changes. Third, we conducted separate analyses on all major demographic subgroups of the sample to ensure that any conclusions relative to psychometric adequacy of the scales applied generally, at least to the sex, social class, ethnic, and religious affiliation groupings of the sample employed in this study. Fourth, we tested both five- and three-item versions of every scale, recognizing that many research programs have limited space and therefore seek the fewest items necessary to adequately tap constructs. Fifth, we examined the validity of our measures, reporting results from the published literature and presenting correlational analyses from data for fifth and eighth graders.

The findings of our study are quite straightforward. Of the 13 scales tested (two versions each of 6 scales and one version of the empathy scale), 11 had strong psychometric properties. In other words, in every year of assessment (across pubertal development and transitions to middle and high school) and for every subgroup of the sample (males, females, Whites, non-Whites, poor, not poor, Mormons, non-Mormons), these 11 measures of positive adolescent functioning (self-esteem, perspective taking, social initiative, peer connection, communication with father) were internally consistent (Cronbach's alpha) and otherwise had acceptable distributional properties (skewness and kurtosis). Of the two exceptions to these findings, one occurred because several subgroups had alphas below .70 on the empathy scale. The other exception occurred because several subgroups had high kurtosis coefficients on the communication-with-mother scale. In addition, our tests of construct validity indicate that all of the scales, except the measure of peer connection, are significantly associated with theoretically related measures of background or well-being, such as grades and antisocial behavior.

Naturally, it will be important to test these scales in different samples. Although random, the sample employed in this study was regional (Rocky Mountains), and the findings therefore cannot be generalized to adolescents in other parts of the United States or in other cultures. The internal consistency found across subgroups in this sample, however, suggests confidence that the scales would hold up well in diverse samples. For some of the constructs, such as social initiative or communication with parents, it will also be useful to employ alternate methods of assessment, such as observer, teacher, and/or parent report. However, several of the scales index internal processes (self-esteem, perspective taking, empathy) that are best measured from the perspective of adolescents.

Establishing the reliability of these measures is just the first step in assessing positive adolescent functioning. A variety of further tests of validity will also be required. Specifically, tests of construct validity should be made to ensure that these separate measures are related highly enough with each other to support their common identification as measures of competence. Preliminary inspection of correlations among the scales tested in this study using the full sample indicate that the scales are consistently and significantly correlated with each other, typically to a magnitude of .20 to .40. This is as expected since most of the scales tested derive from established instruments designed to measure adolescent competence of some form or another. For a future report, more elaborated analyses are being pursued to assess this evidence of construct validity across time and subgroup as was done here for the reliability and other psychometric analyses.

Further, analyses are being conducted to assess construct validity in the context of theoretically informed conceptual frameworks. For example, as suggested earlier, rather than simply correlating the several indices of positive adolescent functioning to assess their construct validity, we will hypothesize a higher order model of positive adolescent functioning (e.g., interpersonal, intrapersonal, and institutional domains of competence; see, e.g., Gresham & Reschly, 1987; Rose-Krasnor, 1997) and test it by means of structural equation modeling. Such analyses will help determine whether the several measures of positive adolescent functioning studied here (as well as others) actually are components of a broader, more parsimonious model of competence that, itself, might vary over time and subgroup.

Following additional validity tests, still other important information will be needed about positive adolescent functioning, such as how it develops, how it can be maximized, the extent to which it is constitutional (versus shaped by social experiences), and the extent to which competence in adolescence portends success or well-being in adulthood. Questions such as these can best be answered using sound and reliable instruments to assess positive adolescent functioning. The findings of this study provide a promising start to the development of these tools.

Author's Note

This study was supported by a FIRST Award from the National Institute of Mental Health (R29–MH47067–03) to Brian K. Barber. Appreciation is expressed to the administrators, teachers, and families of the Ogden (Utah) City School District for participating in this study. For further information, contact Brian K. Barber, Department of Child and Family Studies, Knoxville, TN 37996-1900 (bkbarber1@utk.edu).

Appendix

The seven measures of positive adolescent functioning were developed from the following seven scales. Items retained in the five-item version each have a superscript 5 (^{5}), and items retained in the three-item version have a superscript 3 (^{3}).

Intrapersonal Functioning   *Self-esteem*

1. I am able to do things as well as most people.[5]
2. I certainly feel useless at times.
3. At times I think I am no good at all.

4. On the whole, I am satisfied with myself.[5,3]
5. I feel I do not have much to be proud of.
6. I wish I could have more respect for myself.
7. I take a positive attitude toward myself.[5,3]
8. I feel that I have a number of good qualities.[5,3]
9. All in all, I am inclined to feel that I am a failure.
10. I feel that I'm a person of worth, at least on an equal plane with others.[5]

Note: Response options range from 1 = *strongly agree* to 5 = *strongly disagree*. Relevant items were reverse-coded so that high scores represent high self-esteem. From Rosenberg, 1965.

Perspective Taking

1. Before criticizing somebody, I try to imagine how I would feel if I were in their place.[5]
2. If I'm sure I'm right about something, I don't waste much time listening to other people's arguments.
3. I sometimes try to understand my friends better by imagining how things look from their point of view.[5]
4. I believe that there are two sides to every question and try to look at them both.[5,3]
5. I sometimes find it difficult to see things from the "other guy's" point of view.
6. I try to look at everybody's side of a disagreement before I make a decision.[5,3]
7. When I'm upset at someone, I usually try to "put myself in their shoes" for a while. [5,3]

Note: Response options range from 1 = *does not describe me well* to 5 = *describes me very well*. Relevant items were reverse-coded so that high scores represent high perspective taking. From Davis, 1996.

Empathy

1. When I see someone being taken advantage of, I feel kind of protective towards them.[3]
2. When I see someone being treated unfairly, I sometimes don't feel very much pity for them.
3. I often have tender, concerned feelings for people less fortunate than I.[3]
4. I would describe myself as a pretty soft-hearted person.
5. Sometimes I don't feel very sorry for other people when they are having problems.
6. Other people's misfortunes do not usually disturb me a great deal.
7. I am often quite touched by things that I see happen.[3]

Note: Response options range from 1 = *does not describe me well* to 5 = *describes me very well*. Relevant items were reverse-coded so that high scores represent high empathy. From Davis, 1996.

Interpersonal Functioning

Social Initiative

1. I enjoy doing things and talking with peers.[5,3]
2. I get into conversations with adults (e.g., teachers, staff) at the school.[5,3]
3. I share feelings and ideas with peers.[5]
4. I actively participate in topic clubs (e.g., political, history, Honor Society).
5. I talk to teachers and staff about things other than class.
6. I actively participate in the school newspaper or yearbook.
7. I help other students who might need assistance (e.g., lost in the building, sick or hurt).[5]
8. I ask questions in class when I don't understand the material.
9. I actively participate in drama (e.g., school plays) or music (e.g., band).
10. I express liking and caring for my friends.

11. I actively participate in student government.
12. I join in class discussions.[5,3]
13. I am comfortable joking with teachers and staff.

Note: Response options range from 1 = *never/almost never true* to 5 = *very often/always true*. From Barber and Erickson, 2001, as adapted from Bachman, Johnston, and O'Malley, 1993.

Peer Connection

1. How often do you call this friend on the phone?[5,3]
2. If you needed help with something, how often could you count on this friend to help you?[5]
3. How often do you and this friend go over to each other's houses?[5,3]
4. How often do you tell this friend things about yourself that you wouldn't tell most kids?[5]
5. How often do you and this friend go places together, like a movie, skating, shopping, or a sports event?[5,3]
6. When you do a good job on something, how often does this friend praise or congratulate you?

Note: Response options range from 0 = *never* to 4 = *every day*. From Barber and Olsen, 1997.

Communication with Mother

1. I can discuss my beliefs with my mother without feeling restrained or embarrassed.[5]
2. I am very satisfied with how my mother and I talk together.[5,3]
3. If I were in trouble, I could tell my mother.[5,3]
4. I am careful about what I say to my mother.
5. When I ask questions, I get honest answers from my mother.[5]
6. I find it easy to discuss problem with my mother.[5,3]

Note: Response options range from 1 = *strongly agree* to 5 = *strongly disagree*. Relevant items were reverse-coded so that high scores represent high-quality communication. From Barnes and Olson, 1982.

Communication with Father

1. I can discuss my beliefs with my father without feeling restrained or embarrassed.[5]
2. I am very satisfied with how my father and I talk together.[5,3]
3. If I were in trouble, I could tell my father.[5,3]
4. I am careful about what I say to my father.
5. When I ask questions, I get honest answers from my father.[5]
6. I find it easy to discuss problem with my father.[5,3]

Note: Response options range from 1 = *strongly agree* to 5 = *strongly disagree*. Relevant items were reverse-coded so that high scores represent high-quality communication. From Barnes and Olson, 1982.

References

Achenbach, T. M., & Edelbrock, C. (1987). *Manual for the Child Behavior Checklist and Revised Child Behavior Profile*. Burlington: University of Vermont, Department of Psychiatry.

Arnett, J. J. (1999). Adolescent storm and stress, reconsidered. *American Psychologist, 54,* 317–326.

Bachman, G. G., Johnston, L. D., & O'Malley, P. M. (1993). *Monitoring the future: A continuing study of the lifestyles and values of youth 1992.* Ann Arbor, MI: Inter-university Consortium for Political and Social Research.

Baer, J. (1999). The effects of family structure and SES on family processes in early adolescence. *Journal of Adolescence, 22*(3), 341–354.

Barber, B. K. (1996). Parental psychological control: Revisiting a neglected construct. *Child Development, 67,* 3296–3319.

Barber, B. K. (Ed.). (2002). *Intrusive parenting: How psychological control affects children and adolescents.* Washington, DC: American Psychological Association Press.

Barber, B. K., & Erickson, L. D. (2001). Adolescent social initiative: Antecedents in the ecology of social connections. *Journal of Adolescent Research, 16,* 326–354.

Barber, B. K., & Olsen, J. (1997). Socialization in context: Connection, regulation, and autonomy in the family, school, and neighborhood and with peers. *Journal of Adolescent Research, 12*(2), 287–315.

Barber, C. N., Ball, J., & Armistead, L. (2003). Parent–adolescent relationship and adolescent psychological functioning among African-American female adolescents: Self-esteem as a mediator. *Journal of Child and Family Studies, 12,* 361–374.

Barnes, H. L., & Olson, D. H. (1982). Parent adolescent communication scale. In D. H. Olson et al. (Eds.), *Family inventories* (pp. 33–48). St. Paul: University of Minnesota, Department of Family Social Science.

Baumrind, D. (1991). The influence of parenting style on adolescent competence and substance use. *Journal of Early Adolescence, 11,* 56–95.

Beyers, J. M., Loeber, R., Wilkstroem, P. O. H., & Stouthamer-Loeber, M. (2001). What predicts adolescent violence in better-off neighborhoods? *Journal of Abnormal Child Psychology, 29*(5), 369–381.

Bush, K. R., Peterson, G. W., Cobas, J. A., & Supple, A. J. (2002). Adolescents' perceptions of parental behaviors as predictors of adolescent self-esteem in mainland China. *Sociological Inquiry, 72,* 503–526.

Davis, M. H. (1996). *Empathy: A social-psychological approach.* Boulder, CO: Westview Press.

Dillman, D. A. (1978). *Mail and telephone surveys: The total design method.* New York: John Wiley & Sons.

Erikson, E. E. (1968). *Identity: Youth and crisis.* New York: W. W. Norton.

Erkut, S., & Tracy, A. J. (2002). Predicting adolescent self-esteem from participation in school sports among Latino subgroups. *Hispanic Journal of Behavioral Sciences, 24*(4), 409–429.

Gresham, F. M. & Reschly, D. J. (1987). Dimensions of social competence: Method factors in the assessment of adaptive behavior, social skills, and peer acceptance. *Journal of School Psychology, 25,* 367–381.

Halpern-Felsher, B. L., Millstein, S. G., & Irwin, C. E., Jr. (2002). Work Group II: Healthy adolescent psychosocial development. *Journal of Adolescent Health, 31, 6s,* 201–207.

Hartos, J. L., & Power, T. G. (1997). Mothers' awareness of their early adolescents' stressors: Relation between awareness and adolescent adjustment. *Journal of Early Adolescence, 17*(4), 371–389.

Kovacs, M. (1992). *Children's depression inventory.* Niagara Falls, NY: Multi-Health Systems.

Larson, R. (2000). Toward a psychology of positive youth development. *American Psychologist, 55,* 170–183.

Long, E. C. J., Angera, J. J., Carter, S. J., Nakamoto, M. K., & Kalso, M. (1999). Understanding the one you love: A longitudinal assessment of an empathy training program for couples in romantic relationships. *Family Relations: Interdisciplinary Journal of Applied Family Studies, 48*(3), 235–242.

Mandara, J., & Murray, C. B. (2000). Effects of parental marital status, income, and family functioning on African American adolescent self-esteem. *Journal of Family Psychology, 14*(3), 475–490.

McCloskey, L. A., & Lichter, E. L. (2003). The contribution of marital violence to adolescent aggression across different relationships. *Journal of Interpersonal Violence, 18*(4), 390–412.

Rose-Krasnor, L. (1997). The nature of social competence: A theoretical review. *Social Development,* *6*(1), 111–135.

Rosenberg, M. (1965). *Society and the adolescent self-image.* Princeton: Princeton University Press.

Rowan, D. G., Compton, W. C., & Rust, J. O. (1995). Self-actualization and empathy as predictors of marital satisfaction. *Psychological Reports, 77*(3, Pt. 1), 1011–1016.

Steinberg, L. (1990). Autonomy, conflict, and harmony in the family relationship. In S. S. Feldman & G. R. Elliot (Eds.), *At the threshold: The developing adolescent* (pp. 255–276). Cambridge, MA: Harvard University Press.

White, F. A. (2000). Relationship of family socialization processes to adolescent moral thought. *Journal of Social Psychology, 140*(1), 75–92.

Yates, M., & Youniss, J. (Eds.). (1999). *Roots of civic identity: International perspectives on community service and activism in youth.* Cambridge: Cambridge University Press.

11   A Scale of Positive Social Behaviors

Sylvia R. Epps, Seoung Eun Park, and Aletha C. Huston

University of Texas at Austin

Marika Ripke

University of Hawaii

In this chapter, we define positive social behavior as social competence with peers and adults, compliance with rules and adult direction, and autonomy or self-reliance. Social competence or social skills include getting along with peers, being well liked, being generous and thoughtful, and being perceptive about others' feelings and perspectives. Compliance is not merely obedience, but conforming to expectations without constant supervision. High autonomy entails self-reliance, doing things on one's own, and not relying on others for unnecessary help. These positive behaviors are more than the absence of problems; they represent important skills for dealing with both peers and adults.

Historically, policy research on children and youth has emphasized negative behavior. This tendency reflects and also may contribute to the negative images of youth. Few studies have given equal weight to youths' positive behavior. It is important to understand both positive and negative behavior so that adults (parents, teachers, etc.) can make efforts not only to correct problems but also to foster social skills and other kinds of positive behavior.

Positive child social behavior has often been assumed to be the opposite of problem behavior, an assumption that we challenge. Positive or prosocial behaviors can include social skills for relating to peers and adults, empathic and helpful actions, responsibility, autonomy, and self-control. One definition includes voluntary actions that are intended to help or benefit another individual or group (Eisenberg & Fabes, 1998; Eisenberg & Mussen, 1989). Problem behavior, by contrast, is generally defined as behavior that deviates from social norms or indicates distress and unhappiness. The most common measures of problem behaviors

163

suggest two extremes: externalizing and internalizing problems. Externalizing problems involve low levels of behavior control—aggression, defiance, anger, and socially disapproved actions. Internalizing problems are indicated by social withdrawal, sadness, and signs of anxiety (e.g., see Child Behavior Checklist; Achenbach, Edelbrock, & Howell, 1987). Clearly, positive and problem behaviors are not the opposite ends of one dimension, and many have argued that they should be measured separately to reflect their conceptual independence (Aber & Jones, 1997).

Eisenberg and Mussen (1989) suggest that there has been a lag in research on positive social behavior for several reasons. First, modern society has only recently recognized the importance of prosocial behavior and its role in enhancing humanity. The increase in interest led to studies designed to understand how prosocial behaviors develop and the role societal institutions (the education system, religious organizations, and families) play in fostering these behaviors early in life. Another reason for the lack of research is the absence of a widely accepted method of assessing prosocial behavior. For instance, the Positive Behavior Scale that we present in this chapter was developed originally because no available scale was well suited for use with young children in low-income families. Also, until about 30 years ago, there was little interest in studying prosocial behavior, and both definition and measurement issues are complex.

The assessment tools that have been developed for prosocial behavior generally fall into one of five categories: naturalistic observations, situational tests, ratings, sociometric questionnaires, and self-report questionnaires (Eisenberg & Mussen, 1989). Rating scales and questionnaires are the most economical methods of measuring social behavior. Two scales are fairly widely used. The Social Skills Rating System (SSRS) created by Elliot and Gresham (1987) defines social skills as the interaction between individuals and the environment, as the tools used to initiate and maintain vital interpersonal relations. They specify three components of social skills: peer acceptance (is the child accepted by peers?), behavior (behaviors exhibited in specific settings and situations in which punishment is dependent on one's behavior), and social validity (behaviors that in a given situation predict important social outcomes for children; e.g., in school settings important social outcomes may include peer acceptance and popularity) (Elliot & Gresham, 1987). Including both prosocial and negative behavior provides an understanding of the reasoning behind selecting specific behaviors for their measure. This conceptualization serves as an appropriate guideline for developing assessments because it specifies the features of behavior necessary to label it prosocial. The SSRS used by parents, teachers, and children to rate social behavior is on a 3-point scale (*often true, sometimes true, never true*) (Gresham & Elliot, 1987). A significant feature of this scale is the parent's or teacher's report of how important each behavior is for the child's success in a variety of settings.

The other commonly used rating scale for social behavior is the Child Behavior Checklist (Achenbach et al., 1987). It contains a brief scale titled Social Competence, but the overall measure contains much more detail about problem behaviors than about positive behaviors.

A related measure of problem behavior is the Behavior Problem Index (BPI), a 26-item scale designed for children ages 4 years and older (Quint, Bos, & Polit,

1997). It was developed for the 1981 Child Health Supplement to the National Health Interview Survey (Peterson & Zill, 1986) and was also used in the New Chance study and the National Longitudinal Survey of Youth. It is widely used for several reasons, including its ability to measure a broad developmental range and its simplicity in reading and understanding.

Positive Behavior Scale

In this chapter, we examine the psychometric properties of the Positive Behavior Scale, which was developed for a study of young children from low-income families whose mothers were participating in an intervention called New Chance (Quint et al., 1997). The scale was subsequently used in several evaluations of welfare and employment programs for children across a wide age range and in national surveys. We draw on data from two studies. The first is the New Hope project, in which children in low-income families were evaluated on two occasions separated by 3 years. The second is a nationally representative sample of children studied in the Child Development Supplement of the Panel Study of Income Dynamics.

The New Hope Sample

The New Hope project is a longitudinal study of a work-based poverty intervention program for families with low incomes in Milwaukee. Adults (parents) were randomly assigned in a lottery-like process to either a program group (with access to New Hope services) or a control group (with no access to New Hope services, but able to seek other services). To date, data have been collected 2 years (Time 1) and 5 years (Time 2) since the initial treatment phase began, and an 8-year follow-up is in the beginning phase of development.

The sample presented in this chapter consists of families who had at least one child between the ages of 3 and 12 years at the 2-year anniversary of sample enrollment and between ages 6 and 15 years at the 5-year anniversary. Up to two children were selected from these families. Of the 745 eligible parents, 580 (78%) responded at 2 years and 547 (73%) responded at 5 years. The Positive Behavior Scale was completed by parents during an individual interview and by teachers as part of a mailed questionnaire. All interviews were conducted in person unless the family had moved too far from Milwaukee; phone interviews were conducted for people living more than 2 or 3 hours from the city. Children who were 6 years old or older were also interviewed.

When they entered the New Hope study, the average age of the parents was 29 years. About 55% of the sample were African American, 29% Hispanic, 13% White, and 3% of other racial/ethnic backgrounds. The majority of the parents (primarily mothers) had never been married, and 11% were currently married and living with their spouse. At Time 1 (2 years after enrollment), the average family income was $14,000; at Time 2 (5 years after recruitment), it was $22,000.

PSID Sample

Data for the Child Development Supplement (CDS) of the Panel Study of Income Dynamics (PSID) were collected in 1997 (Hofferth, 1998). The PSID, a longitudinal study focusing primarily on the transfer of capital within families and conducted since 1967, was extended in 1997 to obtain measures for children age 12 years and under. The measures assessed each family's home environment, economic status, and a myriad of parenting attitudes and practices, as well as children's cognitive ability, academic achievement, and socioemotional well-being.[1]

The data for the 1997 CDS are from three different samples: the original nationally representative sample of U.S. households from the PSID; an oversample of low-income, mostly African American families; and a refresher sample of immigrant families who had immigrated since the initial sample was collected in 1967. In this study, all analyses were conducted using weighted data (with weights recalibrated for our subsample) and are therefore representative of the U.S. population. Of all families in the PSID with children under 12 years, 2,380 agreed to participate, yielding a total CDS sample of 3,562 children. Up to two children in each family from age 1 to 12 years could be included.

The unweighted estimates of household characteristics show that 51% were girls and 49% were boys. The average age of the head of the family was 36.3 years. About 46% of the sample were White, 41% African American, 7% Hispanic, and 4% Asian, Native American, or other ethnicity. The average number of years of school the head of the family completed was 12.61 years. The average family income was about $44,063. The majority of the sample lived in married two-parent families (60%), with a smaller percentage living in single-parent families (33%) (i.e., never married, separated, divorced, or widowed).

There are important differences between the New Hope and PSID samples. The New Hope sample is drawn from one community and consists primarily of single-parent families with low incomes. Most of the families are ethnic minorities. The PSID is a nationally representative sample with a predominance of Whites and a wider income range, ranging from almost nothing to over $1 million.

Measure of Positive Social Behavior

The Positive Behavior Scale was developed for the New Chance study to assess positive behaviors in a population of educationally and economically disadvantaged children and youth (Quint et al., 1997). Items were adapted from the Block and Block California Child Q Set, and other items were newly developed. The scale, which includes 25 items, is divided into three subscales: social competence and sensitivity (gets along well with other children, shows concern for other people's feelings), compliance and self-control (thinks before

[1] For a more complete discussion of the PSID and the CDS samples see Hofferth and Sandberg (2001).

he/she acts, usually does what he/she is told), and autonomy (tries to do things for him-/herself, is self-reliant). The scale is also intended to measure other constructs, including obedience, persistence, and self-esteem. Parents and teachers use a 5-point scale, ranging from *never* to *all of the time* to describe the frequency with which the child manifests each behavior. The items in the parent and teacher versions are slightly different, reflecting the different contexts in which the child is observed. The complete list of items in the parent version appears in the Appendix.

In the PSID-CDS, parents completed a shortened version of the Positive Behavior Scale with only 10 items, which focused on social competence and compliance. The primary caregiver responded on a 5-point scale ranging from *not at all like my child* to *totally like my child*. The items in the abbreviated version are designated in the Appendix.

Other Measures

Other measures administered to parents and children were examined in this study to provide information about the construct validity and correlates of the Positive Behavior Scale. In both the New Hope and PSID samples, we examined the relationship between positive behavior and problem behavior using parent and teacher reports. The Problem Behavior Scale from the Social Skills Rating System was administered to both parents and teachers in the New Hope study (Gresham & Elliot, 1990). Parents received two subscales: *externalizing* problems and *internalizing* problems. Teachers completed the externalizing, internalizing, and hyperactivity scales.

Parents and teachers reported children's school achievement. Parents' reports were based on their knowledge of recent report cards, as well as an evaluation of their child's performance in reading, mathematics, and written work. Teachers completed the academic subscale of the Social Skills Rating System (New Hope only) (Gresham & Elliot, 1990). They responded to 10 items on a scale of 1 (*lowest 10% of class*) to 5 (*highest 10% of class*) assessing children's performance in comparison to others in the same classroom on reading skills, math skills, intellectual functioning, motivation, oral communication, classroom behavior, and parental encouragement.

In the New Hope study, children responded to the Loneliness and Social Dissatisfaction Questionnaire (or friendship scale), which measures the child's perceptions of peer relations and friendships (Cassidy & Asher, 1992). The items include: "Do you feel alone?" "Do the kids at school like you?" And, "Is it easy for you to make new friends?" All items were coded so that higher scores indicate more satisfaction with friendships.

Children reported their perceptions of their relationship with their parents in the New Hope sample. This measure was adapted from the Child Evaluation of Relationship with Mother/Caregiver measure, which was developed as part of a study of low-income African American families (McLoyd, Jayaratne, Ceballo, & Borquez, 1994). Children aged 6–12 years indicated on a 5-point scale

(1 = *not at all true,* 5 = *very true*) how true 19 statements were about the parent, their relations with the parent, and interactions with the parent (e.g., "Your parent spends a lot of time talking with you").

Children rated their perceived academic competence in New Hope. These items were adapted from the Self and Task Perception Questionnaire and contained questions assessing children's self-concept of ability, expectations for success, extrinsic and intrinsic utility value, and attainment value regarding math and English/reading (e.g., "How good at English are you?" "How useful is what you learn in math?" Eccles, 1983). In the PSID, teachers rated children's competence in academic, physical (athletic), and social skills.

Reliability

The internal consistencies of the total score and of the three subscales were tested using Cronbach's alpha. A higher alpha indicates that the items on the subscales fit together well in a given administration. Alphas greater than .70 are considered adequate. In the New Hope sample, which received all 25 items, the alphas for total positive behavior were all above .90. The internal consistency of the subscales was also high, ranging from .71 to .92. The alpha for the 10-item positive behavior scale in the PSID was .79.

The correlations among subscales in the 2-year and the 5-year follow-ups for the New Hope sample were generally high among the three subscales, ranging from .38 to .96. These analyses could not be completed for the PSID because only 10 items were included.

Parent and teacher reports of child social behavior were minimally related for the New Hope sample. The correlations between their ratings of total positive behavior were .19 (Time 1) and .24 (Time 2). The correlations for the subscales ranged from .01 to .25 (Time 1) and .08 to .25 (Time 2). These weak correlations between parent and teacher report are consistent with other findings on child social behavior.

Parent and teacher reports of child social behavior indicated moderate stability over time. For parents, the relation between total scores at Time 1 and Time 2 was .51, indicating moderate stability over a 3-year period. The correlation between teacher ratings of total positive behavior at the two time periods was .42, a fairly high correlation considering the fact that different teachers made the two sets of ratings and many children had moved from elementary to middle or junior high school. The stability of the subscales was somewhat lower, but most of the correlations were positive and statistically significant.

Validity

In the New Hope sample, there were generally moderate to high correlations between the Positive Behavior Scale and the Problem Behavior Scale at Times 1 and 2. The correlations were higher for teacher ratings than for parent ratings.

The correlation between total positive and problem scores for teachers was −.80 and −.81 at the two times. Correlations among subscales of the two measures were also generally high. For parent ratings, the correlations of total positive and problem behavior were −.50 and −.48 for the two times, and the correlations among subscales were lower as well.

Parent reports of positive behavior were modestly related to school achievement as reported by parents ($r = .30$), but bore little relation to teacher-reported school achievement ($r = .11$). Teacher reports of positive behavior were highly related to teacher-reported achievement ($r = .70$) and modestly related to parent-reported achievement ($r = .37$). This pattern suggests that children's academic achievement had a larger effect on teachers' perceptions of their positive behavior than it did on parents' reports, perhaps accounting in part for the differences between parent and teacher ratings of positive and problem behavior.

There were weak relationships of positive behavior (as rated by parents and teachers) to children's perceived positive relationships with their parents and their satisfaction with friendships, primarily at Time 2. Children with higher scores on positive behavior perceived their relations with their parents as more positive and were more satisfied with their friendships. There were few significant relations of positive behavior to children's perceived academic competence.

In the PSID sample, correlations of the Positive Behavior Scale with other child measures showed significant relationships between positive and problem behaviors. Positive behavior (as rated by parent) was associated with low problem behavior, especially low levels of externalizing behavior, according to parent ratings (−.59). Positive behavior rated by parents was also modestly associated with low teacher ratings of problem behavior (−.23). The correlations with the problem behavior subscales ranged from −.19 to −.61. These results were consistent with the levels of association in New Hope. There were significant relationships between the primary caregiver report of positive behavior and teacher reports of competence in academic, physical, and social skills. The correlation coefficients ranged from .17 to .23, all significant at the .001 level

Differences among Groups

We used one-way analyses of variance to assess gender, ethnic, income, and education differences. In addition, a two-way analysis was conducted to determine gender and age differences.

In general, girls scored higher than boys on positive behavior in both studies. The difference in total positive behavior was significant in New Hope parent ratings at Time 2, New Hope teacher ratings at both times, and in the PSID parent ratings. The largest differences between boys and girls appeared on the compliance subscales; girls were rated considerably more compliant than boys were.

For the New Hope sample, three age groups were formed at Time 1: 3–5, 6–8, and 9–12 years. For parent reports, the patterns of age differences were

Table 1. New Hope Project: Time 1 Parent and Teacher Reports on Positive Behavior, by Age and Gender

Measures	Mean	SD	Mean	SD	Mean	SD
	2- to 5-year-olds		6- to 8-year-olds		9- to 12-year-olds	
			Girls			
Time 1 Parent Report						
Social competence	4.09	0.53	4.08	0.54	4.05	0.53
Compliance	3.54	0.59	3.85	0.49	3.88	0.55
Autonomy	4.23	0.46	4.26	0.54	4.20	0.57
Total positive behavior	3.94	0.46	4.04	0.47	4.02	0.48
Sample size	23		43		57	
Time 1 Teacher Report						
Social competence	4.10	0.70	3.66	0.68	3.78	0.58
Compliance	4.05	0.74	3.79	0.77	3.80	0.61
Autonomy	3.87	0.58	3.56	0.79	3.55	0.69
Total positive behavior	4.03	0.66	3.69	0.67	3.75	0.53
Sample size	23		43		57	
			Boys			
Time 1 Parent Report						
Social competence	4.17	0.56	3.99	0.62	3.93	0.49
Compliance	3.81	0.57	3.59	0.62	3.64	0.62
Autonomy	4.27	0.61	4.33	0.58	4.09	0.64
Total positive behavior	4.08	0.54	3.93	0.52	3.87	0.47
Sample size	18		46		61	
Time 1 Teacher Report						
Social competence	3.76	0.65	3.53	0.69	3.41	0.69
Compliance	3.70	0.71	3.39	0.82	3.27	0.79
Autonomy	3.67	0.67	3.65	0.68	3.39	0.63
Total positive behavior	3.72	0.63	3.47	0.66	3.36	0.66
Sample size	18		46		61	

different for boys and girls[2] (Table 1). Parents rated older girls slightly higher than younger girls, but rated older boys lower than younger boys. Teachers rated older children lower than they did younger children on social competence[3] and total positive behavior.[4] At each age level, they rated girls higher than boys on social competence,[5] compliance,[6] and total positive behavior.[7]

At Time 2, the New Hope age groups were 6–8, 9–12, and 13–16 years. Parents rated girls higher than boys on compliance[8] and total positive behavior,[9] and

[2] There was a significant interaction of age × gender on compliance, $F(2, 241) = 3.34$, $p < .05$.
[3] $F(2, 241) = 3.04$, $p < .05$.
[4] $F(2, 242) = 4.03$, $p < .05$.
[5] $F(1, 241) = 8.65$, $p < .01$.
[6] $F(1, 241) = 16.54$, $p < .001$.
[7] $F(1, 242) = 10.98$, $p < .001$.
[8] $F(1, 476) = 5.20$, $p < .05$.
[9] $F(1, 504) = 4.71$, $p < .05$.

Table 2. New Hope Project: Time 2 Parent and Teacher Reports on Positive Behavior, by Age and Gender

	Mean	SD	Mean	SD	Mean	SD
	5- to 8-year-olds		9- to 12-year-olds		13- to 15-year-olds	
			Girls			
Time 2 Parent Report						
Social competence	3.97	0.49	3.82	0.51	3.90	0.55
Compliance	3.73	0.62	3.80	0.53	3.77	0.62
Autonomy	4.11	0.60	4.10	0.62	4.16	0.64
Total positive behavior	3.96	0.69	3.91	0.51	3.90	0.52
Sample size		91		99		69
Time 2 Teacher Report						
Social competence	3.82	0.71	3.80	0.72	3.45	0.67
Compliance	3.77	0.78	3.92	0.75	3.51	0.74
Autonomy	3.70	0.77	3.65	0.81	3.44	0.71
Total positive behavior	3.80	0.69	3.80	0.67	3.45	0.64
Sample size		91		99		69
			Boys			
Time 2 Parent Report						
Social competence	3.98	0.51	3.87	0.54	3.89	0.44
Compliance	3.64	0.63	3.54	0.69	3.73	0.55
Autonomy	4.03	0.63	4.01	0.64	3.99	0.67
Total positive behavior	3.85	0.53	3.77	0.58	3.85	0.47
Sample size		103		89		59
Time 2 Teacher Report						
Social competence	3.58	0.68	3.46	0.70	3.43	0.84
Compliance	3.47	0.72	3.40	0.79	3.48	0.96
Autonomy	3.53	0.74	3.38	0.74	3.36	0.79
Total positive behavior	3.55	0.64	3.44	0.67	3.43	0.81
Sample size		103		89		59

their ratings did not differ significantly for children of different ages (Table 2). For teacher reports, there were main effects of gender on social competence,[10] compliance,[11] autonomy,[12] and total positive behavior.[13] For the oldest group, who were adolescents, teachers' ratings of girls were lower and more similar to those for boys.[14] Overall, teachers rated younger children more favorably than older children on social competence[15] and total positive behavior.[16]

In the PSID sample, children were grouped in ages 0–2, 3–5, 6–8, and 9–12 years. Parents rated girls higher than boys, but this difference was

[10] $F(1, 476) = 8.61, p < .01$
[11] $F(1, 476) = 15.03, p < .0.01$.
[12] $F(1, 476) = 6.30, p < .05$.
[13] $F(1, 504) = 11.73, p < .001$.
[14] The interaction of age × gender on compliance was $F(2, 476) = 3.51, p < .05$.
[15] $F(2, 476) = 5.04, p < .01$.
[16] $F(2, 504) = 5.02, p < .01$.

Table 3. Panel Study of Income Dynamics: Primary Caregiver Report on Positive Behavior, by Age and Gender

Measures	0- to 2-year-olds (N = 75)		3- to 5-year-olds (N = 819)		6- to 8-year-olds (N = 823)		9-to 12-year-olds (N = 1,088)		All ages (N = 2,805)	
	Mean	SD	Mean	SD	Mean	SD	Mean	SD	Mean	SD
Boys (N = 1,301)	4.14	0.52	4.21	0.48	4.15	0.55	4.15	0.60	4.16	0.55
Girls (N = 1,260)	4.28	0.57	4.23	0.53	4.30	0.56	4.35	0.52	4.28	0.53
All children (N = 2,561)	4.20	0.54	4.22	0.50	4.22	0.54	4.26	0.57	4.23	0.55

minimal for 3–5-year-olds (Table 3). There were no overall differences among age groups. Older boys' scores were equal to or slightly lower than those of younger boys, but older girls had somewhat higher scores than younger girls did.

In both samples, Hispanic children were rated more positively than were children in other ethnic groups (Table 4). In the New Hope sample at both Times 1 and 2, parents and teachers rated Hispanics the highest and Whites the lowest on positive behavior. Hispanics were significantly higher than Whites, while Whites were significantly lower than African Americans and Hispanics (Time 1 parent report only). There were significant differences among groups on all subscales for parent reports at Times 1 and 2 and teacher reports at Time 1. In the PSID sample, Hispanic children displayed more positive behaviors than the other three groups.

We created two education categories in the New Hope data (less than a high school diploma and a high school diploma or more) to determine if children's behavior differed by the level of the education of their parent. There were no significant differences associated with parent education except for teacher ratings at Time 2. Teachers rated children of more-educated parents higher on all three subscales than they did children of less educated parents.

Because the range of education in the PSID sample was larger than that in New Hope, we created four categories describing the education of the head of the household: less than high school, high school, college, and above college. There was a significant association between education and positive behavior. Children who lived with a household head with less than a high school diploma were rated as higher on positive behaviors than were children in the high school or the college groups. Children who lived with a household head in the above-college group did not differ significantly from any other groups.

Families with incomes less than $15,000 were compared to those with incomes higher than $15,000 in the New Hope sample. There were no significant differences associated with family income at Time 1, but at Time 2, children in families with incomes greater than $15,000 were rated higher by parents and teachers.

Table 4. New Hope Project and Panel Study of Income Dynamics: Positive Behavior, by Ethnicity

Measures	African American Mean	SD	Hispanic Mean	SD	White Mean	SD	Others Mean	SD	F
Time 1 Parent Report[1]									
Social competence	4.02	0.51	4.24^a	0.58	4.09^a	0.57	—	—	5.28**
Compliance	3.61	0.59	3.72^a	0.65	3.62^a	0.60	—	—	4.49**
Autonomy	4.31^a	0.52	4.13	0.50	3.89^a	0.54	—	—	5.25**
Total positive behavior	3.95^a	0.45	4.02^b	0.49	3.8^{ab}	0.50	—	—	5.63**
Sample size	315		153		76				
Time 1 Teacher Report[1]									
Social competence	3.55^a	0.72	3.78^a	0.64	3.51	0.64	—	—	5.30**
Compliance	3.48^a	0.78	3.75^a	0.71	3.52	0.71	—	—	4.98**
Autonomy	3.54	0.72	3.55	0.66	3.44	0.67	—	—	0.56
Total positive behavior	3.52^a	0.68	3.72^a	0.65	3.51	0.61	—	—	4.25*
Sample size	240		117		56				
Time 2 Parent Report[1]									
Social competence	3.59^a	0.75	3.7^{ab}	0.68	3.55^b	0.63	—	—	10.58***
Compliance	3.59^a	0.81	3.71^{ab}	0.78	3.55^b	0.74	—	—	8.11***
Autonomy	3.56	0.76	3.53	0.80	3.40	0.68	—	—	0.86
Total positive behavior	3.59^a	0.72	3.67^{ab}	0.68	3.52^b	0.60	—	—	8.20***
Sample size	457		253		108				
Time 2 Teacher Report[1]									
Social competence	3.83	0.52	4.00	0.50	3.79	0.46	—	—	1.73
Compliance	3.62	0.58	3.78	0.67	3.52	0.58	—	—	1.51
Autonomy	4.05	0.62	4.07	0.69	3.98	0.59	—	—	1.23
Total positive behavior	3.81	0.51	3.95	0.55	3.74	0.48	—	—	1.44
Sample size	286		160		77				
Primary Caregiver Report[2]									
Positive behavior	4.24^a	0.57	4.50^{abc}	0.51	4.17^b	0.54	4.23^c	0.50	39.07***
Sample size	454		390		1,747		209		

Note: Dashes indicate that the means were from insufficient sample size. Means in the same row that share superscripts differ at $p < .05$ in the Bonferroni honestly significant difference comparison.
[1]New Hope Project. [2]Panel Study of Income Dynamics.
*$p < .05$. **$p < .01$. ***$p < .001$.

For the PSID sample, four income groups were created using the income-to-needs ratio[17] (Group 1: income-to-needs ratio < 1.0; Group 2: 1.0 <= income-to-needs ratio < 2.0; Group 3: 2.0 <= income-to-needs ratio <= 3.0; Group 4: 3.0

[17] Income to needs is annual family income divided by the federal poverty threshold for that family size and composition.

< income-to-needs ratio). There was a significant relation between income and positive behavior; children in the lowest income group were rated higher than those in other groups.

Summary and Discussion

On the whole, we found the Positive Behavior Scale to be highly reliable. Both the total score and the three subscales have high internal consistency. Parent and teacher reports also indicate moderate stability within contexts over a 3-year period. This stability is particularly striking because the teachers performing the ratings were different, and they were often in different schools. It appears that children's behavior at home and at school remains reasonably consistent over time.

By contrast, social behavior appears to be context specific, a finding that is consistent with other literature. There were weak correlations between parents' and teachers' ratings of children's positive behavior at each time period. Some of the discrepancy may be due to different biases by raters, but some of it probably reflects real differences in behavior as observed by parents and teachers. Children behave differently in different settings. Different settings contain different behavioral requirements, and children adapt their behavior to the environment. For example, at school they may act to gain acceptance from their teachers or peers, whereas at home they may act to gain acceptance from their parents and have their needs met.

Teachers may rate children's positive behavior on the basis of its frequency and their inferences about its possible motives (Eisenberg & Fabes, 1998). Teachers compare children to their classmates, but parents have fewer points of comparison, particularly with children of the same age. Teachers see children in one setting, unlike parents, who see their children in a variety of settings and with a variety of different people.

Parents and teachers may have different expectations and values for children's behavior. For example, parents may focus their expectations on their children getting along with their siblings, being considerate of others, and being happy, all of which are captured by items on the social competence subscale. Teachers may be concerned with their students sticking with their activities until they are finished, waiting their turn, and being prepared for classroom work, all of which are items on the compliance subscale. Teachers' positive behavior ratings were highly correlated with children's achievement and classroom behavior, suggesting that these valued components of school behavior affected their views of children's social qualities. There is also the possibility of a halo effect, given that the teacher ratings of achievement and social behavior are highly correlated.

One question concerns the utility of the subscales. The subscales have relatively high correlations with one another, suggesting that the total score is most useful for many purposes. In fact, it was apparently assumed in the PSID that a subset of the items was sufficient to represent the construct. For some purposes, however, differentiating compliance from autonomy, for example, may yield useful information.

We tested construct validity by examining the relation of positive behavior scores to other characteristics of children as reported by parents, teachers, and children. There was modest evidence for construct validity. Children who were rated high on positive behavior were rated low in problem behavior, particularly externalizing behavior. These associations occurred primarily within raters. That is, parents who rated children high on positive behavior also rated them low on problem behavior. Similarly, teachers' positive behavior ratings were associated with low ratings on behavior problems, but the relations across raters were low. There was evidence, however, that the two measures offered different information; the correlations were not so high that it is reasonable to assume that positive and problem behaviors are mirror images of one another.

Children with positive social behavior skills, particularly compliance, might be expected to perform well in school. In fact, teachers' reports of positive behavior were associated with their perceptions of children's achievement, and parents' reports were less strongly associated with achievement. In the PSID sample, children rated high in positive behavior by their primary caregiver were also rated high in academic competence, physical competence, and social competence by teachers.

Children with good positive behavior skills might also be expected to have more successful relationships with parents and peers and to feel more competent academically. There was little support for this prediction. Children with higher scores on positive behavior (from either parents or teachers) were slightly more likely to report having satisfactory friendships and to report positive relationships with their parents. They did not generally feel more academically competent. These findings suggest that children's own perceptions of their social and academic competence are not highly related to those of either their parents or their teachers. Overall, there was mixed evidence for the construct validity of the measure.

We examined differences among groups based on gender, age, ethnic group, parent education, and family income. On average, girls were rated higher on positive behavior than boys. These gender differences likely reflect societal expectations and are consistent with observational findings. For example, several studies have reported that girls are more likely than boys to comfort, share, and be helpful to others (Feshbach, 1978; Lennon & Eisenberg, 1987; Moore & Eisenberg, 1984; Mussen & Eisenberg, 1977). Gender differences were largest on the compliance subscale and smallest on autonomy, a pattern that is consistent with sex-typed social norms and earlier findings. In an early review of sex differences, Maccoby and Jacklin (1974) concluded that the only consistent observed behavioral difference between boys and girls was on compliance to adults.

Age differences were not clear. There were minimal differences between age groups for parent report and several for teacher report; the patterns were inconsistent in the two samples. Older children were rated less positively than younger ones in New Hope, but more positively in PSID. Whatever the reasons, the absence of large age differences suggests that the measure is useful across a wide age range.

Three ethnic groups were represented in both studies, and consistent patterns of differences associated with ethnic group appeared. In most comparisons, Hispanic children were rated highest and White non-Hispanic children were rated lowest, with African American children falling somewhere in between. These patterns occurred more consistently in parent than in teacher ratings. Although the differences could reflect ethnic differences in standards held by parents or in the tendency to describe one's child in a positive light, their consistency suggests that they are also a valid reflection of group differences. However, there is concern about whether these items measuring "good" social behavior are culturally biased or whether what we are finding reflects true differences between racial and ethnic groups.

Many members of low-income minority communities are concerned about ethnic stereotyping in school, so it is interesting to note that teachers did not manifest negative stereotypes of African American or Hispanic children in comparison to White children. One reason may be familiarity with minority children. The New Hope children attended schools that, in many instances, served large numbers of ethnic minority children. Teachers may have been familiar with the behavior styles of these ethnic groups and may have adapted their expectations accordingly. For example, compliance or autonomy may be manifested somewhat differently for a child from a Hispanic family than for a child from a White family. It is important to note that the ethnic group differences in rating patterns were stable over time.

There were inconsistent differences associated with parent education and income. In New Hope, children from both education groups were rated almost identically by parents both times and by teachers at Time 1. Teachers at Time 2 rated children from higher education families more positively than those from lower education families. A similar pattern occurred for the comparison of lower and higher income families. By contrast, in the PSID, children in families with less than a high school education and those in families living below poverty were rated the highest on positive behaviors by their parents.

The discrepancy could be a result of the differing characteristics of the samples. The New Hope sample lived in one community and had an income constraint; the PSID sample is nationally representative and includes the entire parent education and income ranges of the United States. Most of the differences based on income and education in New Hope appeared in the teacher ratings, and there are no comparable data in PSID. There was some tendency for teachers to perceive children from relatively more advantaged homes more positively than those from homes with very low parent education and income. The differences in the PSID are relatively small. Parents with low levels of education and income may perceive their children more positively, or those with higher levels may be more willing to acknowledge their children's faults. It is also possible that children from low-income families exhibit slightly more positive behaviors at home than do children from families with higher incomes.

In summary, the Positive Behavior Scale is a reliable measure of children's social competence, compliance, and autonomy in home and school settings, at least as they are perceived by important adults in their lives. Individual differences are stable over a long period of time. There is some evidence for validity. The evidence from this scale and similar measures indicates that social behavior and skills are specific to particular environments and settings, suggesting that information should be collected from multiple settings and reporters (including the child) to gain a full understanding of the child's social competence. It might also be possible to improve the usefulness of the scale by adapting it to fit the home and school contexts, yet measure the same constructs. The subscales are highly related, but they represent conceptually distinct constructs that may be useful in some instances.

The patterns of group differences suggest that the scale provides comparable measures across a range of ages, socioeconomic levels, and ethnic groups. Gender differences are possible evidence of validity, given the large literature showing gender differences in observed social behavior. The scale has not been extensively used for samples over the age of 12 years, and more data are needed to extend the scale appropriately for adolescents. More information on its predictive validity for children's social adjustment in school and other settings is also needed.

In conclusion, we recommend that this scale be used to assess positive behavior. It appears worthwhile to include the entire scale with its three subscales whenever possible, but the reduced length 10-item version used in the PSID is reliable and may be adequate for some purposes. Data from two samples, one predominantly from low-income families and one a nationally representative sample, provide consistent evidence that this measure assesses positive behavior, not simply the absence of problem behavior, and is appropriate for parents, teachers, all ethnic backgrounds, and all ages up to about 12 years.

Appendix

Positive Behavior Scale, Parents' Version[a]

---

1. **Social Competence subscales (11 items)**
   The target child:
      a. Is cheerful, happy*
      b. Is warm, loving*
      c. Is curious and exploring, likes new experiences*
      d. Gets along well with other kids*
      e. Can get over being upset quickly*
      f. Is admired and well liked by other kids*
      g. Shows concern for other people's feelings
      h. Is easily calmed when (he/she) gets angry
      i. Is helpful and cooperative
      j. Is considerate and thoughtful of other kids
      k. Tends to give, lend, and share

2. **Autonomy subscales (5 items)**

   The target child:

   l. Does things for (him/her)self, is self-reliant*

   m. Can easily find something to do on (his/her) own

   n. Shows pride when (he/she) does something well or learns something new

   o. Sticks up for (him/her)self, is self-assertive

   p. Is independent, does things (him/her)self

3. **Compliance subscales (9 items)**

   The target child:

   q. Waits his or her turn during activities*

   r. Thinks before he or she acts, is not impulsive*

   s. Usually does what I tell (him/her) to do*

   t. Is able to concentrate or focus on an activity

   u. Is obedient, follows rules

   v. Is calm, easy-going

   w. Sticks with an activity until it is finished

   x. Is eager to please

   y. Is patient when (he/she) wants something

Note: Asterisk indicates item used in the PSID-CDS.

[a] In the teacher version, items are adapted to the school setting.

References

Aber, J. L., & Jones, S. M. (1997). Indicators of positive development in early childhood: Improving concepts and measures. In R. M. Hauser, B. V. Brown, & W. R. Prosser (Eds.), *Indicators of children's well-being* (pp. 395–408).New York: Sage.

Achenbach, T. M., Edelbrock, C., & Howell, C. T. (1987). Empirically based assessment of the behavioral/emotional problems of 2- and 3-year-old children. *Journal of Abnormal Child Psychology, 15,* 629–650.

Cassidy, D., and Asher, S. R. 1992. Loneliness and peer relations in young children. *Child Development, 63,* 350–365.

Eccles (Parsons), J. S. (1983). Expectancies, values, and academic behaviors. In J. T. Spence (Ed.), *Achievement and achievement motives: Psychological and sociological approaches* (pp. 75–146). San Francisco: W. H. Freeman.

Eisenberg, N., & Fabes, R. A. (1998). Prosocial development. In W. Damon (Series ed.) & N. Eisenberg (Vol. Ed.), *Handbook of child psychology: Vol. 3. Social, emotional, and personality development* (pp. 701–778). New York: Wiley.

Eisenberg, N., & Mussen, P. H. (1989). *The roots of prosocial behavior in children.* Cambridge: Cambridge University Press.

Elliot, S. N., & Gresham, F. M. (1987). Children's social skills: Assessment and classification practices. *Journal of Counseling and Development, 66,* 96–99.

Feshbach, N. D. (1978). Studies of empathic behavior in children.In B. A. Mather (Ed.), *Progress in experimental personality research* (Vol. 8, pp. 1–47). New York: Academic Press.

Gresham, F. M., & Elliot, S. N. (1987). The relationship between adaptive behavior and social skills: Issues of definition and assessment. *Journal of Special Education. 21*(1), 167–181.

Gresham, F. M., & Elliot, S. N. (1990). *Social skills rating system manual.* Circle Pines, MN: American Guidance Service.

Hofferth, S. L. (1998). *Report on 1997 data collection for the PSID child development supplement.* Ann Arbor: University of Michigan, Institute for Social Research.

Lennon, R., & Eisenberg, N. (1987). Gender and age differences in empathy and sympathy. In N. Eisenberg & J. Strayer (Eds.), *Empathy and its development* (pp. 195–217). Cambridge: Cambridge University Press.

Maccoby, E. E., & Jacklin, C. (1974). *The psychology of sex differences.* Stanford, CA: Stanford University Press.

McLoyd, V. C., Jayaratne, T. E., Ceballo, R., & Borquez, J. (1994). Unemployment and work interruption among African American single mothers: Effects on parenting and adolescent socioemotional functioning. *Child Development, 65*(2), 562–589.

Moore, B. S., & Eisenberg, N. (1984). The development of altruism. *Annals of Child Development, 1,* 107–174.

Mussen, P., & Eisenberg, N. (1977). *Roots of caring, sharing, and helping: The development of prosocial behavior in children.* San Francisco: W. H. Freeman.

Peterson, J. L., & Zill, N. (1986). Marital disruption, parent-child relationships, and behavioral problems in children. *Journal of Marriage and the Family, 48,* 295–307.

Quint, J. C., Bos, H., &. Polit, D. F. (1997). *New chance: Final report on a comprehensive program for young mothers in poverty and their children.* New York: MDRC.

III   Positive Relationships with Parents and Siblings

12 The Parent–Adolescent Relationship Scale

Elizabeth C. Hair, Kristin Anderson Moore, Sarah B. Garrett, Akemi Kinukawa, Laura H. Lippman, and Erik Michelson

Child Trends

Historically and across diverse cultures, parents have been identified as central influences in the development of their children. Today, despite recent controversy over the role and importance of parents (Harris, 2002), considerable research indicates that the parent–child relationship is important in the lives of infants, children, young adolescents, and teens. Regardless of age, children need parents. Indeed, across multiple studies, it appears that the quality of the parent–child relationship is one of the more important factors in determining what kind of behaviors and attitudes adolescents adopt across domains such as health, education, reproductive behaviors, social interactions, and problem behaviors (Hair, Jager, & Garrett, 2002).

The importance of parents to children's development was briefly the source of considerable controversy in the late 1990s. Harris (2002) argued that the primary influence of parents was genetic. Although she acknowledged that abuse by parents could undermine children's development, she contended that peers are the primary socializing forces in children's lives and that parents could primarily affect their children by influencing the peers with whom the children would interact (Harris, 2002). This contention that parents don't matter energized social scientists, who marshaled a body of evidence illustrating the importance of parents (Collins, Maccoby, Steinberg, Hetherington, & Bornstein, 2000). To summarize the handful of existing high-quality, multivariate studies available, research shows that quality parent–teen relationships are linked to a wide range of positive outcomes, such as mental and emotional well-being, adjustment, and social competence, and to decreased problem behaviors such as substance use, delinquency, and sexual activity (Borkowsky, Ramey, & Bristol-Power, 2002; Hair et al., 2002).

Mental and emotional well-being in adolescence has been associated with quality parent–adolescent relationships. For instance, recent cross-sectional research among youth in grades 7–12 has found that high parent–family connectedness is predictive of decreased emotional distress and suicidality in adolescents (Resnick et al., 1997). This finding is paired with evidence that suggests that child reports of enjoyment of shared activities with parents, the presence of parents at home during the day (e.g., at waking, after school, at dinner, or at bedtime), and high parental expectations for children's school achievement are moderately protective against emotional distress for both younger and older adolescents (Resnick et al., 1997). Similarly, in a longitudinal study of parents and adolescents, high levels of parental support were related to affection for parents, consensus with parents, dating happiness, feelings of community attachment, low psychological distress, happiness, life satisfaction, and an array of other positive outcomes (Amato & Booth, 1997).

The development of social competence and adjustment also appears to be related to high-quality parent–adolescent relationships (Hair et al., 2002). Longitudinal research by Barber and Erickson (2001) shows a supportive parent–child relationship to be the primary family-level predictor of social initiative, a component of social competence, in older teens (14–17 years old); parental support was also indirectly related to social initiative in younger teens. The parent–adolescent relationship is directly associated with self-confidence, empathy, a cooperative personality (Barber & Erickson; Hair et al., 2002), psychological well-being (Franz, McClelland, & Weinberger, 1991), self-reliance, flexibility, positive social orientation, ego resilience, and competent interaction styles in all relationships (Engels, Finkenauer, Meeus, & Dekovic, 2001; Kerns & Stevens, 1996; Zahn-Waxler & Smith, 1992).

The parent–child relationship also appears to be related to positive teen behaviors and outcomes in the academic setting. For instance, lower levels of dropping out of high school have been associated with early mother–adolescent attachment in an all-White population (Garnier & Stein, 1998). In addition, parental involvement and connection with older teens (14–18 years old) predicted higher grades and higher academic expectations (Herman, Dornbusch, Herron, & Herting, 1997).

Problem behaviors, such as school suspensions, delinquent acts, and violent crime, have also been linked to the quality of the parent–child relationship. For instance, longitudinal research in an all-White high school sample suggests that lower levels of parental support are linked with higher levels of adolescent deviant behavior and lower levels of "socially approved, normatively expected" behaviors, such as church involvement and academic achievement (Jessor & Jessor, 1975). Furthermore, a study of more than 12,000 teenagers found a link between a positive parent–child relationship and committing fewer violent behaviors, for both older and younger teens (Blum & Rinehart, 1997; Resnick et al., 1997). Studies of specific populations have supported this pattern, as well. For example, a large sample of mostly Mormon teens showed a link between warm and supportive mother–adolescent relationships and less teen involvement in problem behaviors (Bahr, Maughan, Marcos, & Li, 1998). In the context of adolescent development, problem behaviors, such as violent and deviant acts, are widely viewed as harmful in and of themselves. Such behaviors can also be harmful in the context of the consequences they may bring about, such as school suspensions, expulsions, and poor peer relations (Capaldi & Stoolmiller, 1999; Rodney, Crafter, Rodney, & Mupier, 1999).

Perhaps the most studied outcomes in regard to the parent–adolescent relationship are those concerning alcohol, tobacco, and drug use. The direction of causality, however, is not always clear and may well be bidirectional. Also, some studies do not control for important confounding influences. Nevertheless, multivariate longitudinal studies do find an association. Several studies have revealed that positive relationships or connectedness between parents and adolescent is associated with lower levels of use, or nonuse, of all three of the substances listed above (Blum & Rinehart, 1997; Hundleby & Mercer, 1987; Resnick et al., 1997). The majority of the studies, however, appear to have focused on only one substance-related outcome.

For example, a relationship between positive parent–youth relationships and lower levels of drug use has been found. Attachment between parents and adolescents has been associated with the nonuse of drugs in older teens (Brook, Brook, Gordon, Whiteman, & Cohen, 1989); a quality relationship with parents has been associated with less involvement with drugs and decreased influence of drug-using peers in a White and Hispanic population (Coombs, Paulson, & Richardson, 1991); positive teen–parent relationships have been linked with less drug use in a largely Mormon sample (Bahr et al., 1998); and distress in the mother–adolescent relationship in fatherless homes appears to be related to higher rates of 10th-grader drug use (Farrell & White, 1998).

Precocious sexual activity is another problem behavior that the quality of the parent–adolescent relationship appears to affect (Manlove, Terry-Humen, Romano Papillo, Franzetta, & Ryan, 2002). For instance, adolescents who have high-quality relationships with their parent are less likely to initiate sex or be sexually active (Miller, 1998). If pregnant, teens with quality parent–child relationships have better reproductive health outcomes (Miller, Sabo, Farrell, Barnes, & Melnick, 1998). In analyses of data from the National Longitudinal Study of Adolescent Health (Add Health), parent–adolescent connectedness has been associated with delayed sexual intercourse (Blum & Rinehart, 1997; Resnick et al., 1997); similarly, research on 13- to 18-year-old youth has linked poor-quality parent–child relationships to increased sexual activity for females (Whitbeck, Hoyt, Miller, & Kao, 1992). Finally, research by Jessor and Jessor (1975) suggests that a lack of parental support is linked in high schoolers to the development of characteristics, such as greater deviance, that would lead to sexual activity.

In summary, the quality of the parent–adolescent relationship appears to be associated with fewer negative or problem behaviors and with more positive outcomes, such as academic achievement and social competence. These relationships, however, are not valuable only for these related effects: a high-quality relationship between a teen and his or her parent is a positive and important outcome in itself. Studies consistently find that having a happy family life is a highly rated priority of adolescents and adults.

Measures of Parent–Adolescent Relationships

The quality of the parent–adolescent relationship can be described in many different ways (DeCato, Donohue, Azrin, Teichner, & Crum, 2002). Researchers have discussed it in terms of parent–child attachment, connectedness, degree of communication on key issues, and warmth or affection in the relationship. DeCato and colleagues conducted an in-depth review of a number of available measures to assess satisfaction with the relationship between parents and youth. Their review initially yielded more than 75 different types of measures that included self-reports, rating scales, structured clinical interviews, open-ended questions, projective instruments, Q-sorts, and observational coding schemes. Of these, they reviewed 20 instruments that met the needs of the project on indicators of positive child outcomes: They were closed-ended, self-report scales; they focused on the satisfaction of the relationship between a specific youth and parent or included subscales that measured satisfaction with the parent–adolescent relationship; and they were developed and used with preadolescents (10–12 years old), adolescents (13–17 years old), or parents of preadolescents and adolescents. Of the 20 instruments, only 5 collected information from the perspective of the adolescent. These included the Adolescent's Perception of Deprivation–Satisfaction Scale (Rushing, 1964), Child–Parent Relationship Scale (Swanson, 1950), Index of Child's Perceptions of Parent's Dissatisfaction (Farber & Jenne, 1963), Parental Control Measure (Prinz, Foster, Kent, & O'Leary, 1979), and Youth Happiness with Parent Scale (DeCato, Donohue, Azrin, & Teichner, 2001).

The DeCato et al. (2002) review presented detailed information on each of these five measures. To summarize, the authors noted that the Adolescent's Perception of Deprivation–Satisfaction Scale was easy to understand; however, it did not have tested psychometric properties, and it required that the adolescents have siblings and relationships with both parents in order to respond to the measure. In addition, the DeCato review reported that the questions may be outdated for today's youth. For the Child–Parent Relationship Scale, the authors concluded that the scale did an adequate job of measuring global satisfaction with the parent–youth relationship. However, its psychometric properties had not been demonstrated in a current sample, and its questions may not be relevant to today's youth. The Index of Child's Perceptions of Parent's Dissatisfaction evaluated a youth's perceptions of parental satisfaction with him or her in several key areas, such as curfew, schoolwork, and chores. It did not, however, assess youths' satisfaction with their parents' behavior. Also, important for our purposes, it does not assess parent–child relationships, and psychometric properties for the measure were not provided. The largest drawback to the fourth measure in the DeCato review, parental control, is its singular focus on parental discipline without attention to any other aspect of the parent–youth relationship. The fifth scale, the Youth Happiness with Parent Scale (YHPS), demonstrated adequate psychometric properties in a sample of conduct-disordered youth (Cronbach's alpha = .78), and was correlated positively with the youths' overall happiness with their parents and negatively with the youths' problem behaviors. Additionally, the 11-item scale attempts to measure multiple aspects of the parent–adolescent relationship (e.g., communication, friends and activities, curfew, household rules, schoolwork, rewards, discipline, chores, alcohol and drugs, illicit behaviors, as well as overall happiness). The major weakness is that the YHPS has only been evaluated and used in a clinical sample of behaviorally disordered and substance-abusing male youth.

Add Health uses a self-report measure of four items for the quality of the parent–adolescent relationship (Resnick et al., 1997). This measure has demonstrated high internal consistency (Cronbach's alpha = .83). On the negative side, the items are all very general in nature (e.g., "How close do you feel towards your mother/father?" "How much do you feel your mother/father cares about you?" "How satisfied are you with your relationship with your mother/father?" "To what degree do you feel loved and wanted by family members?") and do not evaluate any specific behaviors between the youth and the parent. There is some indication that this measure does not distinguish among specific demographic characteristics, such as race, as expected. It also appears to be highly skewed (U.S. Department of Health and Human Services: Office of the Assistant Secretary for Planning and Evaluation, 2001).

The measure we selected for this study, from the National Longitudinal Survey of Youth, 1997 cohort (NLSY97), is designed to tap into both the global aspects of the parent–youth relationships, such as identification with the parent (e.g., "I think highly of him/her"), as well as whether the youth feels supported by the parent (e.g., "How often does s/he criticize you or your ideas?").

Method

In this study, we analyzed data from the NLSY97, which collects information over time from a nationally representative sample of adolescents ($N = 8,984$) age 12–16 years in 1997. The survey is funded by the Bureau of Labor Statistics of the U.S. Department of Labor, and is intended to examine school progress, labor force behavior, and the transition from school to work. The NLSY97 also collects information on a broad array of child and family interactions and relationships. Data are collected annually from youth; in Round 1 (1997) they were also collected from one parent or parent figure. Our study uses data from Round 1 (1997) for the parent–adolescent relationship scales. Data from Rounds 2 and 3 (1998, 1999) are used to examine the stability of the parent–youth relationship. Finally, youth outcome measures are drawn from Round 4 (2000) data.

Sample

We focus on the respondents who were ages 12 (31.9%), 13 (34.3%), and 14 (33.8%) at the end of 1996 ($n = 4,724$), these being the ages that received the full battery of questions on the parent–child relationship. For those households that had more than one youth respondent ($n = 656$), a single respondent was randomly selected for analysis. Our final analytic sample is 4,548 youth. Just over 50% of the respondents were White, 25% African American, 21% Hispanic, and 3% of another racial/ethnic background. Fifty-one percent of the sample was male. Participants represent a range of socioeconomic status. Nearly 17% of family incomes were below 100% of the poverty threshold, 16% were at 100%–200% of the threshold, 25% at 200%–400% of the threshold, and 16% at 400% of the threshold or greater. However, almost 26% of respondents had missing data on income. The majority of respondents lived with two biological parents (50%) or a single biological parent (31%). Smaller percentages lived with a biological parent and an unrelated parent figure (13%), or in "other" family structures (5%).

Measure of Parent–Child Relationship

Eight questions were employed to investigate the parent–adolescent relationship. Some of the questions were adapted from items developed for the Iowa Youth and Families Project, a study of the relationship between economic hardships, psychological well-being, and family relations in rural farm families (Conger & Elder, 1994). Other questions are from the National Survey of Children. Respondents received these items and other questions in the form of a self-administered, laptop computer–based questionnaire. On average, it took 13.41 seconds to answer each question about the relationship with the mother and 10.99 seconds for each question about the relationship with the father. The first three questions addressed the youth's identification with the parent(s); responses were measured on a 5-point Likert scale ranging from *strongly disagree* to *strongly agree*. The subsequent five questions addressed perceived parental supportiveness; responses were measured on a 5-point Likert scale, ranging from *never* to *always*. Each question was coded from 0 to 4 points. These items were not subject to formal cognitive pretesting for the NLSY97.

Together, these eight items provide a broad perspective on the parent–adolescent relationship. The eight-item scale includes all parent–child relationship measures asked in the survey (see Appendix). The three-item scale uses the identification items; the five-item scale complements the three-item scale, using the remaining five items that assess supportiveness and behavior.[1] The four-item scale uses the four items with the largest loadings on a factor analysis of the eight-item scale. This scale includes two questions from the three identification items and two questions from the five supportiveness items. We analyzed all four different variations on the parent–child relationship scale. For the purposes of this study, however, we will focus on two: the eight- and four-item versions. These scales differ from the five- and three-item versions in that they comprise both identity and behavior items. It is also worth noting that in the abbreviated four-item version, all items measure behaviors or attitudes

---

[1] For more information on the five- and three-item scales, contact the authors.

that are positive in nature (e.g., helping youth with things that are important to him/her).

For both scales, scores were calculated for respondents who answered at least 75% of the items. In the case of missing responses on, at most, 25% of the items, raw scores were weighted as follows: raw score × ([# of total items]/[# of total items − # items missing]); for example, the score of a respondent who missed two questions on the eight-item scale would be (raw score) × (8/[8 − 2]). This procedure assigns to the missing responses the respondent's average response across the questions answered. The small percentage of respondents who answered fewer than 75% of the items on a given scale were coded as missing on that scale.

We limit our analyses to the measure for residential parents since the missing data on nonresidential parents are quite high owing to a skip-pattern problem in the questionnaire.

Cut Point

To establish an indicator of quality parent–child relationships, a reasonable cut point needed to be created. For the parent–child relationship scale, previous analyses and clinical validity work are not available. Consequently, other criteria were used to develop a cut point. The possible range of scores for the eight-item version was 0 to 32; the possible range for the four-item scale was 0 to 16. In determining the cut point for a quality relationship, we decided that a youth would need to respond, on average, with a 3 on the 4-point response options to be characterized as having a high-quality relationship with his or her parent. A 3 on the identification items corresponds to a response of *agree*. The same score corresponds to *usually* on the five supportiveness items. This would translate to a value of 24 on the eight-item scale, and a value of 12 on the four-item scale.

It is, of course, possible to achieve these scales' values in a variety of ways. Some of the possibilities include a combination of very high scores and a 0, which would suggest rather mixed feelings or, possibly, random responses. To explore such possibilities, we examined the response patterns of youth with scores between 22 and 26 on the eight-item scale. Over 47% of the youth who scored a 24 on the relationship scale answered "3" to at least half of the items, and another 23% of the youth answered "4" to over half of the items. In addition, around 85% of the youth who scored 24 did not answer "0" to any of the questions. In contrast, for those youth who scored 23, only 31% answered "3" to at least half of the items, only 4% answered "4" to over half of the items, and over 21% answered "0" to at least one question. Accordingly, a cutoff of 24 seemed appropriate.

Procedures

We employed two procedures to examine the general data quality of the relationship scale. First, we examined the distribution of the responses to confirm that there was variation. It was anticipated that the distribution of responses would be positively skewed. Second, we examined the level of nonresponse or missing data on both versions of the scale

We employed Cronbach's alpha to test the internal consistency of the items that comprise the scale. A higher level on the alpha indicates that the scale items hang together well in a given administration (Carmines & Zeller, 1985). Reliability was examined for both scale versions. Internal reliabilities greater than .70 are considered adequate.

We examined demographic patterns, construct validity, and prospective validity to test the overall validity of the relationship scale. To examine the demographic patterns, we looked at the percentage of youth who reported a positive relationship with their parents by several categories, including age, gender, and family structure. For construct validity, we examined whether another measure of the parent–adolescent relationship was related to the relationship scales through zero-order correlations and regression models with demographic controls. To investigate prospective validity, we first examined how the mean of the scale functioned over time for each relationship scale. Then we tested whether the parent–adolescent relationship scales predicted, as expected based on the research literature, outcomes for youth 4 years later. These analyses were conducted for both versions of the scale.

Results

We found substantial variation in the distribution of scores for the eight-item mother–adolescent relationship scale, though there was, as expected, a concentration of higher scores (indicating more positive relationships). The same tendency was found with the eight-item scale for the adolescent's relationship with the father. There was also variation in the four-item version of the scale, with scores across the full range of the scale and some concentration on the higher end of the scale. The values for skewness for the mother–adolescent scales were negative for both versions (e.g., -0.94 for the eight-item scale, -0.85 for the four-item version), indicating distributions somewhat skewed toward higher scores. For the father–adolescent relationship scales, the level of skewness remained about the same for both versions of the scale (e.g., -1.00 for the eight-item scale, -0.83 for the four-item version). The four-item version and the eight-item version of the scale had similar skewness and kurtosis values.

The level of nonresponse was very low for the mother–adolescent relationship scale. The questions should have been asked of all youth living with their biological mother ($n = 4{,}214$) or mother figure ($n = 334$). The scores for the eight-item scale were missing for only two respondents: one youth declined to answer all of the eight items, and one declined to answer three of the eight items and was therefore eliminated according to our convention requiring responses on at least 75% of the items. Additionally, nine respondents received weighted scores on the eight-item scale because they did not respond to either one or two of the eight items for the scale. Three respondents received weighted scores on the four-item scale because they did not respond to one item of the four.

The number of missing responses was also very low for the father–adolescent relationship scale. From our sample, youth living with a father ($n = 2,738$) or father figure ($n = 713$) should have answered the questions. The "father figure" category included individuals such as stepfathers and cohabiting partners of the mother or mother figure. The eight-item scale score is missing for only one respondent because this youth answered "don't know" to four out of eight questions. Ten respondents received weighted scores on the eight-item scale because they did not respond to either one or two of the eight items. Similarly, six respondents received weighted scores for the four-item scale.

Reliability

Most versions of the relationship-with-resident-mother scale were found to have an acceptable level of internal consistency, with Cronbach's alpha ranging from .72 to .74. The level of internal consistency for the relationship with resident father scale was generally high, with a Cronbach's alpha of .82.

The reliability of the scales was also examined across demographic characteristics. The internal consistency of both the mother and father scales tended to be higher for females than for males. The level of internal consistency also increased with the age of the adolescent. For the race/ethnicity subgroups, the internal consistency of the mother and father scales was lower for non-Hispanic Black and Hispanic youth than for youth of other race/ethnicity groups.

We also conducted a factor analysis on the eight items included in the longest version of the scale. For the whole sample, as well as for each race/ethnicity and socioeconomic group, all items grouped into a single factor. It should be noted, however, that two variables that tapped into the negative side of the parent–youth relationship (i.e., parent criticizes youth's ideas, parent makes and cancels plans with the youth) consistently had factor loadings less than .30, the lowest among the eight items. These two items and two other items with relatively low loadings were dropped to create the four-item scale.

Demographic Patterns

The demographic patterns for our relationship scale functioned as we expected (Table 1). For the eight-item version of the scale, the percentage of youth reporting positive relationships with their parents decreased among older adolescents. In addition, a higher percentage of girls than boys rated their relationships with their mothers as positive; likewise, a higher percentage of boys than girls rated their relationships with their fathers as positive. Furthermore, a higher percentage of positive relationships were reported in families with two biological parents present. A similar pattern was found for the four-item version of the scale.

Table 1. Percentage of Youth, Ages 12–14, Who Reported Positive Relationships with Their Residential Mother and/or Father in 1997, by Child and Family Characteristics[a]

	8-item scale		4-item scale	
Characteristic	Resident mother	Resident father	Resident mother	Resident father
Age as of 12/31/96				
12	76.07	70.75	69.42	62.95
13	69.16	64.41	60.62	56.41
14	65.02	59.97	58.89	52.68
Race				
White	71.35	67.05	63.31	58.81
Black	68.75	57.84	63.55	49.79
Hispanic	67.77	63.17	62.21	57.34
Other race	62.76	58.50	58.39	54.46
Gender				
Male	68.69	68.19	60.02	61.79
Female	71.51	61.79	66.00	52.70
Poverty[b]				
Missing information	70.20	63.44	62.69	56.63
0–99%	67.43	55.50	60.73	47.86
100–199%	66.48	58.64	62.31	48.23
200–399%	71.77	67.83	64.34	61.09
400% or more	71.76	70.36	63.19	62.04
Family Structure				
Two parents: 1 biological/1 other	67.04	49.77	60.09	42.84
Single parent/other	65.73	61.82	59.91	54.48
Two parents: 2 biological	73.21	69.35	65.41	61.48
Parental education				
Less than HS degree	65.52	59.43	59.52	53.73
HS degree, some college	69.61	62.95	62.79	55.52
College degree or higher	72.85	70.55	64.71	61.78

Note: All original analyses of the National Longitudinal Survey of Youth 1997 (U.S. Department of Labor, Bureau of Labor Statistics) conducted by Child Trends.
[a] "Positive" relationship was defined as a score of 24 or greater on the 8-item relationship scale (range: 0–32), and as a score of 12 or greater on the 4-item relationship scale (range: 0–16).
[b] About 26% of respondents in this age group are missing information for poverty level.

Validity

The self-administered questionnaire of NLSY97 features a question that tapped into the construct of the parent–adolescent relationship but that we did not include in our eight-item scale. It was a single youth-report item about the parent figure: "When you think about how s/he acts towards you, in general, would you say that s/he is very supportive, somewhat supportive, or not very supportive?" With this item, we assessed the construct validity of the parent–adolescent relationship scale using two methods.

First, we employed simple zero-order correlations to examine the association between the single-item measure and our longer parent–adolescent relationship scales. All of the zero-order correlations were in the expected direction and were statistically significant. The correlations were relatively strong for both the mother and the father versions of the eight-item scale (.55 and .63, respectively). The four-item scales have similar correlations (.53 and .62, respectively).

In addition, we ran regression models where the one-item supportiveness measure predicted the scale versions of the parent–adolescent relationship. For each model, we controlled for a standard set of demographic characteristics that included the youth's age, gender, race/ethnicity, as well as socioeconomic status, family structure, and parental education. Even after controlling for demographic characteristics, the one-item supportiveness measure was the strongest predictor of the different scales of the parent–adolescent relationship, with most of the standardized betas between .50 and .61. These analyses followed a pattern similar to the zero-order correlations; the eight- and four-item versions for both the mother and father relationships were predicted well by the single item.

As expected, the mean score on the relationship scale decreased between 1997 and 1999 for each relationship type (e.g., on the eight-item scale, from 25.15 to 24.44 for the mother–adolescent relationship) and for each version of the scale (e.g., on the four-item scale, from 12.07 to 11.67 for the mother–adolescent relationship). Adolescents rated their relationships with their parents as more positive in 1997 than they did in the subsequent rounds of the survey. The proportion of the sample that reported having positive relationships with their parents also declined. On the eight-item scale, reports of a positive relationship with the residential mother fell from almost 70% of the sample in 1997 to just over 53% in 1999; reports of a positive relationship with the residential father fell from almost 64% to 46.5% in the same period. A similar pattern emerged for the four-item scale: reports declined from about 63% to 48% of the sample for positive mother-youth relationships, and about 56% to 40% for positive father–youth relationships in the same time period. Because we expected this decline over time in the quality of the relationships and because relationship quality measurements were made more than a year apart, we did not conduct test–retest reliability analyses.

Descriptive statistics showed the percentage of youth who would be characterized as having positive relationships with their parents for each scale (as determined by the cut point) across the years. In 1997, the eight-item scale demonstrated that slightly less than 70% of the youth reported having positive relationships with their mothers and/or fathers; the four-item scale provided a stricter estimate (63%). A similar pattern was found in 1998 (57% vs. 50% for mothers, 49% vs. 42% for fathers, respectively) and 1999 (53% vs. 48% for mothers, 46.5% vs. 40% for fathers, respectively).

In assessing the predictive validity of the relationship scales, we ran logistic regressions in which a positive parent–adolescent relationship (as defined by the cutoff variable) in 1997 was the predictor. Youth outcomes (reported in 2000) of delinquency, substance use, sexual activity, and school suspensions, and good grades in eighth grade were the dependent variables. For each model, we controlled for our standard set of demographic characteristics, described above. We also included a variable reporting on past behaviors as a control for each problem behavior outcome (e.g., for use in the delinquency models we employed 1997 reports of having committed delinquent acts).

As expected, a positive mother– or father–adolescent relationship in 1997, as measured by the eight-item scale, consistently predicted less delinquency, less sexual activity, fewer suspensions, and better grades, net of demographic control variables and a past behavior control (when available). The eight-item scale did not predict less substance use (Table 2). For the four-item scale, a positive mother–adolescent relationship predicted all outcomes except less substance use. The four-item positive father–adolescent relationship scale predicted less delinquency and sex, and higher grades, but did not significantly predict fewer suspensions or less substance use (Table 3). In all cases, the direction of the prediction was in the expected direction: Positive relationships with parents were related to less delinquency, sexual activity, and suspensions, and to higher academic grades.

To further test the predictive validity of the scales, we ran each logistic model for specific demographic subgroups (e.g., regarding race/ethnicity, poverty, and gender). In examining the odds ratios[2] for each racial/ethnic group, it was apparent that both versions of the parent–adolescent relationship scales consistently produced significant associations within the sample of White adolescents (Table 4). This was especially true in regard to the mother–adolescent relationship scale. On the other hand, there were only sporadic significant associations for the Black and Hispanic adolescent samples. However, the directions of the odds ratios (e.g., fewer behavior problems, less sexual activity, and better grades) followed a pattern similar to those of the White sample.

The same basic pattern was found for poverty level (Table 5). The odds ratios for the sample of adolescents above the poverty threshold were consistently significant; however, few significant associations were found for the sample below the poverty threshold. Although the odd ratios for adolescents in families below the poverty threshold were not significant, their directions followed the expected pattern of association with fewer behavior problems and better grades.

In contrast, considering gender subgroups, most versions of the relationship-with-mother scales produced significant associations for both male and female adolescents (Table 6). For instance, positive relationships with mothers were related to less delinquency and sexual activity, fewer suspensions, and better grades for both genders. However, positive relationships with fathers seemed to work best in the female adolescent sample. Positive relationships between female adolescents and fathers were related to lower levels of delinquency, sexual activity, and suspensions, and to better grades. For male adolescents, only sporadic significant findings were present.

---

[2] With odds ratios, values greater than 1 represent a positive association, values less than 1 indicate a negative association, and values equal to 1 show no association.

Table 2. Logistic Regressions of 8-Item Resident Parent–Youth Relationship in Regard to Round 4 Outcomes

Variable	Delinquency		Substance use		Sexual activity		Suspensions		Good grades	
	Mother	Father	Mother	Father	Mother	Father	Mother	Father	Mother	Father
Age as of 12/31/96	0.7***	0.81***	1.26***	1.29***	1.70***	1.69***	0.80**	0.86+	1.12*	1.09
Gender: Male	0.82+	1.93***	0.87*	0.87+	0.95	1.02	2.43***	2.48***	0.45***	0.41***
Race										
Black	0.75**	0.79+	0.40***	0.45***	1.25*	1.27+	1.00	0.71	0.41***	0.43***
Hispanic	0.82+	0.93	0.77*	0.83	0.87	0.93	0.55***	0.57*	0.72*	0.81
Other race	0.66*	0.66*	0.58***	0.54***	0.61*	0.48***	0.87	1.07	1.19	1.56*
White	1.00	1.00	1.00	1.00	1.00	1.00	1.00	1.00	1.00	1.00
Poverty										
Missing information[a]	1.07	1.06	1.01	0.94	1.07	1.04	1.01	0.83	1.07	1.10
0–99%	1.23	0.94	0.93	0.72*	1.29+	1.07	1.02	1.45	0.75	0.94
100–199%	1.08	0.97	0.84	0.75*	1.29*	1.21	1.00	1.10	0.86	0.97
200–399%	1.10	1.10	0.89	0.88	1.11	1.12	0.81	0.79	0.97	1.09
400% or more	1.00	1.00	1.00	1.00	1.00	1.00	1.00	1.00	1.00	1.00
Family Structure										
Two parents: 1 biological/ 1 other	1.43***	1.46***	1.41**	1.46***	1.71***	1.56***	1.53*	1.33	0.39***	0.44***
Single parent/other	1.30**	1.63***	1.36***	1.45***	1.63***	2.06***	1.24	1.56*	0.59***	0.64**
Two parents: 2 biological	1.00	1.00	1.00	1.00	1.00	1.00	1.00	1.00	1.00	1.00
Parental Education[b]										
Less than HS degree	1.00	1.00	1.00	1.00	1.00	1.00	1.00	1.00	1.00	1.00
HS degree, some college	0.95	0.90	1.22+	1.18	0.77*	0.74*	0.68*	1.00	2.24***	2.13***
College degree or higher	1.01	0.94	1.40*	1.37*	0.49***	0.49***	0.37***	0.54*	5.51***	5.35***
Past Behaviors										
1997 or earlier control	2.70***	2.77***	4.00***	4.12***	1.66***	1.67***	3.00***	3.77***	—	—
Resident Parent–Youth Relationship										
Positive relationship[c]	0.68***	0.76**	0.93	0.95	0.74***	0.77**	0.60***	0.67**	1.47***	1.71***
Chi-square	390.05***	324.48***	605.64***	482.33***	496.29***	372.33***	251.85***	217.34***	506.91***	407.04***
DF	15	15	15	15	15	15	15	15	14	14
N	4,181	3,177	4,177	3,171	4,135	3,142	3,956	3,027	4,415	3,364

Note: These data are from the National Longitudinal Survey of Youth 1997, consisting of young men and women who were ages 12 to 14 on December 31, 1996. All original analyses of the National Longitudinal Survey of Youth 1997 (U.S. Department of Labor, Bureau of Labor Statistics) conducted by Child Trends.
[a] Missing refers to 25%–26% of the sample.
[b] In the case of two-parent families, parental education refers to the parent with the highest level of education.
[c] Positive relationship for the 8-item scale is defined as a score of 24 or greater (out of 32 points).
+ p < 0.1. * p < .05. ** p < .01. *** p < .001.

Table 3. Logistic Regressions of 4-Item Resident Parent–Youth Relationship in Regard to Round 4 Outcomes

Variable	Delinquency		Substance use		Sexual activity		Suspensions		Good grades	
	Mother	Father	Mother	Father	Mother	Father	Mother	Father	Mother	Father
Age as of 12/31/96	0.78***	0.82***	1.26***	1.29***	1.70***	1.69***	0.81**	0.88	1.13*	1.09
Gender: Male	1.74***	1.92***	0.87*	0.88+	0.95	1.03	2.39***	2.44***	0.46***	0.40***
Race										
Black	0.75**	0.79+	0.40***	0.45***	1.25*	1.28+	1.00	0.71	0.41***	0.42***
Hispanic	0.83	0.93	0.77*	0.83	0.88	0.93	0.56**	0.58*	0.71*	0.81
Other race	0.67	0.68*	0.59***	0.54***	0.62**	0.49***	0.89	1.09	1.18	1.52*
White	1.00	1.00	1.00	1.00	1.00	1.00	1.00	1.00	1.00	1.00
Poverty										
Missing information[a]	1.06	1.06	1.01	0.95	1.07	1.04	1.01	0.84	1.07	1.10
0–99%	1.22	0.94	0.93	0.72+	1.29+	1.07	1.01	1.48	0.75	0.95
100–199%	1.09	0.96	0.84	0.75*	1.30*	1.20	1.03	1.10	0.85	1.00
200–399%	1.10	1.10	0.89	0.88	1.11	1.12	0.81	0.80	0.96	1.08
400% or more	1.00	1.00	1.00	1.00	1.00	1.00	1.00	1.00	1.00	1.00
Family Structure										
Two parents: 1 biological/1 other	1.44***	1.48***	1.41**	1.47***	1.72***	1.57***	1.53*	1.37+	0.39***	0.43***
Single parent/other	1.32**	1.62***	1.37***	1.45**	1.64***	2.06***	1.25	1.55*	0.60***	0.64**
Two parents: 2 biological	1.00	1.00	1.00	1.00	1.00	1.00	1.00	1.00	1.00	1.00
Parental Education[b]										
Less than HS degree	1.00	1.00	1.00	1.00	1.00	1.00	1.00	1.00	1.00	1.00
HS degree, some college	0.95	0.89	1.22+	1.18	0.77*	0.74*	0.68*	1.00	2.23***	2.15***
College degree or higher	1.01	0.93	1.40*	1.37*	0.49***	0.49***	0.37***	0.53*	5.50***	5.45***
Past Behaviors										
1997 or earlier control	2.73***	2.80***	4.02***	4.12***	1.67***	1.66***	3.07***	3.81***	—	—
Resident Parent–Youth Relationship										
Positive relationship[c]	0.72***	0.81*	0.96	0.96	0.79***	0.78**	0.70**	0.82	1.65***	1.71***
Chi-square	384.27***	320.41***	605.02***	482.28***	490.68***	372.46***	243.77***	211.47***	522.58***	411.35***
DF	15	15	15	15	15	15	15	15	14	14
N	4,181	3,177	4,177	3,171	4,135	3,142	3,956	3,027	4,415	3,364

Note: These data are from the National Longitudinal Survey of Youth 1997, consisting of young men and women who were ages 12 to 14 on December 31, 1996. All original analyses of the National Longitudinal Survey of Youth 1997 (U.S. Department of Labor, Bureau of Labor Statistics) conducted by Child Trends.

[a] Missing refers to 25%–26% of the sample.

[b] In the case of two-parent families, *parental education* refers to the parent with the highest level of education.

[c] Positive relationship for the 4-item scale is defined as a score of 12 or greater (out of 16 points).

+$p < 0.1$. *$p < .05$. **$p < .01$. ***$p < .001$.

Table 4. Odds Ratios of Parent–Youth Relationship by Race/Ethnicity with Demographic and Past Behavior Controls[a]

	Delinquency		Substance use		Sexual activity		Suspensions		Good grades	
Scale version	Mom	Dad	Mom	Dad	Mom	Dad	Mom	Dad	Mom	Dad
White										
8-item	0.71***	0.83+	0.87	1.02	0.67***	0.76**	0.55***	0.62**	1.50***	1.73***
4-item	0.77**	0.83+	1.10	0.99	0.76**	0.77**	0.65**	0.78	1.66***	1.71***
n	2094	1779	2091	1775	2076	1760	1998	1708	2212	1889
Black										
8-item	0.67*	0.53*	0.97	0.74	1.10	0.85	0.60+	0.77	1.20	1.92
4-item	0.64*	0.77	0.56***	0.97	0.87	0.74	0.73	0.71	1.27	1.71
n	1,058	595	1,057	594	1,036	582	997	564	1,106	625
Hispanic										
8-item	0.46***	0.60*	1.15	0.85	0.75	0.79	0.96	0.85	2.19*	2.37*
4-item	0.47***	0.70	1.06	0.69+	0.70+	0.76	0.89	1.31	2.26*	2.10*
n	876	665	877	665	871	662	814	623	936	704

Note: All original analyses of the National Longitudinal Survey of Youth 1997 (U.S. Department of Labor, Bureau of Labor Statistics) conducted by Child Trends. Data are for individuals who were ages 12–14 years on December 31, 1996.
[a] Controls include child (age, gender, race, past behaviors related to measured outcomes) and family characteristics (SES, parental education, family structure).
$+p < 0.1.$ $*p < .05.$ $**p < .01.$ $***p < .001.$

Summary and Discussion

The four- and eight-item versions of the parent–adolescent relationship scale generally exhibit excellent data quality. Also, they demonstrate variability in the distribution of responses: Not all youth rated their parents positively. Furthermore, the two versions of the scale had quite similar skewness and kurtosis values, and each had very little missing data. This finding suggests that young adolescents were able and willing to answer questions about the quality of their

Table 5. Odds Ratios of the Parent–Youth Relationship Variable by Poverty Level with Demographic and Past Behavior Controls[a]

	Delinquency		Substance use		Sexual activity		Suspensions		Good grades	
Scale version	Mom	Dad	Mom	Dad	Mom	Dad	Mom	Dad	Mom	Dad
Below 100%										
8-item	0.48**	0.77	1.04	1.05	0.65*	0.62+	0.69	0.46*	1.41	1.57
4-item	0.74	0.86	1.11	1.19	0.61*	0.63+	1.48	0.91	1.24	0.77
n	687	357	686	356	678	354	611	316	722	377
Above 100%										
8-item	0.71***	0.75**	0.90	0.93	0.75***	0.78**	0.57***	0.71*	1.46***	1.71***
4-item	0.72***	0.80*	0.93	0.93	0.82**	0.79**	0.61***	0.79	1.67***	1.78***
n	3,494	2,820	3,491	2,815	3,457	2,788	3,345	2,711	3,693	2,987

Note: All original analyses of the National Longitudinal Survey of Youth 1997 (U.S. Department of Labor, Bureau of Labor Statistics) conducted by Child Trends. Data are for individuals who were ages 12–14 years on December 31, 1996.
[a] Controls include child (age, gender, race, past behaviors related to measured outcomes) and family characteristics (SES, parental education, family structure).
$+p < 0.1.$ $*p < .05.$ $**p < .01.$ $***p < .001.$

Table 6. Odds Ratios of the Parent–Youth Relationship Variable by Gender with Demographic and Past Behavior Controls[a]

Scale version	Delinquency		Substance use		Sexual activity		Suspensions		Good grades	
	Mom	Dad	Mom	Dad	Mom	Dad	Mom	Dad	Mom	Dad
Males										
8-item	0.69***	0.84	0.91	0.98	0.69***	0.89	0.58***	0.85	1.71***	1.28
4-item	0.70***	0.83+	0.99	1.09	0.76**	0.83+	0.69*	1.14	1.90***	1.16
n	2,140	1,662	2,138	1,659	2,115	1,645	2,032	1,591	2,264	1,765
Females										
8-item	0.65***	0.64*	0.96	0.94	0.79*	0.68***	0.68+	0.41**	1.31*	2.05***
4-item	0.76*	0.77+	0.95	0.85	0.82+	0.73**	0.76	0.36***	1.48***	2.21***
n	2,041	1,515	2,039	1,512	2,020	1,497	1,924	1,436	2,151	1,599

Note: All original analyses of the National Longitudinal Survey of Youth 1997 (U.S. Department of Labor, Bureau of Labor Statistics) conducted by Child Trends. Data are for individuals who were ages 12–14 years on December 31, 1996.
[a] Controls include child (age, gender, race, past behaviors related to measured outcomes) and family characteristics (SES, parental education, family structure).
$+p < 0.1.$ $*p < .05.$ $**p < .01.$ $***p < .001.$

relationships with their parents. In fact, postinterview remarks indicate that respondents in the NLSY97 found the questions in the self-administered questionnaire (which houses these relationship questions) to be the most engaging and enjoyable in the survey.

These scales appear to be reliable measures of the parent–adolescent relationship overall. The Cronbach's alphas and factor analyses for the scales suggest that the items hang together well as a construct.

Evidence also indicates that the parent–adolescent relationship scales are valid measures. Both scales follow the expected patterns for the demographic characteristics of age, gender, and family structure. Regarding construct validity, the zero-order correlations and regression models for the mother- and father–adolescent relationship scales were predicted well by the single item that measured the same construct.

Moreover, as expected, the mean score for the parent–adolescent relationship was found to decrease over time for both versions of the scale, as the young adolescents entered their middle and late teens. In addition, the percentage of adolescents who reported a positive relationship with their parents also decreased as the young adolescents aged.

Both versions of the scale did well on predictive validity for the whole sample. Based on the research literature, we would expect the quality of the parent–adolescent relationship to be negatively related to problem behaviors such as delinquency, substance use, and sexual activity. The eight-item measure for both parents predicted less delinquency, less sexual activity, and fewer suspensions 4 years later. In addition, it predicted better grades at the end of eighth grade. The shorter, four-item version of the scale, though not as comprehensive, did nevertheless predict fewer problem behaviors and better grades.

The predictive validity for the four- and eight-item scale, however, did not perform as well when we examined it by specific subgroups. For instance, both versions of the scale seem to function better in a White adolescent sample and in a sample above the poverty threshold. For Black adolescents, Hispanic adolescents, and adolescents in poverty, coefficients were generally in the hypothesized direction but typically fell short of statistical significance. To ensure that the poverty analyses were not mimicking the racial/ethnic group findings, we repeated our analyses for the sample of White adolescents below the poverty threshold and for Blacks and Hispanics above the poverty threshold. These results looked more like the poverty threshold sample findings than the racial/ethnic subgroup findings. The sample of White adolescents below the poverty threshold had sporadic significant findings. Furthermore, the sample of Black and Hispanic adolescents above the poverty threshold produced more significant findings than the sample of Black and Hispanic youth below the poverty threshold, but less than the sample of White adolescents above the poverty threshold. Thus, the scale works best among nonpoor White adolescents, somewhat less well for nonpoor Black and Hispanic adolescents and poor White adolescents, and least well for poor Black and Hispanic adolescents.

Additional work on how to strengthen these measures for specific subgroups is needed. It is possible that there are other factors of the parent–youth relationship that are more crucial to producing these outcomes in low-income and minority subgroups. It would be beneficial to add these factors to a measure of the parent–youth relationship. Indeed, there is evidence that at least one other parent–youth relationship measure has been effective in disadvantaged and minority populations (Moore & Chase-Lansdale, 2001). It is also possible that there is too little variation in the dependent variables for disadvantaged youth or that these scales predict other positive outcomes (e.g., thriving), rather than negative outcomes such as delinquency and substance use.

One limitation of the analyses presented in this chapter is the fact that the parent-youth relationship measures were asked only of young adolescents, ages 12–14 years. The items were repeated with similar success in subsequent rounds when the youth were older (1998, 1999), so they seem to be appropriate for teens. However, their appropriateness for younger children needs to be established, or modified items need to be developed.

In addition, this parent-youth relationship measure focuses only on resident parents. There is no inherent reason that the measure would not work with nonresident parents; in fact, some of the items were chosen to explore relationship issues found among nonresident parents, such as the question about "mak[ing] plans . . . and cancel[ing] for no good reason." However, due to skip patterns in the NLSY97, the questions were not asked of all nonresident parents, so definitive tests could not be conducted for nonresident parents. Nevertheless, preliminary analyses of the eight-item scale for adolescents who had seen their nonresidential parent (primarily fathers) within the last 12 months show that the scale seems to function well for this group. However, the full range of psychometric analyses presented in this study has not been conducted on this subsample.

In conclusion, these parent–adolescent relationship measures from the NLSY97 seem to be reliable and valid measures of an important construct. They seem well measured for Whites and nonpoor adolescents, in particular. Further work might strengthen the scale for use among minority and low-income adolescents.

The eight-item measure works best; however, based on the preceding analyses, the four-item scale would be a good alternative. Both of these scales were more successful measures than the five- and three-item versions that we also investigated. The eight- and four-item versions have variability in their distribution, have little missing data, are reliable overall and across demographic subgroups, follow expected demographic patterns, and enjoy construct validity. Additionally, they demonstrate predictive validity for the whole sample. The major drawback to these measures is that their predictive nature does not seem to work well within specific subgroups of the population (e.g., non-White adolescents and adolescents living below the poverty threshold). Beyond being a reliable and valid measure, the construct of quality parent–adolescent relationships is an important aspect of children's lives in and of itself; either version of the relationship scale is therefore recommended for use in national data systems interested in the well-being of children and youth. These parent-adolescent relationship measures may also be useful tools for programs, evaluators, or longitudinal researchers interested in tracking the development of children and youth.

Authors' Note

The authors are grateful for the funding provided by the National Institute for Child Health and Human Development Family and Child Well-being Research Network (Grant number 5U01 HD 30930-06) to complete this article. This chapter uses data from the National Longitudinal Study of Youth 1997, which is funded by the Department of Labor, Bureau of Labor Statistics.

Correspondence concerning this article can be addressed to Elizabeth Hair, Child Trends, 4301 Connecticut Avenue NW, Suite 350, Washington, DC 2000 (ehair@childtrends.org).

Appendix

Parent–Adolescent Relationship Scale

	Number of items			
	8	4	5	3
Identification with parents[a]				
I think highly of him/her.	•			•
S/he is a person I want to be like.	•	•		•
I really enjoy spending time with him/her.	•	•		•
Perceived parental supportiveness[b]				
How often does s/he praise you for doing well?	•	•	•	
How often does s/he criticize you or your ideas?	•	•	•	
How often does s/he help you do things that are important to you?	•		•	
How often does s/he blame you for her/his problems?	•		•	
How often does s/he make plans with you and cancel for no good reason?	•		•	

[a] 5-point response options range from 0 (*strongly disagree*) to 4 (*strongly agree*).
[b] 5-point response options range from 0 (*never*) to 4 (*always*).

References

Amato, P., & Booth, A. (1997). *A generation at risk: Growing up in an era of family upheaval.* Cambridge, MA: Harvard University Press.

Bahr, S. J., Maughan, S. L., Marcos, A. C., & Li, B. (1998). Family, religiosity, and the risk of adolescent drug use. *Journal of Marriage and Family, 60*(4), 979–992.

Barber, B. K., & Erickson, L. D. (2001). Adolescent social initiative: Antecedents in the ecology of social connections. *Journal of Adolescent Research, 16*(4), 326–354.

Blum, R., & Rinehart, P. M. (1997). Reducing the risk: Connections that make a difference in the lives of youth. *Youth Studies Australia, 16*(4), 37–50.

Borkowsky, J., Ramey, S., & Bristol-Power, M. (Eds.). (2002). *Parenting and the child's world: Influences on academic, intellectual, and social-emotional development.* Mahwah, NJ: Lawrence Erlbaum.

Brook, J. S., Brook, D. W., Gordon, S., Whiteman, M., & Cohen, P. (1989). The psychosocial etiology of adolescent drug use: A family interactional approach. *Genetic, Social and General Psychology Monographs, 116*(2), 111–267.

Capaldi, D. M., & Stoolmiller, M. (1999). Co-occurrence of conduct problems and depressive symptoms in early adolescent boys: III. Prediction to young-adult adjustment. *Development and Psychopathology, 11*(1), 59–84.

Carmines, E. G., & Zeller, R. A. (1985). Reliability and validity assessment. In J. L. Sullivan (Ed.), Quantitative applications in the social sciences. Beverly Hills, CA: Sage.

Collins, W. A., Maccoby, E. E., Steinberg, L., Hetherington, E. M., & Bornstein, M. H. (2000). Contemporary research on parenting: The case for nature and nurture. *American Psychologist, 55*(2), 218–232.

Conger, R. D., & Elder, G. H., Jr. (1994). *Families in troubled times: Adapting to change in rural America.* New York: Aldine de Gruyter.

Coombs, R. H., Paulson, M. J., & Richardson, M. A. (1991). Peer vs. parental influence in substance use among Hispanic and Anglo children and adolescents. *Journal of Youth and Adolescence, 20*(1), 73–88.

DeCato, L. A., Donohue, B., Azrin, N. A., & Teichner, G. A. (2001). Satisfaction of conduct disordered and substance abusing youth with their parents. *Behavior Modification, 25*(1), 44–52.

DeCato, L. A., Donohue, B., Azrin, N. A., Teichner, G. A., & Crum, T. (2002). Adolescents and their parents: A critical review of measures to assess their satisfaction with one another. *Clinical Psychology Review, 22*, 833–874.

Engels, R. C., Finkenauer, C., Meeus, W., & Dekovic, M. (2001). Parental attachment and adolescents' emotional adjustment: The associations with social skills and relational competence. *Journal of Counseling Psychology, 48*(4), 428–439.

Farber, B., & Jenne, W. C. (1963). Family organization and parent–child communication: Parents and siblings of a retarded child. *Monographs of the Society for Research in Child Development, 28*(7, Serial No. 91).

Farrell, A. D., & White, K. S. (1998). Peer influences and drug use among urban adolescents: Family structure and parent–adolescent relationship as protective factors. *Journal of Consulting and Clinical Psychology, 66*(2), 248–258.

Franz, C. E., McClelland, D. C., & Weinberger, J. (1991). Childhood antecedents of conventional social accomplishment in midlife adults: A 36-year prospective study. *Journal of Personality and Social Psychology, 60*(4), 586–595.

Garnier, H. E., & Stein, J. A. (1998). Values and the family: Risk and protective factors for adolescent problem behaviors. *Youth & Society, 30*(1), 89–120.

Hair, E. C., Jager, J., & Garrett, S. B. (2002). *Background for community-level work on social competency in adolescence: Reviewing the literature on contributing factors.* Washington, DC: Child Trends.

Harris, J. R. (2002). Beyond the nurture assumption: Testing hypotheses about the child's environment. In M. Bristol-Power (Ed.), *Parenting and the child's world* (pp. 3–20). Mahwah, NJ: Lawrence Erlbaum.

Herman, M. R., Dornbusch, S. M., Herron, M. C., & Herting, J. R. (1997). The influence of family regulation, connection, and psychological autonomy on six measures of adolescent functioning. *Journal of Adolescent Research, 12*(1), 34–67.

Hundleby, J. D., & Mercer, G. W. (1987). Family and friends as social environments and their relationship to young adolescents' use of alcohol, tobacco, and marijuana. *Journal of Marriage and Family, 49*(1), 151–164.

Jessor, S. L., & Jessor, R. (1975). Transition from virginity to nonvirginity among youth: A social-psychological study over time. *Developmental Psychology, 11*(4), 473–484.

Kerns, K. A., & Stevens, A. C. (1996). Parent–child attachment in late adolescence: Links to social relations and personality. *Journal of Youth and Adolescence, 25*(3), 323–342.

Manlove, J., Terry-Humen, E., Romano Papillo, A., Franzetta, K., & Ryan, S. (2002). *Background for community-level work on positive reproductive health in adolescence: A review of antecedents, programs, and investment strategies.* Washington, DC: Child Trends.

Miller, B. C. (1998). *Families matter: A research synthesis of family influences on adolescent pregnancy.* Washington, DC: National Campaign to Prevent Teenage Pregnancy.

Miller, K. E., Sabo, D. F., Farrell, M. P., Barnes, G. M., & Melnick, M. J. (1998). Athletic participation and sexual behavior in adolescents: The different world of boys and girls. *Journal of Health and Social Behavior, 39*(2), 108–123.

Moore, M. R., & Chase-Lansdale, P. L. (2001). Sexual intercourse and pregnancy among African American girls in high-poverty neighborhoods: The role of family and perceived community environment. *Journal of Marriage and Family, 63*, 1146–1157.

Prinz, R., Foster, S., Kent, S., & O'Leary, D. (1979). Multivariate assessment of conflict in distressed and nondistressed mother–adolescent dyads. *Journal of Applied Behavior Analysis, 12*, 691–700.

Resnick, M. D., Bearman, P. S., Blum, R. W., Bauman, K. E., Harris, K. M., Jones, J., et al. (1997). Protecting adolescents from harm: Findings from the National Longitudinal Study of Adolescent Health. *Journal of the American Medical Association, 278*(10), 823–832.

Rodney, L. W., Crafter, B., Rodney, H. E., & Mupier, R. M. (1999). Variables contributing to grade retention among African American adolescent males. *Journal of Educational Research, 92*(3), 185–190.

Rushing, W. A. (1964). Adolescent-parent relations and mobility aspirations. *Social Forces, 43*, 157–166.

Swanson, G. E. (1950). The development of an instrument for rating parent–child relationships. *Social Forces, 29*, 84–90.

U.S. Department of Health and Human Services: Office of the Assistant Secretary for Planning and Evaluation. (2001). *Trends in the well-being of America's children and youth.* Washington, DC: U.S. Government Printing Office.

Whitbeck, L. B., Hoyt, D. R., Miller, M., & Kao, M. Y. (1992). Parental support, depressed affect and sexual experience among adolescents. *Youth & Society, 24*(2), 166–177.

Zahn-Waxler, C., & Smith, K. D. (1992). The development of prosocial behavior. In M. Hersen (Ed.), *Handbook of social development: A lifespan perspective* (pp. 229–256). New York: Plenum Press.

13 Positive Indicators of Sibling Relationship Quality: The Sibling Inventory of Behavior

Brenda L. Volling and Alysia Y. Blandon

University of Michigan

Most people grow up in a family with at least one brother or sister. The relationship between siblings can be marked with rivalry and conflict, but can also be one of the closest and most intimate relationships a person has in childhood, adolescence, and adulthood (Buhrmester & Furman, 1990; Volling, 2003). Unlike parent–child relationships and children's peer relationships, there is far less empirical research devoted to the study of sibling relationships, which is surprising given that it is the longest-lasting relationship of an individual's life. The sibling relationship exists long before one has met a spouse and long after one's parents have died. There has been considerably more research on children's sibling relationships over the past decade (see Brody, 1998, for a review). Warm, nurturant, and close sibling relationships play an important role in the development of children's social competence with peers, their ability to resolve conflicts in a constructive manner, and their social and emotional understanding (Dunn & Munn, 1985; Herrera & Dunn, 1997; Howe, 1991).

Several bodies of research now indicate that the quality of the sibling relationship is related to several indicators of children's social development. Whether the relationship between siblings is described as nurturant, warm, supportive, and emotionally close or is deemed aggressive, conflictual, and hostile appears to have important implications for the two children involved. Most notable in this regard are the links between sibling relationship quality and the child's *social competence*, or ability to manage and sustain relationships with peers. Herrera and Dunn (1997), for instance, reported that young children using constructive conflict resolution strategies, such as mitigating a conflict or conciliating, were more likely to use similar conflict resolution strategies with a friend several years later.

Although there are clear links between the positive involvement a child enjoys with a sibling and peer competence, it is also the case that sibling relationships can contribute to the development of peer aggression and rejection by one's peers. Several studies have found relations between the aggression, hostility, and coercive interaction between siblings and the children's use of aggression with peers and peer rejection (e.g., Stormshak, Bellanti, Bierman, & the Conduct Problems Prevention Research Group, 1996). In their study of 6- to 8-year-old aggressive children, Stormshak et al. found that those children with warm and close sibling relationships received higher scores on emotional control and those children reporting high levels of sibling conflict at home were actually more aggressive and less socially competent at school. More important, however, it was the children experiencing both high warmth *and* a moderate degree of conflict with their siblings who were more socially competent with their peers, more emotionally controlled, and more attentive at school. Children with sibling relationships characterized by high conflict and low warmth tended to use more peer aggression.

In addition to the child's social competence, other research reveals associations between the quality of the sibling relationship and children's *psychological adjustment*. In a sample of seventh graders, Conger, Conger, and Scaramella (1997) reported that manipulative and excessive control by a sibling was detrimental to the child's self-confidence and predicted increases in both externalizing and internalizing behavior problems 2 years later. Widmer and Weiss (2000) examined whether a caring and supportive sibling relationship with an older brother or sister would protect a younger sibling from the deleterious effects of living in a high-risk neighborhood and experiencing adjustment problems. When the younger sibling perceived the older adolescent sibling as successful and supportive, these children had fewer depressive symptoms and lower delinquent attitudes and reported more school engagement. Moreover, 9- to 11-year-old African American children were more self-regulated if their sibling relationships were described as harmonious and involving little conflict (Brody, Stoneman, Smith, & Gibson, 1999).

Another line of research indicates that a warm, intimate relationship with one's sibling is related to children's *social cognition* (i.e., social and emotional understanding) both in early childhood (e.g., Youngblade & Dunn, 1995) and middle childhood (Howe, Aquan-Assee, Bukowski, Lehoux, & Rinaldi, 2001). Howe and her colleagues reported that preschoolers' use of internal state language with a toddler sibling was related to the child's comforting, helping, and confiding 4 years later, as well as to warmth in the sibling relationship years later (Howe, Aquan-Assee, & Bukowski, 1995). Similarly, Howe et al. (2001) found that sibling relationship warmth was related to fifth- and sixth-grade children's emotional understanding and self-disclosure with their sibling. Finally, the extent to which young siblings were engaged in pretend play, a mature form of play wherein children share imaginary roles, was associated with the young child's emotional understanding, that is, their ability to recognize emotional states and understand the emotions of others (Youngblade & Dunn, 1995).

In sum, the research to date shows clearly that the quality of the sibling relationship can have both detrimental and beneficial effects on the social and emotional development of children in early and middle childhood, as well as in adolescence. Emotional closeness and warmth in children's sibling relationships contribute to the development of children's prosocial behaviors and social understanding, whereas aggression and hostility between siblings predict children's use of such behavior with their peers and future behavior problems. Not only do warm sibling relationships contribute to children's social and emotional development directly, they also may act as a protective factor for high-risk children by buffering them from the effects of adverse life events.

Measures of Sibling Relationship Quality

Observation and questionnaires are the two most prominent methods for assessing the quality of the sibling relationship. Observational paradigms are common in early childhood because of the limited utility in collecting self-reports or interview data from such young children (e.g., Volling, McElwain, & Miller, 2002). Because of increased interest in the sibling relationship and its effects on developmental outcomes in childhood and adolescence, there are now several questionnaires available to assess sibling relationship quality. For instance, the Sibling Relationship Questionnaire (Furman & Buhrmester, 1985), the Sibling Relationship Inventory (Stocker & McHale, 1992), and the Sibling Qualities Scale (Cole & Kearns, 2001) have been used predominantly with children in elementary school and the period of adolescence. Parents have also completed the Sibling Relationships in Early Childhood Questionnaire (Volling & Elins, 1998), the Parental Expectations and Perceptions of Children's Sibling Relationships Questionnaire (Kramer & Baron, 1995), and the Sibling Behaviors and Feelings Questionnaire (Mendelson, Aboud, & Lanthier, 1994) to assess very young children's sibling relationships in the toddler and preschool years. More recently, the Adult Sibling Relationship Questionnaire (Stocker, Lanthier, & Furman, 1997), the Lifespan Sibling Relationship Scale (Riggio, 2000), and the Brother–Sister Questionnaire (Graham-Bermann & Cutler, 1994) have been developed to assess sibling relationships in late adolescence and early adulthood. This chapter focuses on the Sibling Inventory of Behavior (SIB; Schaefer & Edgerton, 1981), given that it is one of the earliest inventories to have been developed to assess sibling relationship quality and has, as a result, a long history of use and psychometric testing.

Sibling Inventory of Behavior

The SIB was developed by Schaefer and Edgerton (1981) to assess sibling relationships in families with and without a handicapped child. It was developed using mothers' and fathers' reports in a sample of 52 maritally intact families (39 with a handicapped child), with children ranging in age from 3 to 8 years. The SIB consisted of 28 items that assessed one sibling's behavior toward the other and was designed to measure eight dimensions of sibling behavior. This included four 4-item scales assessing empathy and concern (Cronbach's alpha = .81), kindness (α = .74), leadership and involvement (α = .80), and acceptance (α = .78), in addition to four 3-item scales assessing anger (α = .75), unkindness and teasing (α = .79), avoidance (α = .64), and embarrassment (α = .89). As for reliability, the alpha coefficients indicated the scales were internally consistent, and correlations between mothers' and fathers' reports ranged from .33 (avoidance) to .80 (empathy/concern), with a median of .64. Validity of the SIB scales was examined by correlating the scales with teachers' ratings of the children's classroom behavior. Parents' ratings of empathy/concern (r = .45, p < .01), kindness (r = .37, p < .05) and leadership/involvement (r = .30, p < .05) were significantly correlated with teachers' ratings of the older siblings' considerateness of others in the classroom.

Hetherington and Clingempeel (1992) modified and expanded the SIB by adding 21 items for use in their study of marital transitions following divorce by studying sibling relationships in married families, divorced single-mother families, and stepfamilies in which the mother remarried. At the start of the study, a target child between the ages of 9 and 13 years was identified, along with a closest age sibling. Both parents completed questionnaires, and children were interviewed about their sibling relationships. Factor analyses of the 49 items resulted in six sibling relationship scales that closely resembled the original eight reported by Schaefer and Edgerton (1981): (a) involvement/companionship, (b) empathy/concern, (c) rivalry, (d) avoidance, (e) aggression, and (f) teaching/directiveness. Hetherington and Clingempeel reported that alpha coefficients of parents' and children's reports across the three waves of data collection ranged from .86 to .93 (M = .91) for involvement/companionship, from .64 to .89 (M = .78) for empathy/concern, from .61 to .89 (M = .78) for rivalry, from .75 to .88 (M = .81) for avoidance, from .77 to .90 (M = .86) for aggression, and from .60 to .81 (M = .73) for teaching/directiveness. Composites of *positivity* (sum of empathy/concern, involvement/companionship, and teaching/directiveness/guidance) and *negativity* (sum of aggression, rivalry, and avoidance) in the sibling relationship were created from mothers', fathers', and children's reports. Intercorrelations between parents' and children's reports across family type and the three waves of data collection were significant, from .45 to .69 for *positivity* and from .32 to .56 for *negativity*. Correlations across the three waves of data collection indicated remarkable stability in mothers', fathers', and children's reports of positivity and negativity in sibling relationship quality across time.

The SIB was revised and shortened again by Hetherington and her colleagues for use in the Nonshared Environment of Adolescent Development (Hetherington, Henderson, & Reiss, 1999), a longitudinal study designed to examine family relationship functioning across diverse family forms, including nonstepfamilies and stepfamilies, with both full and half siblings. The study included two waves of data collection separated by approximately 3 years. The 49 items of the SIB were shortened to 32, and principal components analyses confirmed a six-scale structure using mothers', fathers', and both siblings' self-reports on the SIB. This included (a) a 5-item empathy/concern scale, (b) a 6-item companionship/involvement scale, (c) a 6-item rivalry scale, (d) a 5-item conflict/aggression scale, (e) a 5-item avoidance scale, and (f) a 4-item teaching/directiveness scale. Cronbach's alphas across scales were acceptable for empathy (median $\alpha = .88$), rivalry (median $\alpha = .77$), aggression (median $\alpha = .80$), avoidance (median $\alpha = .85$), teaching/directiveness (median $\alpha = .67$) and companionship/involvement (median $\alpha = .88$). Again a factor analysis indicated that the scales formed two larger factors, *positivity* (sum of teaching, companionship, and empathy) and *negativity* (sum of aggression, avoidance, and rivalry). Cross-time correlations from Wave 1 and Wave 2 indicated relatively high stability in individual differences over time, with correlations ranging from .59 for companionship and .72 for rivalry and empathy. Intercorrelations of the older and younger siblings' reports were also quite high for rivalry ($r = .81$), aggression ($r = .89$), companionship ($r = .90$), empathy ($r = .79$), avoidance ($r = .54$), and teaching ($r = .34$), with intersibling correlations of .56 for the positivity composite and .91 for the negativity composite.

The six scales from the SIB emerge reliably across studies and show adequate internal consistency and cross-time correlations, as well as impressive associations across respondents (e.g., parents, siblings). The research conducted by Hetherington and her colleagues has focused predominantly on samples of preadolescents and adolescents, demonstrating the utility of this measure for this age group, using both parents' reports and children's self-reports. The remainder of this chapter demonstrates the psychometric properties of the 32-item SIB based on both mothers' and fathers' reports of young children's sibling relationships in the preschool years.

Method

Because there are so few studies examining the quality of sibling relationships, there is *no nationally representative data set* to our knowledge that currently includes a psychometrically sound measure of sibling relationship quality. The data used in this report come from a longitudinal study of parent–child and sibling relationships in early childhood (Volling et al., 2002). Because the study was intended to capture parent–child and sibling interaction with young children, laboratory observations were the main, and preferred, means to gather information on the quality of these relationships. The sample to be discussed is small, White, and middle class, and includes 60 families at the initial time, but only 37 in the longitudinal follow-up. Therefore, caution is prudent in interpreting the findings and generalizing them to more ethnically and socioeconomically diverse families.

Sample

Families that participated in the study were initially recruited from birth announcements, local day care centers, and through referrals by other study participants. The families were required to meet three eligibility criteria: (a) intact marital status, (b) participation of both mothers and fathers, and (3) at least two children in the family, with the youngest child nearing 12 months of age and the older sibling between the ages of 2 and 6 years. Of the families meeting these criteria, 69% agreed to participate. All parents were the biological mothers and fathers of the two children. Participating families were primarily European American ($N = 56$), with one Native American couple and three interracial couples. Parents had been married for an average of 7 years (range = 3–16 years). On average, fathers were 35.6 years old and had completed 17.4 years of education, whereas mothers were, on average, 33.2 years old and had completed 16.5 years of education. The mean family income was $73,607 ($SD$ = $41,791$). The age of the younger sibling (toddler) in all families was 16 months, the mean age of the older sibling was 50 months (range = 2–6 years), and the average age space between siblings was 35 months (range = 11–68 months). Most of the toddlers in the study were second born ($n = 44$), and the remaining 16 toddlers were third through fifth born. For families with more than two children, the older sibling closest in age to the 16-month-old was asked to participate. The sample included 20 girl/girl dyads (younger/older), 14 boy/boy dyads, 10 girl/boy dyads, and 16 boy/girl dyads.

Approximately 3 years later, when the younger sibling was 4 years old, 37 of the initial families returned for a follow-up visit to assess sibling and friend relationships. An additional 21 families were recruited at this time to increase the sample size to 58. Younger children, at this time, ranged in age from 46 to 60 months (SD = 3.29 months), and their older siblings ranged in age from 5 to 10 years (SD = 7.3 years). The average age space between siblings was approximately 3 years (range: 1–6 years).

Design and Procedure

Families were initially recruited when their younger child was approaching 12 months of age and were observed in a series of observational paradigms designed to assess parent–child and sibling interaction when the younger child was 12, 13, and 16 months of age. At the 16-month assessment point, both mothers and fathers completed the 32-item SIB to assess the older siblings' behavior toward the younger sibling. Several of the SIB items are more applicable to older children (e.g., baby-sits, teaches, shares secrets) than to preschool children. However, for present purposes, we included all 32 items when creating scales in order to maintain measurement equivalence so that findings could be compared across studies.[1]

Three years later when the younger child was 4 years old, both older and younger siblings were invited to participate in a laboratory visit designed to assess the quality of sibling interaction. Again, mothers and fathers completed

---

[1] For the current research, we used the same wording as the original SIB items, but explained to parents how to interpret them in line with the developmental ages of their children.

the 32-item SIB, but this time they completed it with respect to the older siblings' behavior directed to the younger sibling *and* the younger siblings' behavior directed to the older sibling. At the 4-year visit, sibling dyads were also videotaped in two interactive sessions: a 20-minute free play session and a 5-minute sharing task. During the free play session, both children could explore and play with any toys available in the laboratory playroom. During the more structured, sharing task, children were seated at a table and introduced to a new toy (e.g., Play-doh camera) and instructed to play with the toy until the experimenter returned. The purpose of this situation was to see how children handled a situation involving limited resources. Videotapes of free play and sharing task interaction were reliably coded for the following individual and dyadic behaviors: (a) manage/teach (child indirectly attempts to control and teach the other child by using suggestions or requests); (b) affection (child demonstrates affectionate behavior toward the other sibling); (c) social play sophistication (the complexity of the children's play interactions, with low scores indicating solitary play and high scores more complex levels of social pretend play); and (d) shared positive affect (children engage in mutual joy or pleasure) (McElwain & Volling, 2002). Composites for each of the four interactive codes were created by averaging scores across the free play and sharing task. For present purposes, we used the observations of sibling interaction as a means of examining the construct validity of the SIB scales by correlating the parents' reports of positive sibling relationship quality at both 16 months and 4 years, with actual sibling *behavior* observed during the 4-year laboratory visit.

At the 4-year time point, both mothers and fathers completed the aggressive behavior scale from Achenbach's (1991) Child Behavior Checklist, a well-standardized measure of children's behavior problems. Internal consistency (Cronbach's alpha) for mothers' reports was .83 and .87 for younger and older siblings, respectively, and for fathers' reports, .80 and .83 for younger and older siblings, respectively.

Measures of Sibling Relationship Quality

The Appendix lists the 32 items that make up the SIB and denotes which items correspond to the six scales. Each item is answered on a 5-point Likert scale, ranging from 1 (*never*) to 5 (*always*). In this chapter, we focus on the 6-item *companionship* scale, the 5-item *empathy* scale, and the 4-item *teaching/directiveness* scale. These three subscales can be summed together to form one 15-item *positive involvement* scale. When describing the properties and psychometrics of these scales, we will present results using the three subscales along with the composite scale of positive involvement. Data are available for 60 mothers and fathers at 16 months and for 57 mothers and 52 fathers at 4 years.

Table 1 provides the descriptives of the scales for both mothers' and fathers' reports at both the 16-month and 4-year time points for the older siblings' behavior and the mothers' and fathers' reports of the younger siblings' behavior at 4 years. Examination of Table 1 indicates substantial variation in the distribution

Table 1. Descriptive Statistics for the Sibling Inventory of Behavior

	Range	Mean	SD	Skewness	Kurtosis
16-month parent reports					
Older Sibling					
Mother					
Positive involvement scale	28–74	50.84	8.40	−.15	.38
Companionship	11–29	19.12	3.59	−.04	.08
Empathy	11–25	19.08	2.87	−.26	.34
Teaching	6–20	12.69	2.78	−.07	−.30
Father					
Positive involvement scale	25–64	48.93	8.49	−.54	−.05
Companionship	9–26	18.72	3.51	−.47	−.05
Empathy	10–24	18.30	3.44	−.55	−.10
Teaching	6–17	11.92	2.48	−.21	−.56
4-year parent reports					
Younger Sibling					
Mother					
Positive involvement scale	36–71	52.04	6.79	−.07	.90
Companionship	17–30	22.93	2.95	−.14	−.21
Empathy	13–25	18.82	2.80	−.13	−.18
Teaching	4–15	9.32	2.45	.18	.25
Father					
Positive involvement scale	37–71	51.55	6.69	.68	1.46
Companionship	16–30	22.89	2.79	.16	.67
Empathy	9–25	17.94	3.22	.22	.48
Teaching	4–17	8.87	2.48	.46	1.26
Older Sibling					
Mother					
Positive involvement scale	36–64	52.61	6.48	−.47	.06
Companionship	13–28	21.25	2.92	−.73	.76
Empathy	12–24	18.49	2.89	−.02	−.75
Teaching	9–16	12.88	2.02	−.14	−.81
Father					
Positive involvement scale	36–71	52.04	6.79	−.07	.90
Companionship	14–30	21.79	3.16	−.11	.28
Empathy	13–25	17.89	3.05	.29	−.49
Teaching	8–17	12.37	2.23	.02	−.06

of the scores for both mothers and fathers across both time points and for both siblings.

Reliability

We examined the internal consistency of the various scales using Cronbach's alpha for the scales as completed by mothers and fathers for both older and younger siblings. Internal consistency is greater than .70 for all scales, with the exception of the teaching scale (mean $\alpha = .66$, range = .54 to .75). The alpha for the teaching scale would be expected to be lower, in general, given that there are fewer items on this scale. Also, teaching is not necessarily descriptive of the typical interaction characterizing preschool siblings and may be better at describing the transactions occurring between siblings in the period of middle childhood or adolescence. In this case, we might anticipate the internal consistency of this scale to reach the levels reported earlier by Hetherington and her colleagues. Our observations of preschoolers indicated, however, that they were quite capable of directing or managing the interaction, even if it did not involve sophisticated teaching techniques.

We also examined consistency in scale scores by correlating mothers' and fathers' reports at 16 months and then again at 4 years. The correlations across parents are moderately high, ranging from .26 to .65, indicating considerable consistency in parents' reports of the siblings' behavior toward the other sibling. The lower correlations between mothers' and fathers' reports for the teaching scale (.26 for both siblings at 4 years) may again be due to the fact that teaching interactions are more characteristic of sibling relationships in middle childhood and adolescence than they are of preschool sibling relationships.

Finally, we examined the cross-time correlations between mothers' and fathers' reports of the older siblings' behavior toward the younger sibling at 16 months and at 4 years to determine whether there was any consistency in scores over time in the 37 families that were seen at both time points. These cross-time correlations showed more consistency in fathers' reports of sibling relationship quality than in mothers' reports. Statistically significant correlations between father's reports ranged from .42 to .50 for all but the companionship scale, whereas the only statistically significant correlation between mothers' reports was for empathy ($r = .34$). Companionship is the only scale where there does not appear to be stable individual differences across either mothers' or fathers' reports for either sibling.

Validity

In order to examine the concurrent validity of the scales, we correlated mothers' and fathers' reports of the sibling relationship at 4 years with actual sibling behaviors (e.g., manage/teach, shared positive affect) observed during videotaped observations at the 4-year visit. Although there were no significant relations between mothers' reports of the older or younger siblings' behaviors at 4 years and the observed sibling behaviors, several associations were significant or reached significance when examining the fathers' reports of sibling relationship quality. Fathers' reports of the older siblings' empathy were modestly related ($r = .27$, $p < .07$), and their reports of the older siblings' teaching ($r = .32$, $p < .05$) were significantly correlated with the shared positive affect expressed in the sibling dyad. The overall positive involvement score was also modestly correlated with the extent of shared positive affect expressed between siblings during the sibling interaction tasks ($r = .26$, $p < .08$). Similarly, fathers' reports of the older siblings' teaching ($r = .29$, $p < .05$) and the overall positive involvement score ($r = .27$, $p < .07$) were correlated with the older siblings' managing and teaching behavior during sibling interaction with their younger sibling. Similarly, fathers' reports of the younger siblings' companionship were significantly correlated with the extent of shared positive affect expressed in the sibling dyad ($r = .39$, $p < .01$) and the younger siblings' attempts to manage the sibling interaction ($r = .37$, $p < .01$). The overall positive involvement score for fathers' reports of the younger sibling showed similar relations to positive affect shared between siblings ($r = .39$, $p < .01$) and the younger sibling's attempts to manage and "teach" their older sibling ($r = .37$, $p < .01$).

To examine the predictive validity of parents' reports of the sibling relationship, correlations were also run between mothers' and fathers' reports at 16 months of the older siblings' behavior and observed sibling interaction at 4 years during the laboratory visit. These analyses only included a subsample of the families who remained in the follow-up study ($n = 37$). Mothers' reports of the older siblings' companionship ($r = .36$, $p < .05$) and overall positive involvement ($r = .35$, $p < .05$) at 16 months were significantly related to the amount of affection the older sibling showed toward the younger sibling approximately 3 years later at the 4-year follow-up visit. Similarly, mothers' reports of the older siblings' teaching of the younger sibling at 16 months ($r = .31$, $p < .08$), as well as her reports of overall positive involvement ($r = .32$, $p < .08$), were modestly related to the complexity of sibling play, indicating that sibling play was more sophisticated and involved more joint pretend at 4 years when older siblings had been more directive and managed sibling interaction with their younger siblings at 16 months. Fathers' reports of the older siblings' empathy ($r = .44$, $p < .01$), companionship ($r = .29$, $p < .10$), and teaching ($r = .31$, $p < .07$), as well as overall positive involvement with their younger sibling ($r = .40$, $p < .05$), were related to the older siblings' manage and teach behaviors toward their younger siblings during the 4-year laboratory visit.

Links to Children's Well-being

We also examined both the concurrent relations between parents' reports on the SIB at 4 years with parents' reports of children's behavior problems at 4 years, along with the predictive relations between the parents' reports of the older siblings' SIB scores at the 16-month time point and their problematic behaviors at the 4-year time point. We specifically chose to look at the children's aggressive behavior problems, given the significance of aggression for children' social competence and its role in the coercive, destructive sibling conflicts noted by others (e.g., Garcia, Shaw, Winslow, & Yaggi, 2000). We would expect there to be inverse associations between the positive indicators of sibling relationship quality and children's aggression. Table 2 summarizes the correlations between mothers' and fathers' reports of the older and younger siblings' aggressive behavior problems at 4 years and their reports on the positive relationship indicators of sibling relationship quality. Although several of the correlations are marginal, particularly with respect to the younger siblings' behavior, there appears to be a consistent pattern among the correlations, in general, indicating that children with aggressive behavior problems are less likely to develop sibling relationships involving high levels of positive involvement, companionship, empathy, and teaching.

Table 2. Correlations of Older and Younger Sibling SIB Scale
Scores with Aggressive Behavior Problems at 4 Years (n = 54)

	Aggressive behavior problems at 4 years	
	Older sibling	Younger sibling
SIB Scales at 16 Months		
Mother		
Positive involvement	−.28	
Companionship	−.20	
Empathy	−.27	
Teaching	−.29+	
Father		
Positive involvement	−.37*	
Companionship	−.34*	
Empathy	−.30+	
Teaching	−.36*	
SIB Scales at 4 Years		
Mother		
Positive involvement	−.18	−.21
Companionship	−.02	−.19
Empathy	−.25+	−.25+
Teaching	−.18	−.06
Father		
Positive involvement	−.31*	−.24+
Companionship	−.13	−.27*
Empathy	−.30*	−.21
Teaching	−.34*	.06

Note: $+p < .10$. $*p < .05$. $**p < .01$.

One final means of addressing the predictive validity of the SIB scales was to correlate mothers' and fathers' reports of the older siblings' behaviors toward their 16-month-old toddlers with parents' reports of the older siblings' aggressive behavior problems approximately 3 years later, when the younger sibling was 4 years of age. Table 2 indicates that there is only one marginal relation between mothers' reports of the older siblings' teaching of the toddler at 16 months and the older siblings' aggressive behavior problems at the 4-year assessment. However, correlations between the older siblings' aggressive behavior problems at the 4-year assessment and the fathers' reports at 16 months of the older siblings' overall positive involvement, companionship, and teaching were significant. The correlation between the older siblings' aggression at the 4-year assessment and fathers' reports at 16 months of this child's empathy for the younger toddler was marginally significant.

Gender and Age Differences

To examine whether the positive dimensions of sibling relationship quality differed for boys and girls, we ran 2 × 2 (older sibling gender × younger sibling

gender) analyses of variance (ANOVAs) on mothers' and fathers' reports of
sibling relationship quality at both 16 months and again at 4 years. At 16 months,
several main effects for the older child's gender were found. For mothers' reports,
this included the overall positive involvement scale, $F(1, 60) = 4.20$, $p < .05$;
companionship, $F(1, 57) = 4.12$, $p < .05$; and teaching, $F(1, 60) = 5.33$, $p < .05$.
In all cases, older female siblings were more positively involved ($Ms = 52.5$
and 48.0 for females and males, respectively), experienced more companionship
($Ms = 19.9$ and 17.0), and did more teaching ($Ms = 13.4$ and 11.7) of their younger
siblings than did older male siblings.

Similar gender effects were found when examining the fathers' reports of the
older siblings' behavior at the 16-month time point. Significant main effects for
the older siblings' gender were found for fathers' reports of overall positive involvement, $F(1, 59) = 4.15$, $p < .05$, and empathy, $F(1, 59) = 4.93$, $p < .05$. The
main effect for the older siblings' gender for fathers' reports of older sibling
companionship was marginally significant, $F(1, 59) = 3.64$, $p = .06$. Older female siblings were judged by their fathers to be more positively involved ($Ms =$
50.7 and 46.1 for females and males, respectively), more empathic ($Ms = 19.1$
and 17.1), and expressed more companionship ($Ms = 19.4$ and 17.6) in their
relationships with a younger sibling than did older male siblings.

There were no significant main effects for the younger siblings' gender or
significant older-sibling-by-younger-sibling interactions for either mothers' or
fathers' reports of the older siblings' behavior to their 16-month-old toddler sibling, indicating that older sisters' behaviors did not differ depending on whether
they had a younger brother or a younger sister at 16 months.

The 2×2 (older sibling gender $\times$ younger sibling gender) ANOVAs conducted with the 4-year data revealed a very different picture. There were no
significant main effects or interactions involving either sibling's gender when
we examined mothers' reports of the older and younger siblings' behaviors
at 4 years, and fathers' reports of the younger sibling's behavior at the 4-year
time point. Only one statistically significant interaction was found for fathers'
reports of the older siblings' teaching, $F(1, 51) = 6.95$, $p < .01$. As one might
expect, older sisters were far more likely to teach their younger sisters, with
older brothers far less likely to teach their younger sisters. Younger brothers, on
the other hand, were just as likely to be taught by their older brothers as their
older sisters. However, given that only one interaction was found to be significant, caution needs to be exercised in interpreting gender differences in sibling
interaction at this age.

Summary and Discussion

Based on the earlier review of studies using the SIB in relatively modest
samples of adolescents and children in middle childhood, the SIB scales appear
to be psychometrically sound. The SIB is perhaps the oldest of the sibling relationship questionnaires currently available and has been used quite extensively
by researchers interested in obtaining both children's self-reports and parents'

reports of sibling relationship quality. The vast majority of research using this instrument has been conducted on preadolescents and adolescents, and this earlier research finds these scales are internally consistent for both parent and child reports, and have fairly high correlations across respondents in the family, as well as over time, in many cases, several years later.

Neither the SIB nor any of the many sibling relationship questionnaires are currently included in nationally representative data sets, which precluded the possibility of analyzing the psychometric properties of any sibling relationship inventory using large survey samples. As a result, the current analyses were conducted on a smaller, local data set that had information on the SIB from multiple respondents (both the mother and the father) on two children (both the younger and the older sibling) in the family and across two time points (both toddlerhood and preschool). This allowed us to examine whether the internal consistency of the scales was acceptable across multiple respondents for two different-age children at two different time points. All the scales, with the exception of the teaching scale, showed adequate internal consistency across parents' reports, across the siblings, and across both time points. In no case did the internal consistency appear to be affected by how old the child was, which child was being assessed, or which parent was completing the items. In general, then, the reliability of these scales is robust with respect to Cronbach's alpha estimates, and the results presented here on parents' reports of younger children mirror those results reported by others using adolescent samples.

In the present study, we analyzed only the positive dimensions of sibling relationship quality by including the empathy, companionship, and teaching scales, along with a composite scale of positive sibling involvement that we created. The teaching scale was the only scale where the internal consistency was lower than .70, but this is most likely due to the fact that this scale has fewer items than the others and because teaching is not as typical of sibling interactions in early childhood as it is in the later years of childhood and adolescence. Although the focus of this chapter was on the positive indicators of sibling relationship quality, we also provided all 32 items that make up the SIB. Earlier research indicates that conflict and warmth in the sibling relationship may need to be examined together in order to get the most complete picture of the manner in which sibling relationship quality will affect children's outcomes. It is unrealistic to think that siblings will never argue or fight with each other. Indeed, the research suggests that being able to resolve sibling conflict constructively might actually enhance children's social competence and their abilities to interact successfully with their school-age peers. Some level of conflict is perhaps needed for children to learn how to handle conflict. Sibling conflict bodes poorly for children, however, when it involves aggression, hostility, and coercive control, and there is little warmth expressed between siblings. Perhaps the best advice for those interested in studying sibling relationships in childhood and adolescence is to suggest that positive indicators, such as companionship and empathy, be included with indicators of sibling conflict and rivalry, and that these be examined together (e.g., high companionship and moderate conflict) and not treated as separate independent dimensions of the sibling relationship.

Limitations and Future Directions

Because we were analyzing data from a much smaller data set, we were confronted with serious issues concerning statistical power. This was a particular concern whenever we presented findings using the longitudinal data where we were able to include only the 37 families with data at both time points. For this reason, many of the reported associations only reached marginal significance. However, we did have actual observations of the children's behavior when interacting with their siblings during a laboratory session to which parental reports could be related. All associations found, whether significant or marginally significant, were in the expected direction, and all provided evidence that parents' reports of positive indicators of sibling relationship quality were correlated with positive indicators of *actual observed sibling behavior* during a laboratory session and inversely related to the parents' reports of children's aggressive behavior problems at the 4-year time point.

Because of the small sample size, because these were all families with toddler and preschool children when the study started, and because the sample is relatively homogeneous with respect to ethnicity and socioeconomic status, we did not include many control variables in our analyses. The few gender effects indicated that parents reported older female siblings to be more companionate, express more empathy, teach more, and overall be more positively involved with their younger 16-month-old toddler siblings than did older male siblings. By 4 years, however, the only significant finding with respect to gender was that older sisters were much more likely, according to their fathers, to teach their younger sisters than were older brothers, whereas younger brothers appeared to be taught equally by their older brothers and older sisters.

The fact that the majority of these families (over 95%) were White and middle class did not allow us to address diversity with respect to ethnicity or to examine children from different socioeconomic backgrounds. Brody and his colleagues (Brody & Murry, 2001; Brody et al., 1999) are one of the few groups of investigators to examine children's sibling relationships in African American families. Although these investigators did not use the SIB, they did use another well-respected measure of sibling relationship quality, the Sibling Relationship Questionnaire (Furman & Buhrmester, 1985), and reported good internal consistency (alphas at .80 or above) on the prosocial and antagonistic scales of this measure. Moreover, the quality of the sibling relationship was related to African American children's social and emotional outcomes, indicating that sibling relationship quality is an important contributor to the development of self-regulation and behavior problems in these families as well. Indeed, the role of siblings may be even more relevant for children in low-income, single-mother, ethnically diverse families than in middle-class White families. Some have argued (e.g., Taylor, Chatters, & Mays, 1988) that African American families rely more on siblings as sources of support. Given recent changes in welfare policies, it may indeed be an older sibling—not a paid child care provider—who is caring for younger children in the family when low-income mothers are entering the work force. In many cases, older children in the family may be the only consistently reliable means of child care on which these mothers can rely. Whether sibling caregiving has negative effects or possible benefits for children living in different family circumstances cannot be adequately addressed at this time because of the exclusion of these constructs in existing databases. Any large-scale study examining children always has at least one, if not many, measures of mothering, but rarely, if ever, considers the possibility that fathers, the children's older siblings, grandparents, or even the siblings of the parents themselves (i.e., aunts, uncles) could and probably do care for and "parent" these children. Whether this is due to lack of research funding or a theoretical bias where mothers are viewed as the only legitimate caregivers of children, the fact remains that we cannot know the effects of these other caregivers unless investigators include measures that allow us to do so.

Even though the sibling relationship is one of the longest lasting relationships an individual will have, we still know far too little about the development of sibling relationships throughout childhood, adolescence, and adulthood. Only when survey researchers begin to include measures of sibling relationship quality as consistently as they now include measures of mother–child relationship quality, will we have a nationally representative database allowing researchers to address the contributions of siblings to children's developmental outcomes.

Appendix

Sibling Inventory of Behavior Items

Companionship/Involvement
    Accepts (Child 1) as a playmate
    Gets ideas for things they can do together
    Has fun at home with (Child 1)
    Treats (Child 1) as a good friend
    Makes plans that include (Child 1)
    Shares secrets with (Child 1)
Empathy/Concern
    Is pleased by progress (Child 1) makes
    Wants (Child 1) to succeed
    Shows sympathy when things are hard for (Child 1)
    Is concerned for (Child 1's) welfare and happiness
    Tries to comfort (Child 1) when (s/he) is unhappy or upset
Teaching/Directiveness
    Teaches (Child 1) new skills
    Helps (Child 1) adjust to a new situation
    Baby-sits and cares for (Child 1)
    Tries to teach (Child 1) how to behave
Rivalry
    Tattles on (Child 1)
    Is jealous of (Child 1)
    Is nosy and has to know everything about (Child 1)
    Takes advantage of (Child 1)
    Blames (Child 1) when something goes wrong
    Is very competitive against (Child 1)
    Resents (Child 1)

Conflict/Aggression
    Teases or annoys (Child 1)
    Gets angry with (Child 1)
    Fusses and argues with (Child 1)
    Hurts (Child 1's) feelings
    Has physical fights with (Child 1) (not just for fun)
Avoidance
    Is embarrassed to be with (Child 1) in public
    Stays away from (Child 1) if possible
    Acts ashamed of (Child 1)
    Frowns or pouts when (Child 1) has to be with (him/her)
    Tries to avoid being seen with (Child 1)

References

Achenbach, T. M. (1991). *Manual for the Child Behavior Checklist/4–18 and 1991 profile.* Burlington: University of Vermont, Department of Psychiatry.

Brody, G. H. (1998). Sibling relationship quality: Its causes and consequences. *Annual Review of Psychology, 49,* 1–24.

Brody, G. H., & Murry, V. M. (2001). Sibling socialization of competence in rural, single-parent African American families. *Journal of Marriage and Family, 63,* 996–1008.

Brody, G. H., Stoneman, Z., Smith, T., & Gibson, N. M. (1999). Sibling relationships in rural African American families. *Journal of Marriage and Family, 61,* 1046–1057.

Buhrmester, D., & Furman, W. (1990). Perceptions of sibling relationships during middle childhood and adolescence. *Child Development, 61,* 1387–1398.

Cole, A. K., & Kearns, K. A. (2001). Perceptions of sibling qualities and activities of early adolescents. *Journal of Early Adolescence, 21,* 204–227.

Conger, K. J., Conger, R. D., & Scaramella, L. V. (1997). Parents, siblings, psychological control and adolescent adjustment. *Journal of Adolescent Research, 12,* 113–138.

Dunn, J., & Munn, P. (1985). Becoming a family member: Family conflict and the development of social understanding in the second year. *Child Development, 56,* 480–492.

Furman, W., & Buhrmester, D. (1985). Children's perceptions of the qualities of sibling relationships. *Child Development, 56,* 448–461.

Garcia, M. M., Shaw, D. S., Winslow, E. B., & Yaggi, K. E. (2000). Destructive sibling conflict and the development of conduct problems in young boys. *Developmental Psychology, 36,* 44–53.

Graham-Bermann, S. A., & Cutler, S. E. (1994). The Brother-Sister Questionnaire: Psychometric assessment and discrimination of well-functioning from dysfunctional relationships. *Journal of Family Psychology, 8,* 224–238.

Herrera, C., & Dunn, J. (1997). Early experiences with family conflict: Implications for arguments with a close friend. *Developmental Psychology, 33,* 869–881.

Hetherington, E. M., & Clingempeel, W. G. (1992). Coping with marital transitions: A family systems approach. *Monographs of the Society for Research in Child Development, 57* (2–3, Serial No. 227).

Hetherington, E. M., Henderson, S. H., Reiss, D. (1999). Adolescent siblings in stepfamilies: Family functioning and adolescent adjustment. *Monographs of the Society for Research in Child Development, 64*(4), 222.

Howe, N. (1991). Sibling-directed internal state language, perspective-taking and affective behavior. *Child Development, 62,* 1503–1512.

Howe, N., Aquan-Assee, J., & Bukowski, W. M. (1995). Self-disclosure and the sibling relationship: What did Romulus tell Remus? In K. J. Rotenberg (Ed.), *Disclosure processes in children and adolescents* (pp. 78–99).Cambridge: Cambridge University Press.

Howe, N., Aquan-Assee, J. Bukowski, W. M., Lehoux, P. M., & Rinaldi, C. M. (2001). Siblings as confidants: Emotional understanding, relationship warmth, and sibling self-disclosure. *Social Development, 10*, 439–454.

Kramer, L., & Baron, L. A. (1995). Parental perceptions of children's sibling relationships. *Family Relations, 44*, 95–103.

McElwain, N. L., & Volling, B. L. (2002). Relating individual control, social understanding, and gender to child–friend interaction: A relationships perspective. *Social Development, 11*, 362–385.

Mendelson, M. J., Aboud, F. E., & Lanthier, R. P. (1994). Kindergartners' relationships with siblings, peers, and friends. *Merrill-Palmer Quarterly, 40*(3), 416–435.

Riggio, H. R. (2000). Measuring attitudes toward adult sibling relationships: The Lifespan Sibling Relationship Scale. *Journal of Social and Personal Relationships, 17*(6), 707–728.

Schaefer, E. S., & Edgerton, M. (1981). *The Sibling Inventory of Behavior.* Chapel Hill: University of North Carolina.

Stocker, C. M., Lanthier, R. P., & Furman, W. (1997). Sibling relationships in early adulthood. *Journal of Family Psychology, 11*(2), 210–221.

Stocker, C. M., & McHale, S. M. (1992). The nature and family correlates of preadolescents' perceptions of their sibling relationships. *Journal of Social and Personal Relationships, 9*, 179–195.

Stormshak, E. A., Bellanti, C. J., Bierman, K. L., & Conduct Problems Prevention Research Group. (1996). The quality of sibling relationships and the development of social competence and behavioral control in aggressive children. *Developmental Psychology, 32*, 79–89.

Taylor, R. J., Chatters, L. M., & Mays, V. M. (1988). Parents, children, siblings, in-laws, and non-kin as sources of emergency assistance to black Americans. *Family Relations, 37*, 298–304.

Volling, B. L. (2003). Sibling relationships. In M. H. Bornstein, L. Davidson, C. L. M. Keyes, K. A. Moore, & the Center for Child Well-being (Eds.), *Well-being: Positive development across the life course* (pp. 205–220). Mahwah, NJ: Lawrence Erlbaum.

Volling, B. L., & Elins, J. (1998). Family relationships and children's emotional adjustments as correlates of maternal and paternal differential treatment: A replication with toddler and preschool siblings. *Child Development, 63*, 1209–1222.

Volling, B. L., McElwain, N. L., & Miller, A. L. (2002). Emotion regulation in context: The jealousy complex between young siblings and its relations with child and family characteristics. *Child Development, 73*, 581–600.

Widmer, E. D., & Weiss, C. C. (2000). Do older siblings make a difference? The effects of older sibling support and older sibling adjustment on the adjustment of socially disadvantaged adolescents. *Journal of Research on Adolescence, 10*, 1–27.

Youngblade, L. M., & Dunn, J. (1995). Individual differences in young children's pretend play with mother and sibling: Links to relationships and understanding of other people's feelings and beliefs. *Child Development, 66*, 1472–1492.

IV Positive Attitudes and Behaviors toward Learning and School Environments

14 The Patterns of Adaptive Learning Survey

Eric M. Anderman

University of Kentucky

Tim Urdan

Santa Clara University

Robert Roeser

Stanford University

Achievement goal theory has emerged as one of the most prominent motivational theories over the past 25 years. According to this theory, individuals' perceptions about the purposes of achievement provide an organizing framework. This framework involves cognitions about the value of the task and self-perceptions, explanations about the causes of success or failure on the task, and affective reactions to success and failure. Unlike more narrowly defined performance objectives (e.g., the goal of getting 90% or an A on a test), achievement goals represent beliefs and concerns about the meaning of getting an A on the test. Whereas performance objectives focus on *what* the individual is trying to achieve (Bandura, 1986; Wentzel, 1989), achievement goal theorists are concerned with students' perceptions of *why* they are trying to achieve. What is the perceived purpose of getting a score of 90% on the test? Goals, when defined in this way, represent "more superordinate classes of goals that are behind the particular outcomes individuals strive for" (Dweck, 1992, p. 165). Goal theorists are generally concerned with the quality of motivation rather than the absolute amount of motivation (Ames, 1987, 1992; Ames & Ames, 1984; Covington, 1984; Dweck, 1986; Maehr & Nicholls, 1980; Nicholls, 1989; Urdan, 1997). Two students may be equally motivated to complete an assignment, but they may have different reasons for doing so.

Current research on achievement goals generally includes three types of goals: mastery, performance-approach, and performance-avoidance. Although a fourth type of goal—mastery-avoidance—has been posited (Pintrich, 2000), there is currently little research that has examined that goal. In this chapter, therefore, we focus on the first three goals. Mastery goals represent a concern with understanding, developing competence, and improving. Performance-approach goals involve a desire to *demonstrate* competence, often by outperforming others. Performance-avoidance goals represent a concern with *not* appearing *incompetent* or less competent than others. When pursuing mastery goals, individuals tend to rely on internal frames of reference to judge success and failure at a task, whereas both types of performance goals involve social comparison. Research suggests that the particular achievement goals individuals adopt in a given achievement situation depend in part on stable personality characteristics, such as need for achievement and fear of failure (Elliot, 1997), as well as situational characteristics (Ames, 1992).

How Goals Have Been Measured

Research on achievement goals has generally been conducted using two methodologies: experimental manipulation and questionnaires. Survey measures have varied widely across research programs. Some researchers have measured goals by asking students when they feel most successful (e.g., "I feel most successful when I learn something new" in the 1985 Nicholls, Patashnick, and Nolen study). Other measures, including the one described in this chapter, usually ask students more directly about their goals (e.g., "I want to do better than other students in this class"). In addition, some measures combined different types of goals into a single construct, whereas other measures only included items that divided into unique constructs. For example, the Nicholls et al. (1985) measure includes a scale called "Ego and Social Goals." In this measure, ego goals are merged with social goals to form an "ego and social orientation" scale that includes demonstration-of-ability items ("I feel most successful if I show people I'm smart"), social approval items ("I feel most successful if the teacher likes my work"), and social interaction items ("I feel most successful if I work with friends") (p. 685). More recent measures, including the ones described in this chapter, assess single constructs such as mastery goals or performance-approach goals (Elliot & Church, 1997).

Survey measures of mastery goals have generally been consistent across research programs. These measures typically include items assessing the desire to learn, understand, and master concepts, as well as the goal of improving skills. Measures of performance goals have been less consistent. As previously mentioned, some measures merged social comparative goals with other goals, such as social goals (Nicholls et al., 1985), extrinsic goals, and preference for challenge

(Pintrich & Garcia, 1991). Earlier versions of the Patterns of Adaptive Learning Survey (PALS) included social approval items ("I feel bad when I do well in class and the teacher doesn't say anything about it") and challenge preference items ("I like problems that are easy") in the performance goal scale (Midgley, Maehr, & Urdan, 1993). Before the recent distinction between performance-approach and performance-avoidance goals, some measures of performance goals only included items assessing performance-approach goals, whereas others included both performance-approach and performance-avoidance items but failed to distinguish between the two (Harackiewicz, Barron, Pintrich, Elliot, & Thrash, 2002). The varied and imprecise measurement of goals, particularly performance goals, has created a somewhat unclear pattern of results regarding the effects of pursuing these goals. Fortunately, recent measures of goals, including PALS, have corrected some of these shortcomings (Elliot & Church, 1997; Midgley et al., 2000; Skaalvik, 1997).

For the most part, examinations of mastery goals have yielded consistent results. Briefly, when oriented toward mastery goals, students tend to attribute failure to lack of effort, persist in difficult situations, choose moderately challenging tasks, have relatively positive feelings about school and schoolwork, use deep cognitive processing strategies, use more self-regulating strategies, and be more intrinsically motivated than when low in mastery goal orientation (see Ames, 1992; Anderman & Maehr, 1994; Pintrich & Schunk, 2002; Urdan, 1997, for reviews). Because mastery goals are generally associated with a positive constellation of outcomes, they have sometimes been said to represent an "adaptive" motivational orientation (Dweck, 1986). Despite this characterization, research has often failed to find an association between mastery goals and measures of achievement (Harackiewicz et al., 2002).

For performance goals, in contrast, the picture is much less clear. When performance goal oriented, students have been shown to be more likely to attribute failure to ability, prefer less challenging tasks, use more surface and less deep processing learning strategies, give up when faced with difficulty, and have more negative affect about school than when task goal oriented (see Ames, 1992; Dweck & Leggett, 1988; Midgley, 1993 for reviews). Accordingly, some have labeled a performance goal orientation "maladaptive" (Ames, 1992; Dweck & Leggett, 1988). This characterization may not always be warranted, however.

There are several reasons to be cautious. First, there is now considerable evidence that performance-approach goals often are related positively to beneficial learning outcomes, including academic achievement, task value, and academic self-concept (see Harackiewicz et al., 2002, for a review). However, research has also often yielded null associations between performance goals and outcomes. For example, Nicholls et al. (1985) found no relation between ego-social goals and college plans, satisfaction with learning, perceptions of ability, or grade point average. Nolen (1988) found no relation between ego-social goals and the use of deep processing strategies. Midgley and Urdan (1995, 2001) found no association between performance-approach goals and self-handicapping. Results of a number of studies revealed no association between performance-approach goals and intrinsic motivation (Harackiewicz et al., 2002). Second, past research often did not distinguish between performance-approach and performance-avoidance goals. Performance-avoidance goals are usually negatively related to beneficial learning and performance outcomes, and including avoidance items in some performance goal measures but not others likely produced mixed effects for performance goals across studies. Third, important individual differences may affect the relations between performance goals and various outcomes. Midgley, Kaplan, and Middleton (2001) suggested that performance-approach goals may have more negative consequences for early adolescent students than for college students. Similarly, Urdan and his colleagues (Enos & Urdan, 2002; Urdan & Giancarlo, 2001) found a positive association between performance-approach goals and academic achievement for students with an individualistic sense of self, but not among students with a collectivist sense of self.

Finally, a number of researchers (Ainley, 1993; Barron & Harackiewicz, 2000; Meece & Holt, 1993; Pintrich & Garcia, 1991; Urdan, 1994; Wolters, Yu, & Pintrich, 1996) have found that the interaction of mastery and performance-approach goals reveals few ill effects of being performance-approach goal oriented when simultaneously having a mastery goal orientation. It also reveals some potential benefits of performance-approach goals for individuals low in their mastery goal orientation. Some research indicates that the pursuit of performance-approach goals can slightly weaken the positive relation between mastery goals and strategy use, self-efficacy, and task value (Wolters et al., 1996) and between mastery goals and interest (Elliot & Church, 1997). But most research reveals few interactive effects of mastery and performance-approach goals (see Harackiewicz et al., 2002).

Hundreds of studies examining the effects of achievement goals have been conducted during the past 2 decades. Surveys have been used in a substantial portion of these studies. Recent studies have employed measures that clearly have distinguished between mastery, performance-approach, and performance-avoidance goals, and these measures generally do not include references to other motives (a problem found in previous measures). Research with these improved measures has generally found positive motivational and behavioral correlates of mastery goals, although these goals are often not associated with measures of achievement. Similarly, recent research has typically found a negative pattern of outcomes associated with performance-avoidance goals and a somewhat mixed pattern of associations with performance-approach goals.

Patterns of Adaptive Learning Survey

One of the most widely used survey measures of goals is PALS, which has been under development for more than a decade. In its current form, it contains highly reliable and valid measures of students' personal mastery, performance-approach, and performance-avoidance goal orientations. These measures have been used repeatedly in both cross-sectional and longitudinal samples.[1] Measures for PALS initially were developed in the early 1990s. The various measures have been refined throughout the past decade by reducing the number of items in some of the scales, improving the internal consistencies of scales, honing the questions to focus on the core aspects of the major goal orientations, and developing separate measures for performance-approach and performance-avoidance goal orientations.

Initially, Midgley and Maehr received funding to apply goal orientation theory to the reform of elementary and middle schools. Throughout the course of this 3-year intervention, the PALS measures were utilized and further refined (Maehr & Midgley, 1996). The researchers then conducted the Patterns of Adaptive Learning Study, which used a large sample of early adolescents to examine changes in students' achievement goals. Students were followed from the fifth grade through the ninth grade, completing measures at least once per academic year. The personal goal orientation measures were greatly improved during this study (Midgley, 2002). Near the end of the 1990s, Turner and Midgley conducted an additional longitudinal study of students' achievement goals, across the transition from elementary school to middle school. Students were surveyed twice during the sixth grade (in elementary school), and again twice during the seventh grade (after the transition to middle school) (Turner et al., 2002). This again served as an opportunity to still further examine and refine the psychometric properties of PALS.

A variety of other research programs have incorporated various versions of PALS. Some of these include a study in the People's Republic of China (Mu et al., 1997), a study that included multiple ethnic groups (Urdan & Giancarlo, 2001), and a study of more than 5,000 adolescents who viewed the Channel One television news program (Anderman & Johnston, 1998; Johnston, Brzezinski, & Anderman, 1994).

PALS has been used in both elementary and secondary school classrooms. The measures typically are worded in a general (nondomain-specific) format when used with elementary school samples, since elementary school students generally spend the majority of the day in the same classroom with the same teacher. In contrast, when used with middle or high school students, the items often refer to a specific academic domain (e.g., math, English). In most cases, internal consistency is higher for the domain-specific measures, compared with the general measures.

In our research with PALS, we have used 5-point Likert scales. We have anchored our items at 1 = *not at all true*, 3 = *sometimes true*, and 5 = *very true*. We have generally included the goal orientation measures on surveys that also have included other motivation measures. We tend to mix the personal goal orientation items with each other and with other items that utilize the same anchors and the same introduction.

---

[1] Downloadable manuals and documentation for PALS are available at http://www.umich .edu/~pals/pals/

We suggest that surveys be administered by trained research assistants in students' regular classrooms. We generally tell students that the survey is not a test and that there are no right or wrong answers; we are merely interested in their opinions and beliefs about these issues. We reassure students that the information we collect is confidential and that their parents, teachers, and peers will not see their specific responses to any of the questions. We stress to the students that the survey is very important and that we really value their thoughts on these issues. We also try to explain to the students that some questions may sound very similar to others in the survey, but that this is important for ensuring that we really understand what each student thinks. We include a sample question, which the survey administrator goes over with the students to familiarize them with the Likert scale. In general, we have read the items and instructions aloud to the students.

Reliability

The *mastery goal orientation* scale assesses the extent to which students engage in academic tasks in order to develop their competence. Students who are mastery oriented are interested in extending their current understanding of a given topic. Students' attention is focused on the task because the students' main goal is to master the task at hand. The original version of the scale (Cronbach's alpha = .86) is presented in Midgley et al. (2000). However, the version presented in this chapter ($\alpha = .85$) does not include items that assess intrinsic value and does not refer to specific behaviors (see Appendix).

Students who endorse *performance-approach goal orientation* are interested in demonstrating their competence. Such students are highly focused on the self. The original version contained five items, which referred to how students would feel or what students would want under certain circumstances (e.g., "I would feel really good if I were the only one who could answer the teacher's questions in class"). This scale displayed excellent internal consistency ($\alpha = .86$). The revised version ($\alpha = .89$) primarily refers to students' goals during class (see Appendix). As was the case for the measure of mastery goal orientation, for both performance goal orientation measures the original scales included items that referred to specific behaviors, whereas the revised versions focused specifically on students' goals.

Students who endorse a performance-avoidance goal orientation want to avoid the demonstration of incompetence. Such students do not want to be perceived as "stupid" by their peers and teachers. Performance-avoidance-oriented students are focused on the self. Similar to the measure of performance-approach goals, the original version of the performance-avoidance goal orientation measure ($\alpha = .75$) contained items that referred to how students would feel or what students would want when doing class work (e.g., "The reason I do my work is so others won't think I'm dumb"). The current version ($\alpha = .74$) contains four items and primarily refers to students' goals during class (see Appendix).

Discriminant Validity

The original PALS goal orientation items were subjected to confirmatory factor analyses to determine whether each construct was distinct from the others. Most of those initial analyses were conducted on data collected during the spring of 1996 from a large sample of sixth-grade students. Confirmatory factor analyses were conducted using LISREL 8 (Jöreskog & Sorbom, 1993). Maximum likelihood estimation was used. Data were assessed using covariance matrices and listwise deletion of data. In addition, multiple fit indices were used, as suggested by Hoyle and Panter (1995). These analyses are explained in detail in Midgley et al. (1998).

The items assessing personal mastery goal orientation, performance-approach goal orientation, and performance-avoidance goal orientation were entered into the analysis. A measurement model in which the three goal orientation measures were hypothesized to be distinct, albeit correlated, was tested. The model displayed excellent fit, $\chi^2(132, N = 647) = 389.77$, $p < .001$; GFI $= .94$; TLI $= .93$; CFI $= .94$; RMSEA $= .055$ with $P(0.05) = .94$. When one item that cross-loaded on both the performance-approach and performance-avoidance scales was eliminated, the model fit was improved, $\chi^2(116, N = 647) = 298.55$, $p < .001$; GFI $= .95$; TLI $= .95$; CFI $= .96$; RMSEA $= .049$ with $P(0.05) = .55$. The model was subsequently tested separately for European American and African American students and separately for female and male students (Midgley et al., 1998). Results indicated that the scales operate in the same ways with students from different genders and ethnic groups.

The revised goal orientation items also were examined using confirmatory factor analysis, using LISREL 8. The goal orientation measures again loaded on three distinct factors ($GFI = 0.97$, $AGFI = 0.95$). The factors represented the hypothesized mastery, performance-approach, and performance-avoid goal orientations (Midgley et al., 2000).

Other Psychometric Properties

Various members of our research team have conducted analyses assessing other psychometric aspects of the PALS personal goal orientation scales. All of these analyses indicate that the scales are both reliable and valid. For example, Anderman and Midgley (1997) conducted a longitudinal study examining the stability of the mastery and performance-approach goal orientation scales, using a sample of fifth- and sixth-grade students during a 2-year period over the transition from elementary to middle school. Because much research indicates that students' motivation and beliefs change over the middle school transition, we expected that the scales would not necessarily prove to be stable. Nevertheless, moderate stability was found in scales assessing personal goal orientations in both English and math. Stability was found for both females and males and for both high- and low-ability students. Analyses from a subsequent sample assessed stability within the same school year. Those analyses indicated fairly high stability ($r = .63$ for mastery goals and .61 for performance-approach goals) within the school year (Midgley et al., 1998).

Midgley et al. (1998) also examined the convergent validity of these measures, using a large sample of fifth graders. Specifically, Midgley and colleagues included scales developed by Nicholls and his colleagues, and examined the relations between several PALS measures and Nicholls's scales. Nicholls's scales and the PALS scales were related. Specifically, the correlation between Nicholls's ego-orientation scale and our performance-approach goal orientation scale was .63, and the correlation between his task-orientation scale and our personal mastery goal orientation scale was .67.

In addition, several studies indicate that PALS demonstrates good construct validity. Specifically, the PALS goal orientation measures are related in expected ways to other measures. In a number of studies, we have demonstrated that our measure of personal mastery goals is related positively to perceived academic efficacy (e.g., Roeser, Midgley, & Urdan, 1996). As expected, personal performance-avoidance goals are related negatively to academic efficacy (Middleton & Midgley, 1997). For performance-approach goals, there are mixed results, with some studies finding approach goals positively related to academic efficacy (Midgley & Urdan, 1995), some finding approach goals negatively related to academic efficacy (Anderman & Young, 1994), and some finding no relation between performance-approach goals and academic efficacy (Middleton & Midgley, 1997).

A number of studies have indicated that mastery goals are related positively to the use of adaptive learning strategies (e.g., Meece, Blumenfeld, & Hoyle, 1988; Nolen, 1988). Our analyses with PALS have yielded similar findings (Anderman & Young, 1994; Middleton & Midgley, 1997, 1999; Ryan, Hicks, & Midgley, 1997).

In addition, our analyses indicate that performance-avoidance goals tend to be related to the use of maladaptive strategies, such as self-handicapping. The relations between performance-approach goals and maladaptive strategies are somewhat mixed. For example, in some studies, personal performance-approach goals were unrelated to self-handicapping (Midgley & Urdan, 2001), although in one study, we found a positive relation between personal performance-approach goals and self-handicapping for African American students (Midgley, Arunkumar, & Urdan, 1996). In both our studies and other research, performance-approach goals appear to be related positively to the avoidance of help seeking (Middleton & Midgley, 1999; Ryan & Pintrich, 1997; Ryan et al., 1997).

Finally, we also have examined the relations of mastery and performance goals to various indices of affect. Previous research suggests that mastery goals are related positively to indices of affect, whereas performance goals are related negatively to affect (see Midgley et al., 1998, for a summary). Using PALS, Roeser et al. (1996) found that personal mastery goals were related positively to affect at school, whereas performance-approach goals were unrelated to affect. Midgley et al. (1996) obtained similar results in examining the relations of goal orientations to self-esteem.

Summary

Goal orientation theory is a prominent and greatly researched theory of academic motivation. The personal goal orientation scales developed for PALS by Midgley and her colleagues are among the most reliable and valid measures of these constructs for use with adolescents. This has been demonstrated in a variety of studies in both cross-sectional and longitudinal research. The scales have good discriminant, convergent, and construct validity. They are stable over time, and they are internally consistent.

As noted by Midgley et al. (1998), the PALS goal orientation scales offer several advantages, compared with other goal orientation measures. In PALS, personal achievement goals have been separated from perceptions of the goal structure in the learning environment. Although we also have developed measures of classroom goal structure (Anderman, 1999; Anderman & Midgley, 1997; Turner et al., 2002; Urdan, Midgely, & Anderman, 1998) and school goal structure (Anderman & Young, 1994; Kaplan & Maehr, 1999; Midgley & Urdan, 1995), the PALS personal goal orientation scales clearly separate students' perceptions of personal goals from their perceptions of the classroom and school learning environments.

In addition, because research clearly indicates that performance goals can be construed as both approach and avoidance goals, our measures are consistent with current research indicating that these goals are in fact distinct (Elliot & Harackiewicz, 1996; Middleton & Midgley, 1997; Skaalvik, 1997). In addition, our measures of performance goals do not include items that assess extrinsic goals, social goals, anxiety, or fear.

Motivation is a critical issue in American education, yet we have little nationally representative data on student motivation. Goal orientation theory is perhaps the most prominent of all current motivation theories. The PALS measures are among the best existing motivation measures. They have been demonstrated to be both valid and reliable in samples of various ages, ethnicities, and cultures. Because they do not include items that measure other motivational variables (classroom goal structures, other types of personal goals, other types of motivation), they are "cleaner" than many other measures. They are strongly related to a variety of educational and psychological variables, and they are sensitive to developmental changes in students' goals and beliefs. The inclusion of PALS personal goal orientation scales in nationally representative studies would yield extremely important information concerning students' motivation to learn and achieve and would be of value to many researchers.

Authors' Note

Address all correspondence to Eric M. Anderman, University of Kentucky, 249 Dickey Hall, Lexington, KY 40506-0017 (eande1@uky.edu); Tim Urdan, Santa Clara University, Department of Psychology, 500 El Camino Real, Santa Clara,

CA 95053 (turdan@scu.edu); Robert Roeser, Stanford University, School of Education, Stanford, CA 94305 (rroeser@stanford.edu).

Appendix

Current PALS Personal Goal Orientation Scales

Personal mastery goal orientation   Alpha = .85
   It is important to me that I learn a lot of new concepts this year.
   One of my goals in class is to learn as much as I can.
   One of my goals is to master a lot of new skills this year.
   It's important to me that I thoroughly understand my class work.
   It's important to me that I improve my skills this year.

Personal performance-approach goal orientation   Alpha = .89
   It's important to me that other students in my class think I am good at my class
      work.
   One of my goals is to show others that I'm good at my class work.
   One of my goals is to show others that class work is easy for me.
   One of my goals is to look smart in comparison to the other students in my class.
   It is important to me that I look smart compared to others in my class.

Personal performance-avoidance goal orientation   Alpha = .74
   It's important to me that I don't look stupid in class.
   One of my goals is to keep others from thinking I'm not smart in class.
   It's important to me that my teacher doesn't think that I know less than others in
      class.
   One of my goals in class is to avoid looking like I have trouble doing the work.

References

Ainley, M. D. (1993). Styles of engagement with learning: Multidimensional assessment of their relationship with strategy use and school achievement. *Journal of Educational Psychology, 85,* 395–405.

Ames, C. (1987). The enhancement of student motivation. In M. L. Maehr & D. Kleiber (Eds.), *Advances in motivation and achievement: Vol. 5. Enhancing motivation* (pp. 123–148). Greenwich, CT: JAI Press.

Ames, C. (1992). Classrooms: Goals, structures, and student motivation. *Journal of Educational Psychology, 84,* 261–271.

Ames, C., & Ames, R. (Eds). (1984). *Research on motivation in education: Vol. 1. Student motivation.* San Diego, CA: Academic Press.

Anderman, E. M., & Johnston, J. (1998). TV news in the classroom: What are adolescents learning? *Journal of Adolescent Research, 13,* 73–100.

Anderman, E. M., & Maehr, M. L. (1994). Motivation and schooling in the middle grades. *Review of Educational Research, 64,* 287–309.

Anderman, E. M., & Midgley, C. (1997). Changes in achievement goal orientations, perceived academic competence, and grades across the transition to middle level schools. *Contemporary Educational Psychology, 22,* 269–298.

Anderman, E. M., & Young, A. J. (1994). Motivation and strategy use in science: Individual differences and classroom effects. *Journal of Research in Science Teaching, 31,* 811–831.

Anderman, L. (1999). Classroom goal orientation, school belonging and social goals as predictors of students' positive and negative affect following the transition to middle school. *Journal of Research and Development in Education, 32*, 89–103.

Bandura, A. (1986). *Social foundations of thought and action: A social cognitive theory.* Englewood Cliffs, NJ: Prentice-Hall.

Barron, K. E., & Harackiewicz, J. M. (2000). Achievement goals and optimal motivation: A multiple goals approach. In C. Sansone & J. M. Harackiewicz (Eds.), *Intrinsic and extrinsic motivation: The search for optimal motivation and performance* (pp. 229–254). New York: Academic Press.

Covington, M. V. (1984). The motive for self-worth. In C. Ames and R. Ames (Eds.), *Research on motivation in education: Vol. 1. Student motivation* (pp. 77–113). San Diego, CA: Academic Press.

Dweck, C. S. (1986). Motivational processes affecting learning. *American Psychologist, 41*, 1040–1048.

Dweck, C. S. (1992). The study of goals in human behavior. *Psychological Science, 3*, 165–167.

Dweck, C. S., & Leggett, E. L. (1988). A social-cognitive approach to motivation and personality. *Psychological Review, 95*, 256–273.

Elliot, A. J. (1997). Integrating the "classic" and "contemporary" approaches to achievement motivation: A hierarchical model of approach and avoidance achievement motivation. In M. L. Maehr & P. R. Pintrich (Eds.), *Advances in motivation and achievement* (Vol. 10, pp. 143–179). Greenwich, CT: JAI Press.

Elliot, A., & Church, M. (1997). A hierarchical model of approach and avoidance achievement motivation. *Journal of Personality and Social Psychology, 72*, 218–232.

Elliot, A., & Harackiewicz, J. M. (1996). Approach and avoidance goals and intrinsic motivation: A mediational analysis. *Journal of Personality and Social Psychology, 70*, 461–475.

Enos, S., & Urdan, T. (2002, April). *Understanding cultural and ethnic differences in the pursuit and effects of achievement goals.* Paper presented at the meeting of the American Educational Research Association, New Orleans.

Harackiewicz, J. M., Barron, K. E., Pintrich, P. R., Elliot, A. J., & Thrash, T. M. (2002). Revision of achievement goal theory: Necessary and illuminating. *Journal of Eductional Psychology, 94*, 638–645.

Hoyle, R. H., & Panter, A. T. (1995). Writing about structural equation models. In R. Hoyle (Ed.), *Structural equation modeling: Concepts, issues, and applications* (pp. 158–176). Thousand Oaks, CA: Sage.

Johnston, J., Brzezinski, E. V., & Anderman, E. M. (1994). *Taking the measure of Channel One: A three year perspective.* Ann Arbor: University of Michigan, Institute for Social Research.

Jöreskog, K., & Sorbom, D. (1993). LISREL 8. Chicago: Scientific Software.

Kaplan, A., & Maehr, M. L. (1999). Achievement goals and student well-being. *Contemporary Educational Psychology, 24*, 330–358.

Maehr, M. L., & Midgley, C. (1996). *Transforming school cultures.* Boulder, CO: Westview Press.

Maehr, M. L., & Nicholls, C. (1980). Culture and achievement motivation: A second look. In N. Warren (Ed.), *Studies in cross-cultural psychology* (Vol. 2, pp. 221–267). New York: Academic Press.

Meece, J. L., Blumenfeld, P. C., & Hoyle, R. H. (1988). Students' goal orientations and cognitive engagement in classroom activities. *Journal of Educational Psychology, 80*, 514–523.

Meece, J. L., & Holt, K. (1993). A pattern analysis of students' achievement goals. *Journal of Educational Psychology, 85*, 582–590.

Middleton, M., & Midgley, C. (1997). Avoiding the demonstration of lack of ability: An under-explored aspect of goal theory. *Journal of Educational Psychology, 89*, 710–718.

Middleton, M., & Midgley, C. (1999, August). *Beyond motivation: Middle school students' perception of press for understanding.* Paper presented at the meeting of the American Psychological Association, Boston.

Midgley, C. (1993). Motivation and middle level schools. In M. L. Maehr & P. R. Pintrich (Eds.), *Advances in motivation and achievement: Vol. 8. Motivation in the adolescent years* (pp. 217–274). Greenwich, CT: JAI.

Midgley, C. (2002). *Goals, goal structures, and patterns of adaptive learning.* Mahwah, NJ: Lawrence Erlbaum.

Midgley, C., Arunkumar, R., & Urdan, T. (1996). "If I don't do well tomorrow, there's a reason": Predictors of adolescents' use of academic self-handicapping strategies. *Journal of Educational Psychology, 88,* 423–434.

Midgley, C., Kaplan, A., & Middleton, M. (2001). Performance-approach goals: Good for what, for whom, under what circumstances, and at what cost? *Journal of Educational Psychology, 93,* 77–86.

Midgley, C., Kaplan, A., Middleton, M., Maehr, M. L., Urdan, T., Anderman, L. H., et al. (1998). The development and validation of scales assessing students' achievement goal orientations. *Contemporary Educational Psychology, 23,* 113–131.

Midgley, C., Maehr, M. L., Hruda, L., Anderman, E. M., Anderman, L., Freeman, K. E., et al. (2000). *Manual for the Patterns of Adaptive Learning Scales (PALS).* Ann Arbor: University of Michigan.

Midgley, C., Maehr, M. L., & Urdan, T. (1993). *Manual for the Patterns of Adaptive Learning Survey (PALS).* Ann Arbor: University of Michigan.

Midgley, C., & Urdan, T. (1995). Predictors of middle school students' use of self-handicapping strategies. *Journal of Early Adolescence, 15,* 389–411.

Midgley, C., & Urdan, T. (2001). Academic self-handicapping and performance goals: A further examination. *Contemporary Educational Psychology, 26,* 61–75.

Mu, X., Shi, K., Wang, P., Live, D., Kaplan, A., & Maehr, M. L. (1997). *School motivation of Chinese students: The relevance of goal theory in the People's Republic of China.* Unpublished research report. Ann Arbor: University of Michigan, Leadership and Learning Laboratory.

Nicholls, J. G. (1989). *The competitive ethos and democratic education.* Cambridge, MA: Harvard University Press.

Nicholls, J. G., Patashnick, M., & Nolen, S. B. (1985). Adolescents' theories of education. *Journal of Educational Psychology, 77,* 683–692.

Nolen, S. B. (1988). Reasons for studying: Motivational orientations and study strategies. *Cognition and Instruction, 5,* 269–287.

Pintrich, P. R. (2000). An achievement goal theory perspective on issues in motivation terminology, theory, and research. *Contemporary Educational Psychology, 25,* 92–104.

Pintrich, P. R., & Garcia, T. (1991). Student goal orientation and self-regulation in the college classroom. In M. L. Maehr & P. R. Pintrich (Eds.), *Advances in motivation and achievement: Vol. 7. Goals and self-regulatory processes* (pp. 371–402). Greenwich, CT: JAI Press.

Pintrich, P. R., & Schunk, D. H. (2002). *Motivation in education: Theory, research, and applications* (2nd ed.). Englewood Cliffs, NJ: Prentice-Hall.

Roeser, R. W., Midgley, C., & Urdan, T. C. (1996). Perceptions of the school psychological environment and early adolescents' psychological and behavioral functioning in school: The mediating role of goals and belonging. *Journal of Educational Psychology, 88,* 408–422.

Ryan, A. M., Hicks, L., & Midgley, C. (1997). Social goals, academic goals, and avoiding seeking help in the classroom. *Journal of Early Adolescence, 17,* 152–171.

Ryan, A. M., & Pintrich, P. R. (1997). Should I ask for help? The role of motivation and attitude in adolescents' help seeking in math class. *Journal of Educational Psychology, 89,* 329–341.

Skaalvik, E. M. (1997). Self-enhancing and self-defeating ego orientation: Relations with task and avoidance orientation, achievement, self-perceptions, and anxiety. *Journal of Educational Psychology, 89,* 71–81.

Turner, J. C., Midgley, C., Meyer, D. K., Gheen, M., Anderman, E. M., Kang, J., et al. (2002). The classroom environment and students' reports of avoidance behaviors in mathematics: A multimethod study. *Journal of Educational Psychology, 94,* 88–106.

Urdan, T. (1994). *Extending goal theory: Examining social goals and multiple goals profiles.* Unpublished doctoral dissertation, University of Michigan, Ann Arbor.

Urdan, T. (1997). Achievement goal theory: Past results, future directions. In M. L. Maehr & P. R. Pintrich (Eds.), *Advances in motivation and achievement* (Vol. 10, pp. 99–141). Greenwich, CT: JAI Press.

Urdan, T., & Giancarlo, C. (2001, April). *Differences between students in the consequences of goals and goal structures: The role of culture and family obligation.* Paper presented at the meeting of the American Educational Research Association, Seattle.

Urdan, T., Midgley, C., & Anderman, E. M. (1998). Classroom influences on self-handicapping strate-gies. *American Educational Research Journal, 35,* 101–122.

Wentzel, K. R. (1989). Adolescent classroom goals, standards for performance, and academic achieve-ment: An interactionist perspective. *Journal of Educational Psychology, 81,* 131–142.

Wolters, C., Yu, S. L., & Pintrich, P. R. (1996). The relation between goal orientation and stu-dents' motivational beliefs and self-regulated learning. *Learning and Individual Differences, 8,* 211–238.

15 Ability Self-Perceptions and Subjective Task Values in Adolescents and Children

Jacquelynne S. Eccles and Susan A. O'Neill

University of Michigan

Allan Wigfield

University of Maryland

Individual differences in school performance and other achievement-related behaviors have been a central concern of social and personality theory for more than 50 years. Various theoretical analyses of these differences have been proposed, and a variety of beliefs and perceptions about self and task have been proposed as mediators of achievement-related behavior. Many of these theories focus on individual differences in expectations for success and the subjective valuing of various achievement-related behaviors as the two major predictors of individual differences in achievement. Theorists predict, for example, that doing well in school is facilitated by having high confidence in one's academic abilities and by placing high value on doing well in school. Similar arguments have been proposed for other domains such as sports and instrumental music (see Eccles, Wigfield, & Schiefele, 1998).

Given that doing well and feeling competent in school, work, and other socially valued domains are important outcomes for success in our society and for good mental health, having measures of indicators that predict these outcomes during childhood and adolescence would be useful to policy makers and researchers. In this chapter, we describe the development of measures for two such indicators: *ability self-perceptions* and *subjective task values*. Measurement scales for both indicators, as well as for task difficulty, were initially developed for adolescents (grades 5 through 12). The scales for ability self-concepts and subjective task values were later adapted for use with younger children (grades 1 through 6).

Ability Self-Perceptions

The construct of ability self-perceptions evolved out of classic expectancy-value models of behavior and the work by theorists to operationalize a definition for *expectations for success*. Atkinson (1964) provided one of the first definitions of expectations for success on a task, defining expectancy as the proportion of individuals who have succeeded at the task in the past. Other researchers have argued for a more explicit operational distinction between subjective expectancy and task difficulty, arguing that task difficulty, as defined by Atkinson, is just one of several influences on subjective expectancy (e.g., Bandura, 1994; Eccles et al., 1983; Feather, 1986; Heckhausen, 1977; Weiner, 1974). In addition, all of these researchers have stressed the importance of domain-specific measures of expectancies.

In 1983, Eccles and her colleagues laid out a model of motivated task choice and performance that distinguished between one's self-concept of domain-specific abilities and perceived task difficulty. They predicted that these two beliefs would interact in predicting expectations for success in particular school subjects. Self-concept of domain-specific ability was predicted to relate positively to expectancies, whereas task difficulty perceptions were predicted to relate negatively to expectancies. Subsequently, Eccles and Wigfield (1995) demonstrated that domain-specific expectations for success and ability self-concepts load on the same factor and therefore can be treated empirically as the same construct.

Subjective Task Values

Similar discussions have arisen regarding the concept of task value. Atkinson (1964) defined task value in terms of the incentive value of anticipated success (the anticipated pride one would feel in accomplishment). Over the past 30 years, other individuals have offered broader definitions of task value. Crandall (1969), for example, defined task value in terms of the subjective attainment value (the importance of attaining a goal) and objective task difficulty. Rotter (1982) defined task value as the anticipated reward the individual will receive from engaging in the activity. Similarly, Raynor (1974) argued that the instrumentality of a particular task in allowing one to move along a contingent path toward a desired goal would increase the incentive value of the task.

Building on Rokeach's (1980) work on broader human values, Feather (1982) discussed task value in terms of systems that "capture the focal, abstracted qualities of past encounters, that have a normative or oughtness quality about them, and that function as criteria or frameworks against which present experience can be tested. They are tied to our feelings and can function as general motives" (p. 275). In terms of motivational consequences of these value systems, he assumed that values affect the valence of specific activities or situations for the individual and therefore are linked to action (e.g., approaching or avoiding the activity). The notion that the valence of an activity would affect action is similar to the Lewinian idea that activity choice would be influenced by the relative perceived valences of the options being considered (Lewin, 1938) and to Rokeach's suggestion that we engage in activities that create the effects we like and avoid those activities that create effects we do not like (Rokeach, 1980).

Eccles and her colleagues have offered a broad definition of subjective task value and have specified several components (Eccles et al., 1983). In general, these investigators assume that task value is determined by characteristics of the task itself; by the broader needs, goals, values, and motivational orientations of the individual; and by affective memories associated with similar tasks in the past. The degree to which a particular task is able to fulfill needs, confirm central aspects of one's self-schema, facilitate reaching goals, affirm personal values, and/or elicit positive versus negative affective associations and anticipated states is assumed to influence the value a person attaches to engaging in that task. The researchers therefore predicted that individuals would be more likely to engage in valued tasks. Thus, individuals' values are posited to have both motivational and behavioral consequences.

Eccles and her colleagues argued further that task value should be conceptualized in terms of four major components: attainment value, intrinsic value or interest, utility value, and cost. Attainment value represents the importance of doing well on a task in terms of one's self-schema and core personal values. Intrinsic or interest value is the inherent enjoyment or pleasure one gets from engaging in an activity. Utility value is the value a task acquires because it is instrumental in reaching a variety of long- and short-range goals. Finally, cost is what is lost, given up, or suffered as a consequence of engaging in a particular activity (see Eccles et al., 1983). The first three components are best thought of as characteristics that affect the positive valence of the task. Cost, in contrast, is best thought of as those factors (such as anticipated anxiety and anticipated cost of failure) that affect the negative valence of the activity. It also includes the avoidance goals now emerging in achievement goal theory (Elliott & Church, 1997).

Thus, over time, conceptualizations of constructs linked to expectancy for success and task value have evolved greatly, as have refinements of the components of each construct. Below we summarize the development and confirmation of one set of measures for these two constructs at the domain-specific level, which in this chapter we refer to as ability self-perceptions (ability self-concepts, competence beliefs) and subjective task values.

Factor Analysis of Academic Scales

Data for confirmatory factor analysis of items to assess ability self-perceptions and subjective task values in the domains of mathematics and English come from a 2-year longitudinal study in which adolescents' domain-specific self-perceptions and task values were assessed once each year. The sample was drawn using the mathematics classroom as an intermediate sampling unit. Classrooms at each grade level were chosen randomly from among classrooms whose teachers volunteered to participate in the study. Within each classroom all adolescents were asked to participate. Project staff members supervised the students' completion of the self-report questionnaires. In Year 1, the sample consisted of 742 predominantly White, middle-class adolescents in grades 5 through 12, with approximately 90 adolescents at each grade level. The sample included 366 females and 376 males. In Year 2, the sample contained 575 adolescents in grades 6 through 12 (88% of the 5th through 11th graders from Year 1). In the analyses summarized here, only adolescents with complete data on all measures are included; $N = 707$ for Year 1, and $N = 545$ for Year 2.

The questionnaire given to these adolescents included 29 items grouped under the following nine domain-specific constructs: ability perceptions, performance perceptions, expectations for success, perceived task difficulty, amount of effort required to do well, actual amount of effort exerted, enjoyment in doing task, perceived importance of task, and perceptions of the extrinsic utility value of the subject area. All items focused on the domains of mathematics and English. Responses for all items were made on 7-point Likert scales anchored only at the end points but with numbers indicating 1 through 7.

The psychometric properties of the items and scales are quite good and have been reported elsewhere (see Eccles, Wigfield, Blumenfeld, & Harold, 1984; Eccles et al., 1983, for discussion of development of the questionnaire). Cronbach's alphas ranged from .62 to .92 (see Appendix). There were virtually no missing data on the responses to items. The items had good distributions, with some skewing to the positive end of the scale. These scales can be self-administered either on the computer or on a questionnaire.

Using the Year 1 data, we investigated the factor structure of the nine domain-specific constructs through exploratory factor analyses of the original 29 items. Based on the results, we eliminated 10 items (see Appendix for the final 19 items). To determine whether we could test the models on the whole sample, we assessed the invariance of the covariance matrices of the items for boys and girls, and for younger (5th through 7th grade) and older (8th through 12th grade) adolescents, following procedures described by Jöreskog and Sorbom (1981). Results of the analyses showed that the matrices were reasonably invariant across groups. Thus, the data were collapsed across age and gender.

Using the Year 2 data, we conducted a two-step confirmatory factor analysis of the final 19 items (see Eccles & Wigfield, 1995, for details). First we analyzed the three superordinate categories of ability beliefs, subjective task value beliefs, and task difficulty beliefs individually. The results confirmed a six-factor model. We next analyzed all 19 items simultaneously. As predicted, the six-factor model best fit the relations among all 19 items (see Appendix). This model fit our theoretical predictions regarding the likely factor structure, as well as the pattern of relations among the six factors themselves. We have replicated this factor structure in another sample of fifth through sixth graders that included both European American and African American students (see Eccles et al., 1989; Senior, 1989; Wigfield, Eccles, Mac Iver, Reuman, & Midgley, 1991).

We then used a higher order factor analysis to determine whether these factors could be aggregated into three major higher order constructs: ability/expectancy, subjective task value, and perceived task difficulty. Each item loaded strongly on the appropriate individual factor, and each individual factor loaded strongly on the higher order factor posited to underlie them (see Appendix). The higher order factors are related negatively, as predicted in the Eccles et al. (1983) model. As with the other models, this higher order factor model also provided an excellent fit in the Year 2 data. The pattern of factor loadings and relation between the two higher order factors showed great similarity across the two years. Again, the covariance invariance test shows that the matrices are quite similar each year.

Although the math and English constructs do factor separately, they are highly related and can be collapsed into scales that provide more global school-related constructs for researchers interested in these more general school-related beliefs and their relation to general school achievement. We have used the Michigan Study of Adolescent Life Transitions (MSALT) data to create such scales, and they are relatively reliable (Cronbach's alpha = .68 to .77). These more global scales, however, would not be good for studying the differential performance and course enrollment decisions across the domains of mathematics and English. However, we have now replicated the factor structure for physical science, biological science, computer science, sports, and instrumental music, and are therefore comfortable recommending adaptation of the items for other achievement-related activity domains.

Validity of the Academic Scales

The validity of the academic scales was assessed in three ways: discriminant validity, face validity, and predictive validity. Face validity reflects the logical correspondence between the items themselves and the constructs presumably being measured. As can be seen, there is very close linguistic correspondence between the items themselves and the construct they indicate (see Appendix). Discriminant validity is confirmed by the factor analyses described above.

Predictive validity is confirmed by analyses testing the extent to which these scales relate in the predicated directions to other achievement outcomes. Using the 2-year sample, we assessed the extent to which these scales related to teachers' ratings of the students' prior achievement, to parents' ratings of their children's abilities and interests, and to the courses chosen and grades received later in high school in the domains of math and English (see Eccles, 1984; Eccles et al., 1983; Eccles et al., 1990; Eccles, Meece, Adler, & Kaczala, 1982).

We also conducted similar analyses of predictive validity with a demographically and ethnically more diverse sample that is part MSALT (see Eccles et al., 1989; Wigfield et al., 1997). The MSALT sample was drawn from sixth-grade classrooms in 10 school districts in southeastern Michigan. Eight of the districts were 90% or more European American; 2 of the districts had between 30% and 40% African American students. The full sample included approximately

10% African American students and 85% European American students who came from predominantly working-class and middle-class families. The gender distribution was approximately even. The self-report questionnaires were administered in mathematics classrooms. School record data, teacher reports, parent reports, and classroom observations were also collected.

In both the 2-year and the MSALT samples, there is very high predictive validity, and the scales do an excellent job of explaining the links between gender and differential achievement in mathematics and English. For example, the gender difference in plans to enroll and actual enrollment in advanced mathematics courses in high school is completely explained by the gender difference in the subjective task value attached to advanced mathematical courses, even after family background, prior achievement, and mathematical aptitude are controlled (Eccles, Adler, & Meece, 1984, 1993; Eccles et al., 1983; Eccles et al., 1984; Eccles, Wigfield, Harold, & Blumenfeld, 1993). These associations have been replicated in subsequent samples and hold true for African American youth as well as European American youth (Updegraff, Eccles, Barber, & O'Brien, 1996; Winston, Eccles, Senior, & Vida, 1997), as well as for sports and instrumental music (Eccles & Harold, 1991; O'Neill, in press; O'Neill, Ryan, Boulton, & Sloboda, 2000; Wigfield, O'Neill, & Eccles, 1999).

Most interestingly, the ability self-concept construct and the subjective task value construct sometimes relate differently to performance (course grades) and choice behaviors (the decision to enroll in particular courses). When there is a difference in the pattern of associations, ability self-concept relates most strongly to subsequent performance, and the subjective task value construct relates most strongly to enrollment decisions. For example, in the 2-year sample, only self-concept of math ability predicted subsequent math courses grades (Eccles, Adler, et al., 1984). In contrast, the subjective task values indicators predicted to future course enrollment plans and actual enrollment decisions. We have also found similar patterns for predicting adolescents' participation in sports, enrollment in advanced math courses, and enrollment in advanced physical science courses in the MSALT sample (e.g., Eccles & Barber, 1999).

These differential effects, however, are not always found. In the MSALT sample, math ability self-concept did not predict changes in math grades from one term to the next, once indicators of prior performance were controlled. In contrast, math value did predict increases in math grades. This was truer for the European American than for the African American students (unstandardized coefficients = .22 and .13, respectively; ethnic difference was significant at $p < .10$). In regard to course plans, as predicated by the expectancy-value models, both math value and math ability self-concept significantly predicted plans to take more math courses, and this was equally true for the African American and European American students.

In summary, our first study demonstrates that we can reliably measure the three constructs associated with expectancy value models of achievement behavior: ability self-perceptions, subjective task values, and perceived task difficulty. The six scales (see Appendix) are equally appropriate for boys and girls and for youth from 5th through 12th grade. The scales can be further collapsed into three superordinate scales that relate to each other in the theoretically expected direction. We have replicated this factor structure in subsequent Black and White samples in other school districts in southeastern Michigan. Additional analyses in other data sets have also shown that comparable factor solutions emerge when other domain names are substituted for mathematics. The most powerful scales for predicting subsequent achievement behaviors are the ability/expectancy scale and the three subjective task value scales (interest, importance, utility), which can be used independently or together as a superordinate scale. We believe that these scales are ready for use on national data sets of youth in grades 5 and above.

Scales for Younger Children

Having developed reliable and valid scales to assess self-concepts of abilities and subjective task values for achievement-related domains (particularly school achievement domains), we wanted to determine whether we could assess these same constructs in elementary school–age children and whether we could extend the work to the domains of sports and instrumental music. Data for this effort are part of the longitudinal Michigan Childhood and Beyond Study (Eccles, Wigfield, et al., 1984) investigating the development and socialization of children's beliefs and values about self and tasks, as well as their activity choices. The findings summarized here come from Years 2, 3, and 4 of the study.

The children in this sample are from lower-middle-class to middle-class backgrounds, and more than 95% are White. Children, parents, and teachers were recruited through four school districts in the suburbs of Detroit, and 75% of children solicited agreed to participate and obtained parental permission. In Year 2, the participants included 865 children in first, second, and fourth grades. Thus, over the 3 years of data collection, the sample includes children from grades one through six, as well as three overlapping cohorts of children. The longitudinal sample used in the analyses summarized here includes approximately 615 children (females = 325, males = 290) divided about equally among the three cohorts. The 615 children represent 71% of the original sample. Attrition in the sample was mostly due to children moving far away from the school districts sampled. Every effort was made to relocate children each year, and children continuing to live in the same general area but not attending participating schools are included in the longitudinal sample.

In three consecutive springs, the children completed questionnaires tapping their beliefs about mathematics, reading, instrumental music, and sports, as well as other constructs. Within each of these domains, children answered questions about specific activities. In the academic area, children were asked about mathematics and reading. The music questions concentrated on instrumental music. The sports questions focused on sports in general and included sex-typed sports activities more often done by girls (tumbling) and by boys (throwing and catching a ball).

In the math, reading, and sports activity domains, the five items designed to tap competence beliefs asked the children how good they are at each activity, how good they are relative to the other things they do, how good they are relative to other children, how well they expect to do at each activity, and how good they thought they would be at learning something new in each domain. The four items tapping subjective task values in Year 2 included one item assessing importance, one assessing usefulness, and two assessing interest. At Years 3 and 4, two new values items were added: one asking children how important doing well on the activity is to them compared to other activities they do, and another asking how useful the activity is compared to the other activities they do. For instrumental music, fewer items were included on the questionnaires as follows: three items were used to tap competence beliefs in Year 2, asking the children how good they are, how good they are relative to the other things they do, and how good they thought they would be at learning a new musical instrument. Three items were used to tap subjective task values, one item assessing importance, and two assessing interest. In Years 3 and 4, another item was added for competence beliefs in instrumental music, asking how good they are relative to other children. The wording of these items was essentially the same in each domain. All items in all domains were answered using response scales ranging from 1 to 7. The items have excellent psychometric properties, and the scales themselves have very good reliability and validity (see Eccles, 1984; Eccles et al., 1982; Eccles et al., 1983; Eccles, Wigfield, et al., 1984; Eccles & Wigfield, 1995; Updegraff et al., 1996).

To ensure that these young children understood the constructs being assessed, the items were pilot-tested on 100 children, and the answer scales were illustrated to foster children's understanding of how to use them (see Eccles et al., 1993). All questions were read aloud to the children in Years 2 and 3. In Year 4, the oldest two groups (in grades four and six) did the questionnaires on their own. The distribution of responses was good, with some skewing to the positive end of the scale. In grades one to three, the children did not use all 7 points of the scale with equal frequency; instead their responses clustered around the end and mid points. This, however, did not affect the factor analyses and scale reliability estimates.

Factor Analyses of Children's Scales

Initially, we did factor analyses of the items assessed at Year 2 to determine whether young children's responses had good psychometric properties and yielded the same factors we had obtained on adolescents (Eccles et al., 1993). Within the domains of math, reading, and sports, distinct competence beliefs and task values factors were apparent even among the first graders. The items loading on the competence and values factors were similar, both in the different domains and in the different age groups. Based on these factor analyses, scales defining these constructs were created. The competence belief scales in the domains of math, reading, and sports contained the five items discussed above, and the subjective task values scale contained four items (two items assessing interest, one assessing perceived importance, and one assessing perceived usefulness). Internal consistency reliabilities for these scales ranged from good to excellent, with Cronbach's alphas ranging from .53 to .82. In instrumental music, the competence beliefs scales contained four items, and the subjective task values scale contained three items (one assessing importance and two assessing interest), with Cronbach's alphas ranging from .67 to .86.

We next performed exploratory and confirmatory factor analyses of the items given during Years 3 and 4. In the exploratory factor analyses, Cattell's scree test was used to determine the number of factors that best describe the data. As with the Year 2 data, the analyses at Years 3 and 4 yielded clear competence beliefs and task values factors in each of the domains. In some of the domains (especially the academic domains), there was evidence that the values items formed two factors: usefulness/importance and interest.

Although the items assessing task values did not always factor into separate usefulness/importance and interest factors, we created scales for both of these constructs and analyzed them separately, for three main reasons. First, Eccles et al.'s (1983) theoretical model specifies these as different components, and factor analytic work with older children and adolescents suggests the emergence of these constructs as separate factors (Eccles & Wigfield, 1995). Earlier work with older students (e.g., Eccles et al., 1989; Wigfield et al., 1991) has examined change in the separate values constructs, and we wish to compare results of the present study to that work. Second, our interest construct is somewhat similar to Harter's (1981) curiosity component of intrinsic motivation, and so comparisons to her work are relevant as well. Third, the separate scales were reliable (with the exception of the usefulness and importance scales at Year 2).

Validity of the Children's Scales

We assessed the validity of the children's scales by looking at face, discriminant, and predictive validity. Based on the linguistic overlap between the items and the constructs being assessed, we concluded that the face validity of the scales is quite high. The factor analytic results reported above demonstrate the discriminant validity of the scales.

Predictive validity is provided by the expected gender differences and developmental declines in each scale, the expected relations of the scales to both parent and teacher ratings, and the expected relations of the scales to each other (see further, Wigfield et al., 1997). As predicted, boys had more positive self-perceptions and values than girls for sports and mathematics, and girls had more positive self-perceptions and values than boys in reading and instrumental music. Basically, the self-perceptions and values for all four domains declined over time. The one exception was sports, where interest did not decline. In another set of analyses, we have also found that these developmental declines continue through high school and are related in the expected direction to both gender and parents' ratings of their children's abilities and interests in these domains (Fredricks & Eccles, 2002; Jacobs, Hyatt, Osgood, Eccles, & Wigfield, 2002).

In summary, these scales are quite reliable and have excellent validity. The math and reading scales are also currently being used with 8- to 12-year-olds in the Child Development Supplement of the Panel Study of Income Dynamics (CDS/PSID, a nationally representative sample of adults and their children, and with the upper-elementary school-aged children in the National Institute of Child Health and Human Development's National Child Care Study. Cronbach's alphas for the CDS/PSID sample were .80 or higher for all subgroups and ages.

The instrumental music scales have also been used with a sample of approximately 1,500 elementary and secondary school children in the United Kingdom as part of the 4-year longitudinal Youth Participation in Music Activities study (see further O'Neill et al., 2000; Wigfield et al., 1999). The results confirmed a two-factor model, measuring distinct competence beliefs (Cronbach's alpha = .84) and task values factors (Cronbach's alpha = .95). Predictive validity of the scales has been confirmed by testing the extent to which the scales relate in the predicted direction to measures of participation in instrumental music. Children who reported playing instruments also reported higher ability beliefs and value beliefs than children who had given up playing instruments or considered themselves to be nonplayers. Girls reported higher ability and value beliefs than boys. All groups reported higher value beliefs for instrumental music than ability beliefs. Ability beliefs correlated similarly with both formal (in school) and informal (outside school) instrumental playing, whereas value beliefs correlated higher with informal than formal instrumental playing (see further O'Neill, in press). These results support similar findings obtained with children in the United States (Wigfield et al., 1997).

In conclusion, we have demonstrated that one can create reliable and valid measures of ability self-perceptions and subjective task values in various domains and that these beliefs predict subsequent achievement-related behaviors. As such, these indicators are both useful and important in the area of positive youth development, as researchers and policy makers strive to understand the multiple pathways that lead to positive outcomes for youth.

Appendix

The following items assess adolescents' ability self-perceptions and subjective task values in the domain of mathematics. English, sports, instrumental music, or another achievement-related domain can be substituted for "math" in these items. All items were answered on scales ranging from 1 to 7.

Ability/Expectancy[a]

1. Compared to other students, how well do you expect to do in math this year? (much worse than other students, much better than other students)
2. How well do you think you will do in your math course this year? (very poorly, very well)
3. How good at math are you? (not at all good, very good)

4. If you were to order all the students in your math class from the worst to the best in math, where would you put yourself? (the worst, the best)

5. How have you been doing in math this year? (very poorly, very well)

Perceived Task Difficulty

Task Difficulty[b]

6. In general, how hard is math for you? (very easy, very hard)
7. Compared to most other students in your class, how hard is math for you? (much easier, much harder)
8. Compared to most other school subjects that you take, how hard is math for you? (my easiest course, my hardest course)

Required Effort[c]

9. How hard would you have to try to do well in an advanced high school math course? (not very hard, very hard)
10. How hard do you have to try to get good grades in math? (a little, a lot)
11. How hard do you have to study for math tests to get a good grade? (a little, a lot)
12. To do well in math I have to work (much harder in math than in other subjects, much harder in other subjects than in math).

Perceived Task Value

Intrinsic Interest Value[d]

13. In general, I find working on math assignments (very boring, very interesting).
14. How much do you like doing math? (not very much, very much)

Attainment Value/Importance[e]

15. Is the amount of effort it will take to do well in advanced high school math courses worthwhile to you? (not very worthwhile, very worthwhile)
16. I feel that, to me, being good at solving problems which involve math or reasoning mathematically is (not at all important, very important).
17. How important is it to you to get good grades in math? (not at all important, very important)

Extrinsic Utility Value[f]

18. How useful is learning advanced high school math for what you want to do after you graduate and go to work? (not very useful, very useful)
19. How useful is what you learn in advanced high school math for your daily life outside school? (not at all useful, very useful)

[a]Alpha coefficient = .92
[b]Alpha coefficient = .80
[c]Alpha coefficient = .78
[d]Alpha coefficient = .76
[e]Alpha coefficient = .70
[f]Alpha coefficient = .62

References

Atkinson, J. W. (1964). *An introduction to motivation.* Princeton, NJ: Van Nostrand.

Bandura, A. (1994). *Self-efficacy: The exercise of control.* New York: W. H. Freeman.

Crandall, V. C. (1969). Sex differences in expectancy of intellectual and academic reinforcement. In C. P. Smith (Ed.), *Achievement-related behaviors in children* (pp. 11–45). New York: Russell Sage Foundation.

Eccles, J. S. (1984). Sex differences in achievement patterns. In T. Sonderegger (Ed.), *Nebraska Symposium on Motivation: Vol. 32. Psychology and gender* (pp. 97–132). Lincoln: University of Nebraska Press.

Eccles, J. S. (1993). School and family effects on the ontogeny of children's interests, self-perceptions, and activity choice. In J. Jacobs (Ed.), *Nebraska Symposium on Motivation, 1992: Developmental perspectives on motivation* (pp. 145–208). Lincoln: University of Nebraska Press.

Eccles (Parsons), J., Adler, T. F., Futterman, R., Goff, S. B., Kaczala, C. M., Meece, J. L., et al. (1983). Expectancies, values, and academic behaviors. In J. T. Spence (Ed.), *Achievement and achievement motivation* (pp. 75–146). San Francisco: W. H. Freeman.

Eccles, J. S., Adler, T. F., & Meece, J. L. (1984). Sex differences in achievement: A test of alternate theories. *Journal of Personality and Social Psychology, 46*(1), 26–43.

Eccles, J. S., & Barber, B. L. (1999). Student council, volunteering, basketball, or marching band: What kind of extracurricular involvement matters? *Journal of Adolescent Research, 14,* 10–43.

Eccles, J. S., & Harold, R. D. (1991). Gender differences in sport involvement: Applying the Eccles expectancy-value model. *Journal of Applied Sport Psychology, 3,* 7–35.

Eccles (Parsons), J., Meece, J. L., Adler, T. F., & Kaczala, C. M. (1982). Sex differences in attributions and learned helplessness. *Sex Roles, 8*(4), 421–432.

Eccles, J. S., & Wigfield, A. (1995). In the mind of the actor: The structure of adolescents' achievement values and expectancy-related beliefs. *Personality and Social Psychology Bulletin, 21,* 215–225.

Eccles, J., Wigfield, A., Blumenfeld, P., & Harold, R. (1984). *Psychological predictors of competence development.* Grant proposal to the National Institute for Child Health and Human Development.

Eccles, J. S., Wigfield, A., Flanagan, C. A., Miller, C., Reuman, D. A., & Yee, D. (1989). Self-concepts, domain values, and self-esteem: Relations and changes at early adolescence. *Journal of Personality, 57,* 283–310.

Eccles, J. S., Wigfield, A., Harold, R. D., & Blumenfeld, P. (1993). Ontogeny of children's self-perceptions and subjective task values across activity domains during the early elementary school years. *Child Development, 64,* 830–847.

Eccles. J. S., Wigfield, A., & Schiefele. U. (1998). Motivation to succeed. In W. Damon (Series Ed.) & N. Eisenberg (Vol. Ed.), *Handbook of child psychology: Vol. 3. Social, emotional, and personality development* (5th ed., pp. 1017–1095). New York: Wiley.

Elliott, A., & Church, M. (1997). A hierarchical model of approach and avoidance achievement motivation. *Journal of Personality and Social Psychology, 72*, 218–232.

Feather, N. T. (1982). Human values and the prediction of action: An expectancy-value analysis. In N. T. Feather (Ed.), *Expectations and actions: Expectancy-value models in psychology* (pp. 263–289). Hillsdale, NJ: Lawrence Erlbaum.

Feather, N. T. (1986). Human values, valences, expectations and affect: Theoretical issues emerging from recent applications of the expectancy-value model. In D. Brown & J. Veroff (Eds.), *Frontiers of motivational psychology: Essays in honor of John W. Atkinson* (pp. 146–172). New York: Springer-Verlag.

Fredricks, J. A., & Eccles, J. S. (2002). Children's competence and value beliefs from childhood through adolescence: Growth trajectories in two male-sex-typed domains. *Developmental Psychology, 38*(4), 519–533.

Harter, S. (1981). A new self-report scale of intrinsic versus extrinsic orientation in the classroom: Motivational and informational components. *Developmental Psychology, 17*, 300–312.

Heckhausen, H. (1977). Achievement motivation and its constructs: A cognitive model. *Motivation and Emotion, 1*, 283–329.

Jacobs, J. E., Hyatt, S., Osgood, W. D., Eccles, J. S., & Wigfield, A. (2002). Changes in children's self-competence and values: Gender and domain differences across grades one through twelve. *Child Development, 73*(2), 509–527.

Jöreskog, K. G., & Sorbom, K. (1981). *LISREL VI: Analysis of linear structural relationships by maximum likelihood and least squares methods.* Chicago: National Educational Resources.

Lewin, K. (1938). *The conceptual representation and the measurement of psychological forces.* Durham, NC: Duke University Press.

O'Neill, S. A. (in press). Youth music engagement in formal and informal contexts. In J. L. Mahoney, R. Larson, and J. Eccles (Eds.), *Organized activities as contexts of development: Extracurricular activities, after-school and community programs.* Mahwah, NJ: Lawrence Erlbaum.

O'Neill, S. A., Ryan, K. J., Boulton, M. J., & Sloboda, J. A. (2000, April). Children's subjective task values and engagement in music. Paper presented at the British Psychological Society Annual Conference, Winchester, UK.

Raynor, J. O. (1974). Future orientation in the study of achievement motivation. In J. W. Atkinson and J. O. Raynor (Eds.), *Motivation and achievement* (pp. 121–134). Washington, DC: Hemisphere.

Rokeach, M. (1980). Some unresolved issues in theories of beliefs, attitudes, and values. In M. M. Page (Ed.), *Nebraska Symposium on Motivation* (Vol. 27, pp. 261–304). Lincoln: University of Nebraska Press.

Rotter, J. B. (1982). Social learning theory. In N. T. Feather (Ed.), *Expectations and actions: Expectancy-value models in psychology* (pp. 241–260). Hillsdale, NJ: Lawrence Erlbaum.

Senior, A. M. D. (1989). *Understanding differences in African-American and European-American students' self-concepts of ability.* Unpublished doctoral dissertation, University of Michigan, Ann Arbor.

Updegraff, K. A., Eccles, J. S., Barber, B. L., & O'Brien, K. M. (1996). Course enrollment as self-regulatory behavior: Who takes optional high school math courses. *Learning and Individual Differences, 8*, 239–259.

Weiner, B. (1974). *Achievement motivation and attribution theory.* Morristown, NJ: General Learning Press.

Wigfield, A., Eccles, J. S., Mac Iver, D., Reuman, D. A., & Midgley, C. M. (1991). Transitions during early adolescence: Changes in children's domain-specific self-perceptions and general self-esteem across the transition to junior high school. *Developmental Psychology, 27*, 552–565.

Wigfield, A., Eccles, J. S., Yoon, K. S., Harold, R. D., Arbreton, A. J., Freedman-Doan, C. R., et al. (1997). Changes in children's competence beliefs and subjective task values across the elementary school years: A three-year study. *Journal of Educational Psychology, 89*, 451–469.

Wigfield, A., O'Neill, S. A., & Eccles, J. S. (1999, April). *Children's achievement values in different domains: Developmental and cultural differences.* Paper presented at the Biennial Meeting of the Society for Research in Child Development, Albuquerque, NM.

Winston, C., Eccles, J. S., Senior, A. M., & Vida, M. (1997). The utility of an expectancy/value model of achievement for understanding academic performance and self-esteem in African-American and European-American adolescents. *Zeitschrift für Pädagogische Psychologie, 11*, 177–186.

16 Assessing Academic Self-Regulated Learning

Christopher A. Wolters

University of Houston

Paul R. Pintrich

University of Michigan

Stuart A. Karabenick

Eastern Michigan University

Self-regulated learning concerns the application of general models of regulation and self-regulation to issues of learning, in particular, academic learning that takes places in school or classroom contexts. There are a number of different models of self-regulated learning that propose different constructs and different conceptualizations (see Boekaerts, Pintrich, & Zeidner, 2000), but all of these models share some general assumptions and features. Given these assumptions, a general working definition of self-regulated learning is that it is an active, constructive process whereby learners set goals for their learning and then attempt to monitor, regulate, and control their cognition, motivation, and behavior, guided and constrained by their goals and the contextual features in the environment. In this chapter, we concentrate on the regulation and control phase of self-regulated learning and discuss our instrument development efforts in the three domains of academic cognition, motivation, and, finally, behavior.

Strategies for the Regulation of Academic Cognition

Cognitive control and regulation includes the types of cognitive and metacognitive activities that individuals engage in to adapt and change their cognition. One of the central aspects of the regulation of cognition is the actual selection and use of various cognitive strategies for memory, learning, reasoning, problem solving, and thinking. Numerous studies have shown that the selection of appropriate cognitive strategies can have a positive influence on learning and performance. These cognitive strategies range from the simple memory strategies very young children through adults use to help them remember (Schneider & Pressley, 1997) to sophisticated strategies that individuals have for problem solving and reasoning (see Baron, 1994; Nisbett, 1993). Although the use of various strategies is probably deemed more "cognitive" than metacognitive, the decision to use them is an aspect of metacognitive control and regulation, as is the decision to stop using them or to switch from one strategy type to another.

In our work, we have focused on three general types of cognitive strategies— rehearsal, elaboration, and organization (Weinstein & Mayer, 1986)—and general metacognitive self-regulation. Rehearsal strategies include attempts to memorize material by repeating it over and over or other types of "shallower" processing. In contrast, elaboration strategies reflect a "deeper" approach to learning, by attempting to summarize the material, put the material into one's own words, and so forth. Finally, organizational strategies also involve some deeper processing through the use of various tactics such as taking notes, drawing diagrams, or developing concept maps to organize the material in some manner. Metacognitive self-regulation includes various planning, monitoring, and regulation strategies for learning, such as setting goals for reading, monitoring comprehension as one reads, and making changes or adjustments in learning as one progresses through a task. Sample items for each of these four scales are provided in the Appendix.

Our empirical work on these four general types of strategies has been based in the development of the Motivated Strategies for Learning Questionnaire or MSLQ (e.g., Pintrich, Smith, Garcia, & McKeachie, 1991, 1993). The MSLQ is a self-report instrument that asks students about their cognitive and metacognitive strategies for learning. The MSLQ uses a 7-point Likert scale ranging from 1 (*not at all true of me*) to 7 (*very true of me*), with no specific labels for the other response categories. The MSLQ does not have norms associated with it as it is assumed that students' responses to the items will vary by subject area (reading-English, mathematics, science, social studies, etc.) or by classroom context. In addition, the items include phrases like "in this class" or "in this subject" to increase the likelihood that students will focus their responses on what they do in specific courses or classes. In other words, the MSLQ assumes, at a theoretical level, domain or context specificity in student strategy use and operationalizes it empirically at the course or classroom level.

In our own research, the MSLQ has been used with two general types of samples—students in colleges and universities and students in middle schools or junior high schools. We have not pursued analyses by different ethnic groups because our samples have been from mainly White (95%), middle- or working-class samples in southeastern Michigan. There is a clear need to examine how these measures work with more diverse populations.

In terms of the general structure of the instrument, both exploratory and confirmatory factor analyses on different college samples ($n = >2,000$) demonstrate that the four cognitive strategy factors (see Appendix) of rehearsal, elaboration, organization, and metacognitive self-regulation are supported (e.g., Pintrich, Zusho, Schiefele, & Pekrun, 2001). Estimates of internal consistency, computed using Cronbach's alpha, also are reasonable, ranging across the different studies and samples: rehearsal (.50 to .69), elaboration (.75 to .85), organization (.64 to .81), and metacognitive self-regulation (.71 to .81).

In contrast, studies with younger students in junior high or middle school classrooms ($n = $ >1,000) do not support the four-factor structure (e.g., Wolters & Pintrich, 1998). Factor analyses with these younger students support the creation of one general cognitive strategy scale and one metacognitive strategy scale. Developmentally, it appears that for these younger students, being cognitively engaged in learning the material includes using a combination of rehearsal, elaboration, and organizational strategies, and that they also do not make fine distinctions between these strategies as college students do. Accordingly, for junior high school and younger students, it is recommended that a general cognitive strategy scale that includes all of the cognitive strategy item be used, rather than three separate scales for rehearsal, elaboration, and organization. The Cronbach's alphas for the general cognitive strategy scale are acceptable (.83 to .88) and also for the metacognitive self-regulation scale (.63 to .74) across different studies (Pintrich & De Groot, 1990; Pintrich, Roeser, & De Groot, 1994; Wolters & Pintrich, 1998; Wolters, Yu, & Pintrich, 1996).

Besides the internal consistency of the scales, we also have found evidence of the construct validity of the scales in terms of their relations with other motivational and achievement measures. First, in terms of motivation, in general, we have found that, as theoretically expected, positive motivational beliefs, such as self-efficacy, interest, task value, and mastery goals, are positively related to cognitive strategy use and metacognitive self-regulation (for a summary of these findings, see Pintrich, 1999). As Pintrich points out, we have consistently found that students who believe they are capable (high self-efficacy) are more likely to report using cognitive strategies and being metacognitively self-regulating, with regression coefficients ranging from .10 to .67 across both middle school and high school studies (regressions control for other motivational constructs). In the same manner, students who value and are interested in their schoolwork also report the use of more cognitive and metacognitive strategies, with coefficients ranging from .03 to .73 across different studies. Finally, we also have found that students who are focused on mastery goals and are attempting to learn and understand the material also report higher levels of strategy use and metacognitive self-regulation (coefficients range from .06 to .73). This type of evidence supports the theoretical predictions that students who are more motivated also are more cognitively regulating and demonstrates the construct validity of the cognitive scales.

Finally, we also have found consistent relations between the cognitive strategy and metacognitive scales with various indices of achievement in classrooms. In the college studies, we have found that students who report using more cognitive and metacognitive strategies do score higher on tests in the course, grades on papers, lab performance, as well as receive higher grades (Pintrich, 1989; Pintrich et al., 1991, 1993; VanderStoep, Pintrich, & Fagerlin, 1996). In most cases, the relations are moderate with significant correlations ranging from .15 to .30, and some of the scales do not show strong relations across the studies. The same pattern emerges in the middle school studies with correlations ranging from .11 to .36 (Pintrich & De Groot, 1990; Wolters & Pintrich, 1998; Wolters et al., 1996). At the same time, these studies do show that, even with rather global measures of achievement such as grades or scores on tests, there are consistent, and theoretically predicted, relations between cognitive strategy use, metacognitive self-regulation, and achievement.

In summary, the four scales of cognitive (rehearsal, elaboration, and organization) and metacognitive strategy use seem to provide reliable and valid indicators of students' academic regulation. At the college level it is appropriate to use all four scales, while at the middle school level it is more appropriate to just use two scales, a general cognitive scale and a metacognitive self-regulation scale. Although more research needs to be done with diverse populations and with younger students, the items and scales seem to provide reasonable measures of cognitive self-regulations, albeit they may not be able to make very fine distinctions between different types and levels of self-regulation (Pintrich, Wolters, & Baxter, 2000).

Strategies for the Regulation of Achievement Motivation

Motivation is consistently viewed as a critical determinant of students' learning and achievement within academic settings (Graham & Weiner, 1996; Pintrich & Schunk, 2002). At the same time, learning is an effortful process, and academic tasks are fraught with obstacles that are likely to interfere with students maintaining an adaptive level of achievement motivation. Typical classrooms, for example, are often characterized by multiple tasks occurring at one time, a high level of noise and distractions, and many opportunities for off-task behavior. The challenge to complete academic work at home without the structure or social pressures to continue working that are present in the classroom can be even more difficult. In light of these obstacles, students' ability to actively influence their own motivation is viewed as an important aspect of their self-regulated learning.

In the same manner that learners can regulate their cognition, they can regulate their motivation and affect. Wolters (in press) describes the regulation of motivation as those activities through which individuals purposefully act to initiate, maintain, or supplement their willingness to start, to provide work toward, or to complete a particular activity or goal (i.e., their level of motivation). This form of regulation is achieved by deliberately intervening in, managing, or controlling one of the underlying processes that determine this willingness (i.e., the processes of motivation). At a general level, the regulation of motivation (or motivational regulation) encompasses those thoughts, actions, or behaviors through which students act to influence their choice, effort, or persistence for academic tasks. Although closely related and sometimes difficult to discern, the regulation of motivation is conceptually distinct from motivation itself.

The focus in this chapter is on a set of scales developed by Wolters (1998, 1999b; Wolters & Rosenthal, 2000) that can be used to assess seven strategies for the regulation of academic motivation (see Appendix). These scales include strategies based on self-consequating, environmental structuring, mastery self-talk, performance or extrinsic self-talk, relative ability self-talk, situational interest enhancement, and interest enhancement based on relevance or personal interest. Although this collection does not include all possible such strategies, it does represent a cross section of the ways in which students attempt to manage their motivation or motivational processing (Wolters, 2003).

When using a self-consequating strategy, students establish and provide themselves with an extrinsic consequence for their engagement in learning activities (e.g., Purdie & Hattie, 1996). Students can use concrete rewards and punishments as well as verbal statements as consequences (e.g., Graham, Harris, & Troia, 1998). Environmental structuring describes students' efforts to concentrate attention, to reduce distractions in their environment, or more generally, to arrange their surroundings to make completing a task easier or more likely to occur without interruption (Corno, 1993). This type of strategy can also include students' efforts to manage their own physical and mental readiness for completing a task by taking breaks or by eating or drinking particular foods (Wolters, 1998).

Students also regulate their motivation by emphasizing or articulating particular reasons for wanting to complete an activity in which they are engaged. That is, students use thoughts or subvocal statements to purposefully prompt themselves to recall or make salient some underlying reason they have for wanting to continue working on the activity. Consistent with distinctions within achievement goal theory, students may rely on different types of goals to increase their motivation. Students may subvocalize or think about mastery-related goals such as satisfying their curiosity, becoming more competent or knowledgeable about a topic, or increasing their feelings of autonomy. Alternatively, a student may think about getting high grades, or doing well in a class as a way of convincing themselves to continue working. This type of strategy is labeled performance or extrinsic self-talk. Finally, students may think about more specific performance-approach goals such as doing better than others or showing one's innate ability in order to keep oneself working hard.

Interest enhancement strategies describe activities in which students work to increase their intrinsic motivation for a task through either situational, personal interest, or value. In some studies these interest enhancement strategies have been treated as a single type of more general strategy (Wolters, 1999b), but they can also be differentiated. On the one hand, students can work to improve their situational interest or the immediate enjoyment they experience while completing a task (e.g., Sansone, Wiebe, & Morgan, 1999). On the other hand, interest enhancement also includes students' efforts to increase the relevance or meaningfulness of a task by linking it to their own life or their own personal interests and values.

Two forms of support for the construct validity of the scales used to assess these regulation-of-motivation strategies are discussed below. First, evidence indicating that these motivational strategies accurately represent discrete ways in which students' attempt to manage their motivation is presented. Second, evidence is presented regarding the relations of these motivational regulation strategies to students' motivational beliefs, engagement, use of learning strategies, and classroom performance.

The items used to assess these regulation-of-motivation strategies were developed from responses provided by undergraduate students to an open-ended questionnaire (Wolters, 1998). In this research ($n = 115$), students were presented with a short scenario describing one of four common tasks faced by college students (e.g., reading a textbook chapter, studying for an exam) followed by three common motivational problems (e.g., the material was boring or uninteresting) they might experience with respect to that task. For each of these 12 situations, students reported what they would do if they wanted to get themselves to overcome the problem and continue working on the task. A 14-category coding scheme was developed from motivational and volitional research and used by two independent coders to classify students' written responses. Later, some of the specific behaviors, thoughts, or procedures students reported were used to create a set of Likert-scaled items that tapped into the regulation-of-motivation strategies represented by these categories. Hence, the items used to assess regulation of motivation derive from both important theoretical distinctions within the motivational literature and actual activities reported by college students.

Additional evidence regarding the validity of these items comes from a follow-up study with a subset of the students from Wolters (1998). Forty-eight of these students returned approximately one month after taking the open-ended questionnaire described above for a second experimental session. Students spent approximately the first 20 minutes of this second session studying for their introductory psychology course, then completed a questionnaire that asked them to report on aspects of their motivation and cognition during the short study session they had just finished. The results of this study indicate that students did use a number of regulation-of-motivation strategies during the study session, and that using these strategies to some extent facilitated their engagement in the specific study task in which they were used (Wolters, 1999a).

The items developed from these studies were refined and used in several additional studies examining regulation of motivation within junior high school (Wolters & Rosenthal, 2000), high school (Wolters, 1999b), and college students (Wolters, 2001). The 7-point response scale used ranges from 1 (*not very true of me*) to 7 (*very true of me*) with no labels for the intervening response categories. Although limited in size (see Table 1), the samples of students used in these studies were, as a whole, diverse with respect to gender, ethnicity, and ability level. Data from this series of studies substantiate the view that these items tap into discrete regulation-of-motivation strategies in an internally consistent and reliable manner. Support for this view has been found using factor analyses and Cronbach's alphas within several groups of students. In addition, the motivational regulation scales in these studies typically exhibited moderately strong correlations, indicating that these scales reflect similar, but not overlapping underlying theoretical constructs. In short, there is ample evidence

Table 1. Coefficient Alphas and Number of Items for Regulation-of-Motivation Scales across Five Samples

Sample	n	Mastery self-talk		Situational interest enhancement		Relevance enhancement		Relative ability self-talk		Performance Self-talk		Self-consequating		Environmental structuring	
		Alpha	#	Alpha	#	Alpha	#	Alpha	#	Alpha	#	Alpha	#	Alpha	#
High school	88	.85	4	.87[a]	4	.83[a]	4	.87	5	.84	5	.87	4	.73	4
Junior high	114	.85	5	.82	4	.80	4	.75	4	.79	5	.74	4	.74	4
College 1999	168	.90	6	.75	5	.91	6	.86	4	.88	5	.94	5	.79	5
College 2000	152	.87	6	.88	5	.94	6	.86	4	.82	5	.93	5	.72	5
College 2001	219	.88	5	.88	5	.91	6	—	—	.84	5	.91	5	.74	5

[a] In Wolters (2000) items for these two scales were combined and labeled Interest Enhancement.

indicating that the regulation-of-motivation items tap into discrete underlying strategies within samples of students from early to late adolescence.

The construct validity of these scales is supported by evidence linking them to students' motivational beliefs, motivational engagement, and to their cognitive and metacognitive strategy use. Across several studies, findings indicate positive relations between five of the seven motivational strategies and both task value and a mastery goal orientation (Wolters, 1999b, 2001; Wolters & Rosenthal, 2000). Hence, there is strong evidence that students who express adaptive motivational beliefs are more likely to report using several regulation-of-motivation strategies. In these same samples, the regulation-of-motivation scales were less consistently tied to students' self-efficacy, although the significant correlations that have been found all indicate a positive relation between feeling more confident in one's abilities and use of the regulation strategies. The regulation-of-motivation strategies also showed a less consistent pattern of relations with students' reported focus on wanting good grades or other extrinsic goals. Further, this motivational belief was related negatively to students' reported use of motivational strategies in several instances.

Regulation-of-motivation strategies should help students provide effort and persist at academic tasks and avoid maladaptive academic behaviors such as procrastination. There is some evidence that the regulation-of-motivation scales described here are associated with these behaviors in the expected fashion. For instance, strong positive correlations were found between several of the motivational regulation strategies and a scale reflecting students' self-reported effort and persistence in several studies. In contrast, three of these strategies have consistently exhibited negative relations with a measure of students' procrastination in these same samples. This pattern of findings provides further evidence for the discriminate validity of these strategies.

Overall, prior studies with both younger and older students have provided evidence that students' regulation of motivation is related positively to the more cognitive and metacognitive aspects of their self-regulated learning. For instance, in five different samples students' reported use of metacognitive strategies was related significantly to each of the regulation-of-motivation strategies described here. The strength of these correlations was generally high with most exceeding .40. The pattern of relations between these regulation-of-motivation strategies and students' reported use of cognitive strategies was similar. These findings indicate that students who report using cognitive and metacognitive strategies also tend to report using regulation-of-motivation strategies.

Students' ability to regulate their motivation is one factor that may ultimately play a role in students' achievement or performance within academic settings. Thus far, however, the evidence linking students' regulation of motivation to their achievement is weak. Studies have generally failed to find a positive relation between any of the motivational regulation strategies presented here and students' instructor-assigned grades, regardless of the age level of the students. One explanation for this lack of relation is that any influence regulation of motivation has on achievement is mediated by such factors as effort, persistence, and cognitive engagement. Previous research has not explored this possibility directly, and further work in this area is clearly warranted.

In summary, the scales discussed here seem to provide reliable and valid indicators for seven strategies that students use to regulate their motivation. These scales, furthermore, appear to be appropriate for assessing motivational regulation within younger as well as older adolescent populations. Additional research is needed to determine whether they would be useful for younger populations of students. Research clarifying how to assess other regulation-of-motivation strategies would also be useful.

Strategies for the Regulation of Behavior

Consistent with a triadic model of social cognition (Zimmerman, 1989), regulation of behavior is an aspect of self-regulation that involves individuals' attempts to control their own overt behavior. Individuals can observe their own behavior, monitor it, and attempt to control and regulate it, and as such these activities can be considered self-regulatory for the individual.

In empirical work with the MSLQ, two scales have been developed that reflect behavioral control, one we call effort regulation and the other regulating time and study environment (see Appendix). Students respond to these items using the same response scale as the other items on the MSLQ (see above). Up to now, these items have only been used with college samples because these students have much more autonomy and freedom in terms of their time use and where they study in comparison to younger students, who are often much more externally regulated by teachers, parents, or just the structure of the school day. Accordingly, we only have data on these scales with college students.

Our analyses of these scales show that they separate in factor analyses from the cognitive and metacognitive scales (Pintrich et al., 1991, 1993). In addition, they show reasonable internal consistency. Cronbach's alphas for effort regulation have ranged from .69 to .82 and for time and study regulation from .65 to .76. Although we have not investigated these scales as often in our research, they do show the theoretically predicted relations with adaptive motivational beliefs such as self-efficacy, task value, and goals. Students who have adaptive profiles of motivation, such as higher self-efficacy, higher task value, and mastery goals, are more likely to regulate their effort and time/study environment (correlations range from .12 to .57). In addition, these two scales have shown moderate correlations with achievement measures (correlations range from .10 to .32).

Another behavioral strategy that can be very helpful for learning is help-seeking. When learners run into difficulty completing their academic work their options include seeking assistance from friends, family, classmates, and teachers as well as persistence or abandoning tasks (Feather, 1961, 1963). Help seeking is listed here as a behavioral strategy because it involves the person's own behavior, but it also involves contextual control because it necessarily involves the procurement of help from others in the environment and as such is also a social interaction (Ryan & Pintrich, 1997).

There is now considerable evidence that more motivated, active, engaged, and self-regulated learners are more likely to seek assistance when necessary (Karabenick, 1998). Typically, students' personal mastery goal orientations have been associated with instrumental/autonomous help seeking, whereas help-seeking threat, avoidance, and executive (expedient) help seeking relates to performance avoid goals (e.g., Karabenick, 2003). Children who prefer challenge and independent mastery are more likely to seek such help (e.g., Arbreton, 1998), and high school students who use other self-regulated strategies also seek help from peers, teachers, and adults. In response to poor performance, college students with achievement-oriented "help-relevant" beliefs (Ames, 1983) and those who use a variety of cognitive, metacognitive, and self-regulating learning strategies (Karabenick & Knapp, 1991) will also seek help more frequently. Thus, it appears that good students and good self-regulators know when, why, and from whom to seek help.

Adaptive help seeking is based on actions that would be normative (i.e., ideal) at each phase of the help-seeking process (e.g., Gross & McMullen, 1983): well-calibrated comprehension monitoring, assessing costs and benefits of seeking and not seeking help, instrumental help-seeking goals, identifying and securing appropriate sources of help, and effectively processing help received. Adaptive help seeking also depends on learners' goals. Asking other students for answers to problems would be an example of executive (also called expedient) help seeking that is designed to minimize effort. This may have short-term benefits but not decrease a learner's dependence on others when subsequently faced with similar problems. By contrast, instrumental (also called autonomous) help seeking is that undertaken to increase mastery and competence by obtaining the assistance necessary to further understanding, for example, by asking teachers for explanations rather than solutions.

Recent work has also examined whether students could be characterized not only according to their intentions to seek or avoid seeking help (e.g., Ryan,

1998), or by their help-seeking goals (instrumental vs. expedient), but rather according to more elaborated orientations (Karabenick, 2001, 2002). Somewhat analogous to achievement goals, which incorporate both the purposes of task engagement and standards against which success is measured, orientation as used here is intended to capture affect, cognition, and behavior that, in combination, reflect students' help-seeking experiences. General orientations provide a parsimonious way to summarize different components, or indicators, of the help-seeking process. Consistent with recent analyses of approach and avoidance dimensions in motivation (e.g., Elliot & Thrash, 2002), two rather than one dimension were required to describe students' help-seeking orientations (Karabenick, 2001, 2002).

In our view, help seeking involves more than intentions to seek or avoid help. Rather, it incorporates several components that can be assessed independently and combined to provide more inclusive orientations. Assessment is simplified when the indicators are conceptually independent. For example, just as it is necessary to control for the need for assistance when measuring students' intentions to seek help (Karabenick & Knapp, 1991), indications of helper preference can be made contingent on students' intentions to seek help. That is, students' intentions to seek and to avoid seeking help are measured independent of the type of help (goals and sources) that students would seek if they were to do so. Instrumental and expedient help-seeking goals, as well as preferred source (formal or informal), can also be assessed in a way that maintains their conceptual independence, that is, by asking students to rate why they would seek help (if they did) and from whom.

A recent study that included measures of help seeking involved 852 college students at a large midwestern university (Karabenick, 2001, 2002, submitted). The majority (60%) were females and most (77%) were first-term freshmen and Caucasian (74%) or African American (20%). Measures of help seeking, motivation, achievement goals, and learning strategies were part of a 107-item instrument, with a 5-point (1 to 5) response scale that was anchored with the statements *not at all true* and *completely true*. Measures of help seeking are shown in the Appendix, and descriptive statistics are shown in Table 2. Help-seeking orientations were obtained by computing the means of the component scales. Approach orientation combined students' intentions to seek help, perceived benefits of seeking help, instrumental help-seeking goal, and preferences for obtaining help from teachers. Avoidance orientation combined help-seeking threat, intentions to avoid help, and to seek expedient help. Based on exploratory factor analysis, seeking help from other students was not included in either orientation. All of the help-seeking scales have acceptable levels of internal consistency (Cronbach's alpha). Table 2 also presents stability estimates for each scale and the orientations over a period that began 2 months prior to the final assessment. The correlations indicate that students were relatively consistent over that time but also evidenced variability.

Approach and avoidance help-seeking orientations related in very different ways to students' motivation, achievement goals, and use of learning

Table 2. Help-Seeking Scales Descriptive Statistics (n = 852)

Scale	No. items	Alpha	Mean	SD	2-Month stability
Threat	4	.84	1.5	.7	.48*
Avoidance	3	.69	1.7	.7	.37*
Expedient goal	3	.64	1.9	.8	.49*
Approach	3	.80	3.4	.7	.47*
Benefits	3	.80	3.5	.9	.47*
Instrumental goal	3	.61	3.5	.8	.40*
Formal source	2	.88	3.1	1.0	.38*
Informal source	2	.87	3.1	1.0	.30*
Approach orientation			3.2	.7	.50*
Avoidance orientation			1.8	.7	.52*

*$p < .001$.

strategies. Students with higher approach orientations reported more adaptive motivational beliefs such as greater self-efficacy ($r = .27$, $p < .001$), task value ($r = .43$, $p < .001$), and interest ($r = .31$, $p < .001$), higher levels of mastery approach orientation ($r = .45$, $p < .001$) and lower levels of performance avoidance orientation ($r = -.12$, $p < .001$). These students also more frequently used rehearsal ($r = .31$, $p < .001$), elaboration ($r = .36$, $p < .001$), and metacognitive self-regulation ($r = .50$, $p < .001$) strategies. Conversely, students higher in help-seeking avoidance were less motivated, more test anxious, had lower mastery approach ($r = -.20$, $p < .001$) and higher mastery avoidance ($r = .31$, $p < .001$) and performance achievement goals ($r = .49$, $p < .001$), and tended to use lower level rehearsal rather than higher level learning strategies. These results are consistent with studies of younger learners and suggest the way approach-oriented help seeking is integral to positive approaches to learning: an adaptive self-regulated strategy.

It is important to emphasize, however, that students with higher help-seeking approach orientations are not more likely to seek help, or those with avoidance orientation less help, owing to the nature of relationships between orientations and the need for help. In the study described here, for example, students with higher levels of need reported getting more help overall ($r = .53$). Students higher in help-seeking avoidance orientation reported needing help more ($r = .26$) and reported obtaining more help during the term ($r = .20$). Help-seeking approach orientation was not related to the level of need ($r = .06$), yet was related to reported help obtained ($r = .21$). Thus, both orientations were related to the amount of help actually obtained during the term. Orientations are need contingent, however. Controlling for the level of need, help-seeking avoidance motivation was not related to the total help seeking reported ($r = .06$), whereas help-seeking approach motivation was ($r = .20$). This is just what would be expected since a higher help-seeking approach orientation translates into a greater likelihood of getting needed help, whereas higher levels of help-seeking avoidance orientation result in less help seeking despite greater need.

Conclusions

In this final section, we touch on a few issues that apply more generally to these strategies for assessing students' regulation of their cognition, motivation, and behavior within academic contexts. One issue concerns how these strategies might fit together. As described above, the regulation-of-cognition items were the first to be developed and the scales for assessing the regulation of motivation and behavior later. Consequently, there is sufficient evidence linking the regulation of cognition scales to both the regulation-of-motivation and behavior scales. However, these latter two forms of regulation have not been linked empirically to any great extent, although there is some evidence that they would be positively related (Wolters, 1998).

A second issue concerns whether it is necessary to assess all three areas in order to assess students' self-regulated learning. First, we should note that even when using all of the scales discussed here, some aspects of self-regulated learning are not represented. Second, these scales do not need to be used as a complete set. Individual scales, or sets of scales, can be used as indicators of students' tendency to regulate these different aspects of their academic functioning. The particular scales that are selected should be a function of the specific research questions being investigated.

Another concern that cuts across these three areas of regulation is the domain specificity of the items. Items from the MSLQ and the regulation of motivation were originally intended to tap into students' regulatory behaviors with regard to a specific course. Slight modifications in wording have been used to assess students' functioning within a mathematics, history, English, or science course without a substantial change in reliability (Wolters & Pintrich, 1998; Wolters et al., 1996). An advantage to the items/scales we describe, therefore, is that it is possible to tailor them to the particular courses or subject areas of interest. Having said this, it also is possible to assess this process by tapping into students' more general behaviors without regard to a particular subject area, course, or task. That is, the items can be modified to assess more general beliefs and behaviors. However, the predictive validity and reliability of the scales we describe may fall if they are presented in these more general terms.

Another general concern with the scales presented here is the relative lack of empirical data specifically examining their validity with regard to particular individual differences. In many cases, the sample populations involved in the development and testing of the scales presented here were diverse with regard to gender, age level, and socioeconomic status. Hence, the overall message is that these scales can be used to assess students' regulatory functioning within academic contexts across a broad age range. However, evidence regarding the reliability and validity of these scales with regard to specific ethnic or cultural groups is not readily available and would be a valuable addition to this line of research.

A final issue that cuts across all of the scales discussed here concerns the nature of self-report data on which they are based. Students can accurately self-report some aspects of their cognition, motivation, and behavior, but not all.

The scales presented here assess students' thoughts and actions at a particular level of analysis that has proved useful for understanding and predicting certain academic outcomes. Self-reports may not be appropriate, however, for the more finely detailed analysis of students' functioning necessary to address some research questions. In short, it is important to consider the nature of the information that is made available through these scales when evaluating their appropriateness for any particular study.

As a whole, the strategies presented here provide a reasonably valid and reliable way of assessing many of the regulatory activities that contribute to students' self-regulation of their learning in academic contexts. The scales can be used flexibly to tap into those aspects of this complex process that are of most relevant to a particular study. Thus, they provide a useful set of tools that can be used to address a variety of important research questions focused on understanding students' functioning within academic contexts.

Appendix

Strategies for the Regulation of Academic Cognition

Rehearsal Strategies

> When I study for this class, I practice saying the material to myself over and over.
> When studying for this class, I read my class notes and the course readings over and over again.
> I memorize key words to remind me of important concepts in this class.
> I make lists of important terms for this course and memorize the lists.

Elaboration Strategies

> When I study for this class, I pull together information from different sources, such as lectures, readings, and discussions.
> I try to relate ideas in this subject to those in other courses whenever possible.
> When reading for this class, I try to relate the material to what I already know.
> When I study for this course, I write brief summaries of the main ideas from the readings and the concepts from the lectures.
> I try to understand the material in this class by making connections between the readings and the concepts from the lectures.
> I try to apply ideas from course readings in other class activities such as lecture and discussion.

Organization Strategies

> When I study the readings for this course, I outline the material to help me organize my thoughts.

When I study for this course, I go through the readings and my class notes and try to find the most important ideas.

I make simple charts, diagrams, or tables to help me organize course material.

When I study for this course, I go over my class notes and make an outline of important concepts.

Metacognitive Self-Regulation

During class time I often miss important points because I'm thinking of other things. (REVERSED)

When reading for this course, I make up questions to help focus my reading.

When I become confused about something I'm reading for this class, I go back and try to figure it out.

If course materials are difficult to understand, I change the way I read the material.

Before I study new course material thoroughly, I often skim it to see how it is organized.

I ask myself questions to make sure I understand the material I have been studying in this class.

I try to change the way I study in order to fit the course requirements and instructor's teaching style.

I often find that I have been reading for class but don't know what it was all about. (REVERSED)

I try to think through a topic and decide what I am supposed to learn from it rather than just reading it over when studying.

When studying for this course I try to determine which concepts I don't understand well.

When I study for this class, I set goals for myself in order to direct my activities in each study period.

If I get confused taking notes in class, I make sure I sort it out afterwards.

Strategies for the Regulation of Academic Motivation

Mastery Self-Talk

I tell myself that I should keep working just to learn as much as I can.

I persuade myself to keep at it just to see how much I can learn.

I challenge myself to complete the work and learn as much as possible.

I convince myself to work hard just for the sake of learning.

I tell myself that I should study just to learn as much as I can.

I think about trying to become good at what we are learning or doing.

Relevance Enhancement

I tell myself that it is important to learn the material because I will need it later in life.

I try to connect the material with something I like doing or find interesting.

I think up situations where it would be helpful for me to know the material or skills.

I try to make the material seem more useful by relating it to what I want to do in my life.

I try to make myself see how knowing the material is personally relevant.

I make an effort to relate what we're learning to my personal interests.

Situational Interest Enhancement

I make studying more enjoyable by turning it into a game.

I try to make a game out of learning the material or completing the assignment.

I try to get myself to see how doing the work can be fun.

I make doing the work enjoyable by focusing on something about it that is fun.

I think of a way to make the work seem enjoyable to complete.

Performance/Relative Ability Self-Talk

I think about doing better than other students in my class.

I tell myself that I should work at least as hard as other students.

I keep telling myself that I want to do better than others in my class.

I make myself work harder by comparing what I'm doing to what other students are doing.

Performance/Extrinsic Self-Talk

I remind myself about how important it is to get good grades.

I tell myself that I need to keep studying to do well in this course.

I convince myself to keep working by thinking about getting good grades.

I think about how my grade will be affected if I don't do my reading or studying.

I remind myself how important it is to do well on the tests and assignments in this course.

Self-Consequating

I promise myself I can do something I want later if I finish the assigned work now.

I make a deal with myself that if I get a certain amount of the work done I can do something fun afterwards.

I promise myself some kind of a reward if I get my readings or studying done.

I tell myself I can do something I like later if right now I do the work I have do get done.

I set a goal for how much I need to study and promise myself a reward if I reach that goal.

Environmental Structuring

I try to study at a time when I can be more focused.
I change my surroundings so that it is easy to concentrate on the work.
I make sure I have as few distractions as possible.
I try to get rid of any distractions that are around me.
I eat or drink something to make myself more awake and prepared to work.

Strategies for the Regulation of Academic Behavior

Effort Regulation

I often feel so lazy or bored when I study for this class that I quit before I finish what I planned to do. (REVERSED)
I work hard to do well in this class even if I don't like what we are doing.
When course work is difficult, I give up or only study the easy parts. (REVERSED)
Even when course materials are dull and uninteresting, I manage to keep working until I finish.

Regulating Time and Study Environment

I usually study in a place where I can concentrate on my course work.
I make good use of my study time for this course.
I find it hard to stick to a study schedule. (REVERSED)
I have a regular place set aside for studying.
I make sure I keep up with the weekly readings and assignments for this course.
I attend class regularly.
I often find that I don't spend very much time on this course because of other activities. (REVERSED)
I rarely find time to review my notes or readings before an exam. (REVERSED)

General Intention to Seek Needed Help

If I needed help in this class I would ask someone for assistance.
If I needed help understanding the lectures in this class I would ask for help.
If I needed help with the readings in this class I would ask for help.

General Intention to Avoid Needed Help

If I didn't understand something in this class I would guess rather than ask someone for assistance.

I would rather do worse on an assignment I couldn't finish than ask for help.

Even if the work was too hard to do on my own, I wouldn't ask for help with this class.

Perceived Costs of Help Seeking (Threat)

Getting help in this class would be an admission that I am just not smart enough to do the work on my own.

I would not want anyone to find out that I needed help in this class.

Asking for help would mean I am not as smart as other students in the class.

Others would think I was dumb if I asked for help in this class.

Perceived Benefits of Help Seeking

Getting help in this class would make me a better student.

Getting help in this class would make me a smarter student.

Getting help in this class would increase my ability to learn the material.

Instrumental (Autonomous) Help-Seeking Goal

I would get help in this class to learn to solve problems and find answers by myself.

If I were to get help in this class it would be to better understand the general ideas or principles.

Getting help in this class would be a way for me to learn more about basic principles that I could use to solve problems or understand the material.

Expedient (Executive) Help-Seeking Goal

The purpose of asking somebody for help in this class would be to succeed without having to work as hard.

If I were to ask for help in this class it would be to quickly get the answers I needed.

Getting help in this class would be a way of avoiding doing some of the work.

Seeking Help from Formal Source (Teachers)

If I were to seek help in this class it would be from the teacher.

If I were to seek help in this class I would ask the teacher.

Seeking Help from Informal Source (Other Students)

If I were to seek help in this class it would be from another student.
If I were to seek help in this class I would ask another student.

References

Ames, R. (1983). Help-seeking and achievement orientation: Perspectives from attribution theory. In B. M. DePaulo, A. Nadler, & J. D. Fisher (Eds.), *New directions in helping: Vol. 2. Help seeking* (pp. 165–186). New York: Academic Press.

Arbreton, A. (1998). Student goal orientation and help-seeking strategy use. In S. A. Karabenick (Ed.), *Strategic help seeking: Implications for learning and teaching* (pp. 95–116). Mahwah, NJ: Lawrence Erlbaum.

Baron, J. (1994). *Thinking and deciding.* Cambridge: Cambridge University Press.

Boekaerts, M., Pintrich, P. R., & Zeidner, M. (2000). *Handbook of self-regulation: Theory, research, and applications.* San Diego, CA: Academic Press.

Corno, L. (1993). The best-laid plans: Modern conceptions of volition and educational research. *Educational Researcher, 22,* 14–22.

Elliot, A. J., & Thrash, T. M. (2002). Approach-avoidance motivation in personality: Approach and avoidance temperaments and goals. *Journal of Personality and Social Psychology, 82,* 804–818.

Feather, N. T. (1961). The relationship of persistence at a task to expectations for success and achievement-oriented motives. *Journal of Abnormal and Social Psychology, 63,* 552–561.

Feather, N. T. (1963). Persistence at a difficult task with an alternative task of intermediate difficulty. *Journal of Abnormal and Social Psychology, 66,* 604–609.

Graham, S., Harris, K., & Troia, G. (1998). Writing and self-regulation: Cases from the self-regulated strategy development model. In D. Schunk & B. Zimmerman (Eds.), *Self-regulated learning: From teaching to self-reflective practice* (pp. 20–41). New York: Guilford Press.

Graham, S., & Weiner, B. (1996). Theories and principles of motivation. In D. Berliner and R. Calfee (Eds.), *Handbook of educational psychology* (pp. 63–84). New York: Macmillan Library Reference.

Gross, A. A., & McMullen, P. A. (1983). Models of the help seeking process. In B. M. DePaulo, A. Nadler, & J. D. Fisher (Eds.), *New directions in helping: Vol. 2. Help seeking* (pp. 45–70). New York: Academic Press.

Karabenick, S. A. (Ed.). (1998). *Strategic help seeking: Implications for learning and teaching.* Mahwah, NJ: Lawrence Erlbaum.

Karabenick, S. A. (2001, April). *Help seeking in large college classes: Who, why, and from whom.* Paper presented at the annual meeting of the American Educational Research Association, Seattle, WA.

Karabenick, S. A. (2002, July). *Effects of subjective classroom context on college student help seeking.* Paper presented at the International Congress of Applied Psychology, Singapore.

Karabenick, S. A. (2003). Help seeking in large college classes: A person-centered approach. *Contemporary Educational Psychology, 28,* 37–58.

Karabenick, S. A. (in press). Perceived achievement goal structure and college student help seeking. *Journal of Educational Psychology.*

Karabenick, S. A., & Knapp, J. R. (1991). Relationship of academic help seeking to the use of learning strategies and other instrumental achievement behavior in college students. *Journal of Educational Psychology, 83,* 221–230.

Nisbett, R. (1993). *Rules for reasoning.* Hillsdale, NJ: Lawrence Erlbaum.

Pintrich, P. R. (1989). The dynamic interplay of student motivation and cognition in the college classroom. In C. Ames & M. L. Maehr (Eds.), *Advances in motivation and achievement: Vol. 6. Motivation-enhancing environments* (pp. 117–160). Greenwich, CT: JAI Press.

Pintrich, P. R. (1999). The role of motivation in promoting and sustaining self-regulated learning. *International Journal of Educational Research, 31*, 459–470.

Pintrich, P. R., & De Groot, E. V. (1990). Motivational and self-regulated learning components of classroom academic performance. *Journal of Educational Psychology, 82*, 33–40.

Pintrich, P. R., Roeser, R., & De Groot, E. V. (1994). Intraindividual differences in motivation and cognition in students with and without learning disabilities. *Journal of Learning Disabilities, 27*, 360–370.

Pintrich, P. R., & Schunk, D. H. (2002). *Motivation in education: Theory, research, and applications.* Englewood Cliffs, NJ: Prentice-Hall.

Pintrich, P. R., Smith, D., Garcia, T., & McKeachie, W. J. (1991). *A manual for the use of the Motivated Strategies for Learning Questionnaire (MSLQ).* Ann Arbor: University of Michigan, School of Education, National Center for Research to Improve Post Secondary Teaching and Language.

Pintrich, P. R., Smith, D., Garcia, T., & McKeachie, W. (1993). Predictive validity and reliability of the Motivated Strategies for Learning Questionnaire (MSLQ). *Educational and Psychological Measurement, 53*, 801–813.

Pintrich, P. R., Wolters, C., & Baxter, G. (2000). Assessing metacognition and self-regulated learning. In G. Schraw & J. Impara (Eds.). *Issues in the measurement of metacognition* (pp. 43–97). Lincoln: University of Nebraska, Buros Institute of Mental Measurements.

Pintrich, P. R., Zusho, A., Schiefele, U., & Pekrun, R. (2001). Goal orientation and self-regulated learning in the college classroom: A cross-cultural comparison. In F. Salili, C.-Y. Chiu, & Y.-Y. Hong (Eds.), *Student motivation: The culture and context of learning* (pp. 149–169). New York: Plenum.

Purdie, N., & Hattie, J. (1996). Cultural differences in the use of strategies for self-regulated learning. *American Educational Research Journal, 33*, 845–871.

Ryan, A. M. (1998). *The development of achievement beliefs and behaviors during early adolescence: The role of the peer group and classroom contexts.* Unpublished doctoral dissertation. University of Michigan, Ann Arbor.

Ryan, A., & Pintrich, P. R. (1997). "Should I ask for help?": The role of motivation and attitudes in adolescents' help seeking in math class. *Journal of Educational Psychology, 89*, 329–341.

Sansone, C., Wiebe, D., & Morgan, C. (1999). Self-regulating interest: The moderating role of hardiness and conscientiousness. *Journal of Personality, 67*, 701–733.

Schneider, W., & Pressley, M. (1997). *Memory development between 2 and 20.* Mahwah, NJ: Lawrence Erlbaum.

VanderStoep, S., Pintrich, P. R., & Fagerlin, A. (1996). Disciplinary differences in self-regulated learning in college students. *Contemporary Educational Psychology, 21*, 345–362.

Weinstein, C. E., & Mayer, R. (1986). The teaching of learning strategies. In M. Wittrock (Ed.), *Handbook of research on teaching and learning* (pp. 315–327). New York: Macmillan.

Wolters, C. (1998). Self-regulated learning and college students' regulation of motivation. *Journal of Educational Psychology, 90*, 224–235.

Wolters, C. (1999a). College students' motivational regulation during a brief study period. *Journal of Staff, Program, and Organization Development, 16*, 103–111.

Wolters, C. (1999b). The relation between high school students' motivational regulation and their use of learning strategies, effort, and classroom performance. *Learning and Individual Differences, 11*, 281–299.

Wolters, C. (2001, August). *Motivational problems experienced by college students.* Paper presented at the annual meetings of the American Psychological Association, San Francisco, CA.

Wolters, C. (2003). Regulation of motivation: Evaluating an underemphasized aspect of self-regulated learning. *Educational Psychologist, 38*, 189–205.

Wolters, C., & Pintrich, P. R. (1998). Contextual differences in student motivation and self-regulated learning in mathematics, English, and social studies classrooms. *Instructional Science, 26*, 27–47.

Wolters, C., & Rosenthal, H. (2000). The relation between students' motivational beliefs and attitudes and their use of motivational regulation strategies. *International Journal of Educational Research, 33*, 801–820.

Wolters C., Yu, S., & Pintrich, P. R. (1996). The relation between goal orientation and stu-
    dents' motivational beliefs and self-regulated learning. *Learning and Individual Differences, 8,*
    211–238.
Zimmerman, B. J. (1989). A social cognitive view of self-regulated learning and academic learning.
    Journal of Educational Psychology, 81, 329–339.

17 Identifying Adaptive Classrooms: Dimensions of the Classroom Social Environment

Helen Patrick

Purdue University

Allison M. Ryan

University of Illinois, Urbana-Champaign

Positive educational environments are necessary to facilitate optimally adaptive student outcomes, including learning, motivation, school adjustment, and achievement (Eccles, Wigfield, & Schiefele, 1998). Researchers (e.g., Juvonen & Weiner, 1993) have been noting for some time that school success does not only involve academics. Schools and classrooms are inherently social places, and students go about their work in the presence of many peers. To understand students' success at school, therefore, we must attend to their relationships with others at school and the ways in which the environment promotes different types of social interactions and relationships.

The classroom social environment comprises students' perceptions about how they are encouraged to interact with others (e.g., classmates, the teacher), and it encompasses dimensions of teacher support, promoting mutual respect, promoting student task-related interaction, and promoting performance goals. Recent research has indicated that these dimensions of the classroom social environment are separate, can be measured quickly and reliably, and relate significantly to students' motivation, self-regulated learning, classroom behavior, social relationships, and achievement (Ryan & Patrick, 2001).

The emphasis on the importance of the classroom social environment is apparent in reform recommendations. For example, the National Science Education Standards include explicit reference to teachers creating a social and intellectual environment with support, respect, and collaboration as central features

(National Research Council, 1996). The National Council of Teachers of Mathematics (2000) also explicitly addresses these social norms when it outlines what teachers should strive to create in their class. For example, it advocates that students be:

> encouraged to share their ideas and to seek clarification until they understand.... To achieve this kind of classroom, teachers need to establish an atmosphere of mutual trust and respect.... When teachers build such an environment, students understand that it is acceptable to struggle with ideas, to make mistakes, and to be unsure. This attitude encourages them to participate actively in trying to understand what they are asked to learn because they know that they will not be criticized personally, even if their mathematical thinking is critiqued. (p. 271)

Although the social environment of the classroom is likely to be important to motivation and engagement for students of all ages, it may be particularly important for adolescent students. Adolescence has been identified as a particularly precarious stage regarding changes in achievement beliefs and behaviors (e.g., Carnegie Council on Adolescent Development, 1989, 1995). Certainly, for some adolescent students, the increases in self-reflection, autonomy, and identity exploration lead to new academic interests, increased self-regulated learning, and a commitment to education (Goodenow, 1993). For many children, however, early adolescence marks the beginning of a downward trend in academics. More so than at other ages, young adolescents doubt their abilities to succeed at their schoolwork, question the value of doing their schoolwork, and decrease their effort toward academics (Anderman & Maehr, 1994; Carnegie Council on Adolescent Development, 1989, 1995; Eccles & Midgley, 1989; Eccles et al., 1993).

Research using a stage-environment fit framework indicates that optimal development for adolescents will occur in an educational context that is appropriately matched to their developmental needs (see Eccles et al., 1993, for a review). Nonparental adults are especially important as role models and sources of support during adolescence (Midgley, Feldlaufer, & Eccles, 1989). Adolescence is typically a time of increased self-consciousness and sensitivity (Elkind, 1967; Harter, 1990). Therefore, the promotion of mutual respect within the classroom, with clear norms that involve not making fun of others, may be especially beneficial to adolescents' adaptive social, emotional, and cognitive functioning in the classroom. Adolescents' increased capacity for considering others' perspectives, generating options, reflecting, and evaluating alternatives (Keating, 1990) suggests that interaction in the classroom may be especially beneficial at this stage. Adolescents' increased self-consciousness and sensitivity regarding social comparison (Nicholls, 1990) suggest that promoting competition and ability comparisons may be especially detrimental for adolescents' motivation.

In this chapter, we focus on four important dimensions of the classroom social environment—teacher support, promoting mutual respect, promoting student task-related interaction, and promoting performance goals—and their associations with adaptive outcomes for young adolescent students. We also present survey measures for these social environment dimensions, as well as evidence that these scales are psychometrically sound for use with adolescents (i.e., from fifth grade).

Dimensions of the Classroom Social Environment

Teacher support refers to students' beliefs that their teachers care about them, value them, and establish personal relationships with them (e.g., Goodenow, 1993). Researchers have found positive associations between perceptions of teacher support and students' adaptive motivational beliefs and engagement behaviors. For example, when students view their teacher as supportive they report higher levels of interest, valuing, effort, and enjoyment in their school-work (Fraser & Fisher, 1982; Midgley et al., 1989; Trickett & Moos, 1974), a more positive academic self-concept (Felner, Aber, Primavera, & Cauce, 1985), and greater expectancies for success (Goodenow, 1993). Perceiving the teacher as supportive is also related positively to asking for help with schoolwork when needed (Newman & Schwager, 1993), use of self-regulated learning strategies (Ryan & Patrick, 2001), and a desire to comply with classroom rules (Wentzel, 1994). Perceived teacher support is related negatively to absenteeism (Moos & Moos, 1978) and disruptiveness in the classroom (Ryan & Patrick, 2001).

Promoting mutual respect in the classroom involves a perception that the teacher expects all students to value one another and the contributions they make to classroom life, and will not allow students to make fun of others. Environments that are perceived as respectful are likely to be ones in which students can focus on understanding tasks, without having their attention diverted by concern about what others might think or say if they are incorrect or experience difficulty. Respectful environments are also most conducive to student problem solving, cognitive risk taking, and conceptual understanding (Cohen, 1994; De Lisi & Golbeck, 1999). Perceptions that the teacher promotes mutual respect in the classroom arguably contribute to students' feelings of psychological safety and comfort, including low anxiety and low threat regarding making mistakes. When students are anxious or worried about making mistakes they are less likely to engage in their academic work in an effortful and strategic manner (Turner, Thorpe, & Meyer, 1998). Resource allocation theory suggests this may be due to negative affect increasing task-irrelevant thoughts that overload working memory, thereby reducing the available cognitive capacity (Ellis & Ashbrook, 1987). Thus, a perception that the teacher promotes respect in the classroom is related positively to increased academic efficacy and more self-regulated learning relative to the previous year (Ryan & Patrick, 2001).

Teachers vary in the extent to which they allow or even *promote task-related interaction* among students during academic activities. This interaction may encompass students' sharing ideas and approaches during whole-class lessons, working together in small-group activities, or informal help seeking and help giving during individual work. Whatever the form, however, interaction among students is a critical component of student-centered instructional approaches. When students are encouraged to interact and exchange ideas with each other during academic tasks, they have opportunities to ask or answer questions, make suggestions, give explanations, justify their reasoning, and participate in discussions. These interactions are related to student learning and achievement (e.g., Webb & Palincsar, 1996), consistent with expectations from both Piagetian and Vygotskian theories of learning and development (De Lisi & Golbeck, 1999; O'Donnell & O'Kelly, 1994). Students' perceptions that they are given opportunities to participate actively during lessons and are encouraged to interact with classmates in the pursuit of understanding are also likely to be associated with their motivation. For example, interaction opportunities may foster students' feelings of confidence or efficacy, sustain interest, and support a willingness to persevere with the task when experiencing difficulty or frustration (Patrick & Middleton, 2002). Students should also feel efficacious about their ability to learn and complete activities successfully when interaction among students is promoted, because they have a greater array of resources on which to draw than if they were only working individually. Similarly, students' perception that the teacher encourages them to be actively involved in lessons and participate in discussions is related to their liking and interest in school and specific subject areas (Fraser & Fisher, 1982; Trickett & Moos, 1974).

Promoting performance goals concerns an emphasis on competition and relative ability comparisons between students in the classroom. Research from a goal theory framework has examined this dimension of the classroom and found that when students perceive an emphasis on performance goals they are more likely to exhibit beliefs and behaviors that are less conducive to, and often detrimental to, learning and achievement (see Ames, 1992, for a review). The perception that the teacher promotes performance goals may be particularly harmful to adolescents' motivation, again because of adolescents' heightened self-consciousness and sensitivity (Harter, 1990). In addition, when classrooms are perceived as highly competitive, emphasizing a hierarchy of ability and students' relative position within that hierarchy, students are likely to report engaging in behaviors that are detrimental to learning (see Urdan, Ryan, Anderman, & Gheen, 2002, for a review). For example, classrooms that are perceived as being performance focused are likely to have the highest rates of students' avoiding engaging in tasks, including not seeking help when it is needed (Ryan, Gheen, & Midgley, 1998) and academic self-handicapping (Urdan, Midgley, & Anderman, 1998). Cheating is more prevalent in environments that are seen as emphasizing performance goals (Anderman, Griesinger, & Westerfield, 1998), as is students' disruptive behavior (Kaplan, Gheen, & Midgley, 2002; Ryan & Patrick, 2001).

Measures of Classroom Social Environment

The measures presented in this chapter—teacher support, promoting mutual respect, promoting student task-related interaction, and promoting performance goals—have been used successfully in a number of studies. We report on psychometric analyses from three of those samples. For all samples, students were in their classroom for the academic year. Students in elementary school had the same teacher for all or most of their subjects, whereas students in middle schools had a different teacher for each or most subject(s).

Sample 1 came from a longitudinal study of adaptive adolescent learning and motivation involving students in three school districts in Michigan. The classroom social environment measures were administered in spring 1997 to 587 seventh graders in middle school and in the following year when they were eighth graders. The survey was administered to 341 students in the fall of eighth grade and to 586 students in the spring of eighth grade. The seventh-grade sample was 51% female and 49% male, and 52% of the students received free or reduced-price lunch. The student-reported racial or ethnic background was 53% African American, 36% European American, 8% Hispanic, 2% Asian, & 1% Native American or mixed ethnicity. Family socioeconomic status was similar for both African American and European American students.

Sample 2 came from a longitudinal study conducted with 637 fifth graders in elementary school in the first wave (spring 2000) and, in the second wave (spring 2002) with 780 seventh-grade students in middle school (including some who were not in the original sample). Students came from three school districts in Illinois. The sample was 50% female and 50% male, and almost all of the students were European American.

Sample 3 came from data collected from 1,314 sixth-grade students in elementary school in Michigan, Ohio, and Indiana. The sample was 52% female and 48% male, and 37% of the students received free or reduced-price lunch. The student-reported racial or ethnic background was 29% African American, 65% European American, 4% Hispanic, and 1% Asian.

Measures

The four scales contain 17 items (see the Appendix). In our studies all items were specific to math class. Items are easily altered for different subject areas, however, and we have done so for the scales listed in the Appendix. For two of the scales, we varied the number of items across samples. The scales presented in the Appendix reflect considerations of both internal consistency and efficiency (i.e., fewest numbers of items for acceptable internal consistency).

The scales were administered in surveys to groups of students (e.g., as classrooms) by two researchers. One person read the items aloud while the other monitored the students and answered questions. Students followed along and marked their response to each item.

The scale of *teacher support* includes four items that refer to student perceptions of receiving socioemotional support from, and being understood by, the teacher. It was taken from the Teacher Personal Support subscale of the Classroom Life Measure (Johnson, Johnson, & Anderson, 1983). Responses to these items are measured on a 5-point Likert scale, ranging from 1 (*almost never*) through 5 (*often*).

The measure of *promoting task-related interaction* includes four items about the extent to which students perceive their teacher as encouraging interaction among peers around academic tasks. It was developed by Ryan and Patrick (2001). Responses to this and the following two scales are measured on a 5-point Likert scale, ranging from 1 (*not at all true*) through 5 (*very true*). For the second wave of data collection (i.e., eighth grade) with Sample 1, we added more items to this scale, resulting in an 8-item scale. We report the alphas for both the short and long versions of this scale.

The measure of *promoting mutual respect* includes five items about the extent to which students perceive their teacher as encouraging mutual respect among classmates. It was developed by Ryan and Patrick (2001).

The measure of *promoting performance goals* was taken from the Patterns of Adaptive Learning Survey (Midgley et al., 1996). It refers to the extent to which students perceive their teacher as encouraging competition and comparison among students with respect to academic tasks. We used scales with different numbers of items for different samples. We used a seven-item version for Sample 1 students in seventh and eighth grades, a four-item version for Sample 2 students in fifth and seventh grades, and a five-item version for Sample 3 students in sixth grade. We report the alphas for all versions of this scale.

Data Quality

We examined the distributions of student scores for the four measures of the classroom social environment. There was considerable variability for all measures across the three samples. We anticipated that the distribution of responses to the measures of teacher support and promoting mutual respect would be negatively skewed (i.e., more responses with higher, rather than lower, scores), and those of promoting performance goals would be positively skewed (i.e., more responses with lower, rather than higher, scores). The scale of *promoting mutual respect* was, in fact, negatively skewed, particularly for Samples 2 and 3 (Table 1). This indicates that students' perceptions of their teacher promoting respect in the classroom tend not to be normally distributed, but students tend to view their teacher's actions as more positive. And, as expected, the scale of *promoting performance goals* was positively skewed, particularly for Samples 1

Table 1. Internal Consistency and Skewness for Classroom Social Environment Scales

	Teacher support		Promoting mutual respect		Promoting task-related interaction		Promoting performance goals	
	α	Skew	α	Skew	α	Skew	α	Skew
Sample 1								
Grade 7	.76	−.10	.77	−.47	.79	−.05	.82	.50
Grade 8	.82	−.20	.81	−.39	.85/.90[a]	−.02/.04[a]	.86	.97
Sample 2								
Grade 5	.84	−1.07	.68	−1.43	.71	−.16	.67[b]	.97
Grade 7	.85	−.93	.75	−.89	.80	−.25	.66[b]	1.20
Sample 3								
Grade 6 (fall)	.77	−.66	.72	−1.46	—	—	.72[c]	.09
Grade 6 (spring)	.81	−.54	—	—	.76	−.16	.82[c]	.06

Note: α = Cronbach's alpha.
[a] 8-item version. [b] 4-item version. [c] 5-item version of scale.

and 2. That is, students tended to view their teacher as not promoting high levels of performance goals in the classroom.

Reliability

We used Cronbach's alpha to examine the internal consistency of each of the four scales for all samples. A higher level on the alpha indicates that the scale items are answered in a similar manner within a given administration (Borg & Gall, 1989). Internal consistency coefficients greater than .70 are considered to be adequate. In general, all scales had acceptable internal consistency (Table 1). Across the three samples, the alphas for the measure of *teacher support* ranged from .76 to .85. The alphas for the measure of *promoting mutual respect* ranged from .68 to .81. The only alpha below .70 was with the youngest, fifth-grade sample. The alphas for the measure of *promoting task-related interaction* ranged from .71 to .85. Again, the lowest alpha was with the youngest, fifth-grade sample. We created an eight-item version of this scale, which we used with Sample 1 eighth graders. This longer measure was considerably more internally consistent ($\alpha =$ .90) than the shorter versions. The internal consistency of the *promoting performance goals* scale was highest with Sample 1, when we used seven items ($\alpha =$ .82 and .86). A shorter version with four items, used with Sample 2, produced alphas of .67 and .66. The five-item version, used with Sample 3, resulted in alphas of .72 and .82.

Validity

Exploratory Factor Analysis

To investigate the construct validity of the four classroom social environment scales, we conducted exploratory factor analyses with all scales and samples. Additionally, we conducted separate factor analyses for males and females, and for African American and European American students. We conducted exploratory factor analysis with all samples at all grade levels. All items loaded on the appropriate factor.

In the Appendix we present the items and factor loadings from the exploratory factor analysis conducted with data collected from the eighth graders in Sample 1. Principal axis factor analysis with oblimin rotation was conducted for the entire sample. The analysis yielded four factors with eigenvalues greater than 1.0, which accounted for 56% of the variance. Loadings above .40 are shown. The four factors corresponded to the four hypothesized classroom social environment variables. All factor loadings were above .44 on their primary factor, and no items cross-loaded ($>.40$) on two factors.

Autocorrelations

We examined autocorrelations of the four scales over time with one longitudinal data set. Specifically, we compared students' perceptions of each dimension

Table 2. Correlations among Classroom Social Environment Measures and Student Motivation and Engagement

	1	2	3	4	5	6	7	8
1. Teacher support	—							
2. Promoting task-related interaction	.49	—						
3. Promoting mutual respect	.60	.40	—					
4. Promoting performance goals	−.41	−.14	−.39	—				
5. Social efficacy: teacher	.71	.47	.49	−.45	—			
6. Social efficacy: peers	.17	.15	.20	−.17	.30	—		
7. Academic efficacy	.35	.14	.46	−.29	.47	.42	—	
8. Disruptive behavior	−.41	−.16	−.35	.45	−.35	.04	−.18	—
9. Self-regulated learning	.44	.25	.50	−.22	.41	.20	.50	−.38

Note: Correlations above .13 are significant at the $p < .05$ level.

of the classroom from spring of seventh grade, fall of eighth grade, and spring of eighth grade. Because students were in different classrooms, presumably with different social environments, in seventh and eighth grades we expected that students' scores in seventh grade would be related only modestly to those for the same measures in eighth grade. However, we expected that students' perceptions of the classroom environment would be similar during the same school year, and therefore that the autocorrelations between measures in the fall and spring of eighth grade would be moderately strong.

We examined the autocorrelations of the four classroom social environment measures with Sample 1. As expected, students' perceptions of *teacher support* in fall and spring of eighth grade were correlated moderately with each other ($r = .57$). Furthermore, perceived teacher support in seventh grade was not strongly associated with teacher support in the fall ($r = .21$) or spring ($r = .17$) of eighth grade.

Perceptions of *promoting mutual respect* in fall and spring of eighth grade were also correlated moderately with each other ($r = .54$). Furthermore, the perceptions of promoting mutual respect in seventh grade were not strongly related to this view of the teacher in the fall ($r = .28$) or spring ($r = .24$) of eighth grade.

Perceptions of the teacher *promoting task-related interaction* in fall of seventh grade were not related strongly to perceptions of their eighth-grade teacher in the fall ($r = .18$). This scale was not administered to students in the spring of eighth grade.

Perceptions of the teacher *promoting performance goals* in fall and spring of eighth grade were correlated moderately with each other ($r = .53$). Furthermore, perceptions of promoting performance goals in seventh grade were not strongly related to this view of the teacher in the fall ($r = .33$) or spring ($r = .29$) of eighth grade.

Table 3. Means and Standard Deviations by Gender for Classroom Social Environment Scales

| | Teacher support | | | | Promoting mutual respect | | | | Promoting task-related interaction | | | | Promoting performance goals | | | |
| | Females | | Males | | Females | | Males | | Females | | Males | | Females | | Males | |
	M	SD	M	SD	M	SD	M	SD	M	SD	M	SD	M	SD	M	SD
Sample 1																
Grade 7	3.11	1.13	3.11**	1.14	3.64	1.04	3.60	1.16	3.04	1.07	2.95	1.16	2.23**	.95	2.46**	.96
Grade 8	3.24	1.06	3.13	1.00	3.64	1.09	3.58	1.08	3.13*	1.10	2.88*	1.02	2.05*	.93	2.30*	.99
Sample 2																
Grade 5	3.99**	1.07	3.75**	.91	4.35*	.80	4.20*	.95	3.29	1.01	3.20	1.03	2.17***	.96	2.44***	1.02
Grade 7	3.65	1.00	3.68	.97	3.96	1.02	4.00	.90	3.24	1.01	3.23	1.00	1.83	.88	1.90	.88
Sample 3																
Grade 6 (fall)	3.86	.87	3.78	.96	4.39*	.74	4.31*	.83	—	—	—	—	2.82*	1.00	2.95*	1.00
Grade 6 (spring)	3.73*	.95	3.61*	1.04	—	—	—	—	3.35***	.93	3.10***	1.00	2.92	1.15	2.97	1.13

*p < .05. **p < .01. ***p < .001.

Correlations with Other Constructs

We examined the correlations of the four classroom social environment measures among each other, and with measures of student motivation and engagement. Specifically, the measures of motivation involved student reports of their academic efficacy (Midgley et al., 1996), social efficacy interacting with the teacher (Patrick, Hicks, & Ryan, 1997), and social efficacy relating to peers (Patrick et al., 1997). The measures of engagement involved student reports of their self-regulated learning (adapted from the Motivated Strategies for Learning Questionnaire; Pintrich, Smith, Garcia, & McKeachie, 1993) and their disruptive behavior (Kaplan & Maehr, 1999).

The correlations from one data set (Sample 1, eighth grade) are shown in Table 2. An expected pattern of correlations was found, thus giving further evidence of construct validity. Teacher support, promoting task-related interaction, and promoting mutual respect were positively related to each other, and negatively related to promoting performance goals. The scales of teacher support, promoting task-related interaction, and promoting mutual respect were related positively to social efficacy with teachers and with peers, academic efficacy, and self-regulated learning, and related negatively to disruptive behavior. Promoting performance goals was related negatively to social efficacy with teachers and peers, academic efficacy, and self-regulated learning, and related positively to disruptive behavior.

Qualitative Analysis of Classrooms

Evidence of validity for three of the four scales (teacher support, promoting mutual respect, and promoting performance goals) comes from a recent mixed-method study of classroom psychological environments with Sample 3, which included qualitative analysis of teacher discourse and classroom observations (Patrick, Turner, Meyer, & Midgley, 2003). In this study we analyzed tape-recorded and transcribed teacher discourse and additional observer notes of teacher and student behavior from 8 sixth-grade classrooms. On the basis of qualitative analysis, we identified three different types of classroom environments: those in which the teacher appeared to send consistently supportive messages about learning, respectful social relationships, and management; those in which the messages were consistently nonsupportive; and those in which the teacher messages were ambiguous. After distinguishing among classrooms using the qualitative data, we compared our findings with students' responses to the measures of teacher support, promoting mutual respect, and promoting performance goals, collected later that fall and in the spring. There was strong convergence between the qualitative analysis and students' responses to the scales, as indicated by a multivariate analysis of variance. Tukey post hoc significant difference tests indicated that students in classrooms that appeared to us to be most supportive and respectful rated their classrooms as having most support from the teacher, to be most respectful, and to be least focused on performance goals. Additionally, classrooms that appeared to us to be least supportive and respectful rated their classrooms as having least support from the teacher, to be least respectful, and to be most focused on performance goals.

Descriptive Statistics

Demographic Patterns

We examined whether there were mean-level differences by gender (Table 3) and race (Table 4) in responses to the classroom social environment scales. There were two waves of data collection for each of the three samples, resulting in six sets of data. We used two-way analyses of variance, which allowed us to check for possible gender-by-race interactions; there were none.

We investigated whether there were significant differences in perceptions of *teacher support* by gender. For four of the data sets (Sample 1, seventh and eighth grades; Sample 2, seventh grade; Sample 3, sixth grade fall) there were no significant differences, whereas in two of the data sets (Sample 2, fifth grade; Sample 3, sixth grade spring) females reported greater teacher support on average than did males. This indicates that there were not consistent gender differences, but when there was a difference females tended to view their teacher as more supportive than did males. There were no significant differences in perceptions of teacher support by race.

For three of the data sets (Sample 1, seventh and eighth grades; Sample 2, seventh grade), there were no significant differences in perceptions of the teacher *promoting mutual respect,* whereas in two of the data sets (Sample 2, fifth grade; Sample 3, sixth grade fall), more females than males reported that the teacher promoted respect. This indicates that there were not consistent gender differences, but when there was a difference females tended to view their teacher as promoting more mutual respect in the classroom than males did. In one of the three data sets (Sample 1, eighth grade), African American students reported perceiving more of an emphasis on mutual respect than did European American students; however, there were no significant differences for the other two data sets (Sample 1, seventh grade; Sample 3, sixth grade fall). This indicates that there were not consistent differences by race.

For three of the data sets (Sample 1, seventh grade; Sample 2, fifth and seventh grades), there were no significant differences in perceptions of the teacher *promoting task-related interaction,* whereas in two of the data sets (Sample 1, eighth grade; Sample 3, sixth grade spring), more females than males reported that the teacher promoted task-related interaction. This indicates that there were not consistent gender differences, but when there was a difference females tended to view their teacher as promoting more task-related interaction than males did. In one of the three data sets (Sample 3, sixth grade spring), African American students reported perceiving more of an emphasis on task-related interaction than did European American students; however, the opposite result was found in the second data set (Sample 1, eighth grade). Finally, investigation of the third data set (Sample 1, seventh grade) found no significant differences

Table 4. Means and Standard Deviations by Race for Classroom Social Environment Scales

	Teacher support				Promoting mutual respect				Promoting task-related interaction				Promoting performance goals			
	African American		European American		African American		European American		African American		European American		African American		European American	
	M	SD	M	SD	M	SD	M	SD	M	SD	M	SD	M	SD	M	SD
Sample 1																
Grade 7	3.17	1.09	3.08	1.14	3.63	1.08	3.58	1.07	3.00	1.09	2.92	1.11	2.39	.97	2.28	.94
Grade 8	3.23	1.07	3.14	1.01	3.85***	1.11	3.35***	1.02	2.83**	1.06	3.20**	1.08	2.10	1.01	2.17	.90
Sample 3																
Grade 6 (fall)	3.75	.93	3.85	.89	4.37	.78	4.36	.77	—	—	—	—	2.97*	1.06	2.82*	.97
Grade 6 (spring)	3.67	.99	3.68	1.00	—	—	—	—	3.36**	.96	3.17**	.97	3.05*	1.15	2.88*	1.12

*p < .05. **p < .01. ***p < .001.

between both groups. This indicates that there were not consistent differences by race.

For four of the data sets (Sample 1, seventh and eighth grades; Sample 2, fifth grade; Sample 3, sixth grade fall), males reported that the teacher *promoted performance goals* significantly more than females did. However, two of the data sets (Sample 2, seventh grade; Sample 3, sixth grade spring) indicated no significant differences, although the trend was for the males' means to be higher than the females'. This indicates that there were not consistent gender differences, but when there was a difference males tended to view their teacher as promoting performance goals more than females did. Two waves of Sample 1 (fifth and seventh grades) indicated no difference in students' perceptions of the teacher promoting performance goals for African American and European American students. However, in two waves of Sample 3 (sixth grade, fall and spring), African American students perceived their teacher as promoting performance goals significantly more than European American students did. The differences by race were not sufficiently consistent to indicate a clear difference between perceptions of African American and European American students.

Between-Class Differences in Dimensions of the Classroom Social Environment

We expected that there would be individual differences in student perceptions of their environment and that these perceptions would converge somewhat among students in the same classroom because there is a common experience. Using data from Sample 1 eighth graders, we examined the degree of consensus among students with respect to the classroom social environment. We calculated the intraclass correlation (the ratio of the between-class variance and the total variance) for each measure. These were estimated by running four unbalanced one-way random-effects analyses of variance (ANOVAs), in which class was a random factor with varying numbers of students per class, and each of the four dimensions of the classroom social environment were the outcome variables. The one-way ANOVAs indicated that the intraclass correlations for the student reports about their classroom environment were .26, .35, .39, and .27 for teacher support, promoting mutual respect, promoting task-related interaction, and promoting performance goals, respectively. Thus, whereas there are individual differences regarding student perceptions, there is some degree of concordance among students in a given classroom regarding these four measures.

Summary and Discussion

The results presented in this chapter provide strong evidence that the four scales of the dimensions of the classroom social environment are reliable and valid measures. Factor analyses with separate samples indicated repeatedly that the four dimensions are distinct constructs. Cronbach's alphas for the scales indicated that the items consistently work well together as a construct and are reliable for use with students from fifth through eighth grades. Factor and reliability analyses indicate that the measure works equally well for males and females and for European American and African American students. The scales have considerable variability in their distributions across multiple samples. Furthermore, our research has indicated construct validity through a number of methods. The autocorrelations of the same scales indicate consistency of students' perceptions at different times within the same classroom in the year. However, the correlations among the same measures were much smaller across different classrooms, consistent with the expectation that different environments would be perceived differently by students. Additionally, the expected correlations were found among the social environment measures and several indices of motivation and engagement in the classroom. Additional evidence for construct validity comes from a mixed quantitative and qualitative study that found that students' perceptions of their classroom social environment, measured by these scales, were congruent with observer analyses of the classroom environments. Therefore, based on the evidence presented in this chapter, we believe that these four measures yield reliable, valid, and socially significant information about early adolescent students' classroom perceptions that are linked to a wide range of adaptive student beliefs and behaviors. We recommend that these scales be included in national data collections involving students from the middle grades.

An obvious and much needed area for future research involves addressing the applicability of these classroom environment measures with younger schoolchildren. The classroom dimensions of teacher support, promoting mutual respect, promoting task-related interaction, and not promoting performance goals are arguably vital for students at all grade levels. Use of the scales at lower grade levels may involve researchers adapting these scales through, for example, simplifying vocabulary, having fewer (e.g., three) responses to choose from (e.g., Gottfried, 1990), or representing responses pictorially (e.g., Harter & Pike, 1984). Or it may involve researchers investigating the comparability of similar scales designed specifically for young children, such as the Young Children's Appraisals of Teacher Support Scale (Mantzicopoulos & Neuharth-Pritchett, 2003).

Studies that have used these classroom environment measures have supported theoretical arguments for their association with important learning-related outcomes (e.g., Ryan & Patrick, 2001). That is, students who perceive their teacher as promoting support, respect, and task-related interaction, and not making an ability hierarchy among students salient, tend to hold the most positive beliefs about learning and engage in more adaptive learning-related behaviors. There is a need, however, for future research to investigate longer-term questions, including the longitudinal prediction of "downstream" outcomes (Connell, 2003). For example, in what ways do optimal classroom experiences in elementary and middle school contribute to students' long-term school success (e.g., regular attendance at high school, graduation, college enrollment) and to healthy adjustment in adolescence and early adulthood (e.g., showing responsibility, engaging in low-risk behaviors)? In what ways do positive educational environments and perceptions of teachers' support contribute to students' resilience and compensate for difficulties in other areas of their lives? Are the effects of positive environments for healthy student adjustment cumulative, or is a resiliency effect established with just a small number of particularly supportive teachers or classes?

Authors' Note

Funding for the study involving Sample 1 came from the W. T. Grant Foundation. Funding for the studies involving Samples 2 and 3 came from the Spencer Foundation.

Appendix

Measures of the Classroom Social Environment, with Factor Loadings

Teacher support	
Does your math teacher respect your opinion?	.85
Does your math teacher really understand how you feel about things?	.68
Does your math teacher try to help you when you are sad or upset?	.52
Can you count on your math teacher for help when you need it?	.44
Promoting mutual respect	
My teacher wants students in this class to respect each others' opinions.	.82
My teacher does not allow students to make fun of other students' ideas in class.	.68
My teacher does not let us make fun of someone who gives the wrong answer.	.67
My teacher will not allow students to say anything negative about each other in class.	.66
My teacher wants all students to feel respected.	.55
Promoting task-related interaction	
My teacher allows us to discuss our work with classmates.	.88
My teacher lets us ask other students when we need help in math.	.86
My teacher encourages us to share ideas with one another in class.	.81
My teacher encourages us to get to know all the other students in class.	.59
My teacher encourages us to get to know our classmates' names.	.55
My teacher encourages us to be helpful to other students with their math work.	.46
If you have a problem in math class you can just talk to someone about it.	.80
People in my math class often work out problems together.	.53
Promoting performance goals	
My teacher points out those students who get good grades as an example to all of us.	.77
My teacher tells us how we compare to other students.	.76
My teacher lets us know which students get the highest scores on a test.	.74
My teacher lets us know which students get the lowest scores on a test.	.68
My teacher points out those students who get poor grades as an example to all of us.	.62
My teacher makes it obvious when certain students are not doing well on their math work.	.58
My teacher calls on smart students more than on other students.	.46

Note: Factor loadings < .40 not reported.

References

Ames, C. (1992). Classrooms: Goals, structures, and student motivation. *Journal of Educational Psychology, 84,* 261–271.

Anderman, E. M., Griesinger, T., & Westerfield, G. (1998). Motivation and cheating during early adolescence. *Journal of Educational Psychology, 90*, 84–93.

Anderman, E., & Maehr, M. L. (1994). Motivation and schooling in the middle grades. *Review of Educational Research, 64*, 287–309.

Borg, W. R., & Gall, M. D. (1989). *Educational research: An introduction.* New York: Longman.

Carnegie Council on Adolescent Development. (1989). *Turning points: Preparing America's youth for the 21st century.* New York: Carnegie Corporation.

Carnegie Council on Adolescent Development. (1995). *Great transitions: Preparing adolescents for a new century.* New York: Carnegie Corporation.

Cohen, E. (1994). Restructuring the classroom: Conditions for productive small groups. *Review of Educational Research, 64*, 1–35.

Connell, J. P. (2003, March). *Connectedness to school and school engagement.* Paper presented at the Indicators of Positive Development Conference organized by Child Trends, Washington, DC.

De Lisi, R., & Golbeck, S. L. (1999). Implications of Piagetian theory for peer learning. In A. M. O'Donnell & A. King (Eds.), *Cognitive perspectives on peer learning* (pp. 3–37). Mahwah, NJ: Lawrence Erlbaum.

Eccles, J. S., & Midgley, C. (1989). Stage–environment fit: Developmentally appropriate classrooms for young adolescents. In C. Ames & R. Ames (Eds.), *Research on motivation in education: Vol. 3. Goals and cognitions* (pp. 139–186). New York: Academic Press.

Eccles, J., Midgley, C., Wigfield, A., Buchanan, C. M., Reuman, D., Flanagan, C., et al. (1993). Development during adolescence: The impact of stage–environment fit on young adolescents' experience in schools and families. *American Psychologist, 48*, 90–101.

Eccles, J., Wigfield, A., & Schiefele, U. (1998). Motivation to succeed. In W. Damon (Series Ed.) & N. Eisenberg (Vol. Ed.), *Handbook of child psychology: Vol. 3. Social, emotional, and personality development* (5th ed., pp. 1017–1095). New York: Wiley.

Elkind, D. (1967). Egocentrism in adolescence. *Child Development, 38*, 1025–1034.

Ellis, H. C., & Ashbrook, P. W. (1987). Resource allocation model of the effects of depressed mood states. In K. Fielder & J. Forgas (Eds.), *Affect, cognition, and social behavior* (pp. 25–43).Toronto: Hogrefe.

Felner, R. D., Aber, M. S., Primavera, J., & Cauce, A. M. (1985). Adaptation and vulnerability in high-risk adolescents: An examination of environmental mediators. *American Journal of Community Psychology, 13*, 365–379.

Fraser, B. J., & Fisher, D. L. (1982). Predicting student outcomes from their perceptions of classroom psychosocial environment. *American Educational Research Journal, 19*, 498–518.

Goodenow, C. (1993). Classroom belonging among early adolescent students: Relationships to motivation and achievement. *Journal of Early Adolescence, 13*, 21–43.

Gottfried, A. E. (1990). Academic intrinsic motivation in young elementary school children. *Journal of Educational Psychology, 77*, 631–645.

Harter, S. (1990). Self and identity development. In S. S. Feldman & G. R. Elliot (Eds.), *At the threshold: The developing adolescent* (pp. 352–387). Cambridge, MA: Harvard University Press.

Harter, S., & Pike, R. (1984). The pictorial scale of perceived competence and social acceptance for young children. *Child Development, 55*, 1969–1982.

Johnson, D. W., Johnson, R., & Anderson, D. (1983). Social interdependence and classroom climate. *Journal of Psychology, 114*, 135–142.

Juvonen, J., & Weiner, B. (1993). An attributional analysis of students' interactions: The social consequences of perceived responsibility. *Educational Psychology Review, 5*, 325–345.

Kaplan, A., Gheen, M., & Midgley, C. (2002). The classroom goal structure and student disruptive behavior. *British Journal of Educational Psychology, 72*, 191–211.

Kaplan, A., & Maehr, M. L. (1999). Achievement goals and student well-being. *Contemporary Educational Psychology, 24*, 330–358.

Keating, D. P. (1990). Adolescent thinking. In S. S. Feldman & G. R. Elliot (Eds.), *At the threshold: The developing adolescent* (pp. 54–89). Cambridge, MA: Harvard University Press.

Mantzicopoulos, P., & Neuharth-Pritchett, S. (2003). Development and validation of a measure to assess Head Start children's appraisals of teacher support. *Journal of School Psychology, 41*, 431–451.

Midgley, C., Feldlaufer, H., & Eccles, J. S. (1989). Student/teacher relations and attitudes toward mathematics before and after the transition to junior high school. *Child Development, 60*, 981–992.

Midgley, C., Maehr, M. L., Hicks, L., Roeser, R., Urdan, T., Anderman, E. M., et al. (1996). *Patterns of Adaptive Learning Survey (PALS) Manual.* Ann Arbor: University of Michigan.

Moos, R. H., & Moos, B. S. (1978). Classroom social climate and student absences and grades. *Journal of Educational Psychology, 70*, 263–269.

National Council of Teachers of Mathematics. (2000). *Principles and standards for school mathematics.* Reston, VA: Author.

National Research Council. (1996). *National science education standards.* Washington, DC: National Academy Press.

Newman, R. S., & Schwager, M. T. (1993). Student perceptions of the teacher and classmates in relation to reported help seeking in math class. *Elementary School Journal, 94*, 3–17.

Nicholls, J. (1990). What is ability and why are we mindful of it? A developmental perspective. In R. Sternberg & J. Kolligian (Eds.), *Competence considered* (pp. 11–40). New Haven, CT: Yale University Press.

O'Donnell, A. M., & O'Kelly, J. (1994). Learning from peers: Beyond the rhetoric of positive results. *Educational Psychology Review, 6*, 321–349.

Patrick, H., Hicks. L., & Ryan, A. M. (1997). Relations of perceived social efficacy and social goal pursuit to self-efficacy for academic work. *Journal of Early Adolescence, 17*, 109–128.

Patrick, H., & Middleton, M. J. (2002). Turning the kaleidoscope: What we see when self-regulated learning is viewed with a qualitative lens. *Educational Psychologist, 37*, 27–39.

Patrick, H., Turner, J. C., Meyer, D. K, & Midgley, C. (2003). How teachers establish psychological environments during the first days of school: Associations with avoidance in mathematics. *Teachers College Record, 105*, 1521–1558.

Pintrich, P. R., Smith, D. A. F., Garcia, T., & McKeachie, W. J. (1993). Reliability and predictive validity of the Motivated Strategies for Learning Questionnaire (MSLQ). *Educational and Psychological Measurement, 53*, 801–813.

Ryan, A. M., Gheen, M., & Midgley, C. (1998). Why do some students avoid asking for help? An examination of the interplay among students' academic efficacy, teacher's social-emotional role and classroom goal structure. *Journal of Educational Psychology, 90*, 528–535.

Ryan, A. M., & Patrick, H. (2001). The classroom social environment and changes in adolescents' motivation and engagement during middle school. *American Educational Research Journal, 38*, 437–460.

Trickett, E. J., & Moos, R. H. (1974). Personal correlates of contrasting environments: Student satisfactions in high school classrooms. *American Journal of Community Psychology, 2*, 1–12.

Turner, J. C., Thorpe, P. K., & Meyer, D. K. (1998). Students' reports of motivation and negative affect: A theoretical and empirical analysis. *Journal of Educational Psychology, 90*, 758–771.

Urdan, T. C., Midgley, C., & Anderman, E. M. (1998). The role of classroom goal structure in students' use of self-handicapping strategies. *American Educational Research Journal, 35*, 101–122.

Urdan, T. C., Ryan, A. M., Anderman, E. M., & Gheen, M. (2002). Goals, goal structures, and avoidance behaviors. In C. Midgley (Ed.), *Goals, goal structures, and patterns of adaptive learning* (pp. 55–83). Mahwah, NJ: Lawrence Erlbaum.

Webb, N. M., & Palincsar, A. S. (1996). Group processes in the classroom. In D. C. Berliner & R. C. Calfee (Eds.), *Handbook of educational psychology* (pp. 841–873). New York: Simon & Schuster.

Wentzel, K. R. (1994). Relations of social goal pursuit to social acceptance, classroom behavior, and perceived social support. *Journal of Educational Psychology, 86*, 173–182.

18   Connection to School

Clea McNeely

Johns Hopkins University

In this chapter, I identify two indicators of school connectedness that tap the subdomains of *social belonging* and students' *relationship with teachers*, using questions and data from the National Longitudinal Study of Adolescent Health (Add Health).

Resnick and colleagues (1997) used the term *school connectedness* to describe adolescents' perception of safety, belonging, respect, and feeling cared for at school. In a cross-sectional analysis of risk and protective factors for eight different health risk outcomes among adolescents, Resnick et al. (1997) identified school connectedness as the only school-related variable that was protective for every single outcome. Widespread dissemination of this finding, along with its intuitive appeal, has led to an eagerness on the part of state health departments and school boards to monitor how well they are doing in terms of promoting school connectedness. Despite the interest, however, the empirical evidence of a causal relationship between school connectedness and adolescent development is rather limited.

Several theoretical streams have identified aspects of school connectedness as theoretically important for healthy adolescent development. The social development model (Hawkins & Weis, 1985), derived from integrating social control and social learning theories, posits that when students develop a positive social bond with their school, they are more likely to remain academically engaged and less likely to become involved in antisocial behaviors. Hawkins and Weis (1985) identified three elements of the school social bond: attachment to prosocial peers and school personnel, commitment to conventional academic activities, and belief in the established norms for school behavior. They hypothesized that the school social bond inhibits antisocial behavior primarily through fostering associations with prosocial peers.

Others have used the term *social membership* (Wehlage, Rutter, Smith, Lesko, & Fernandez, 1989) or sense of community (Battistich & Hom, 1997) for the same basic construct that Hawkins and Weis term *social belonging*. The theoretical orientation of these authors is that social belonging is a primary human need. The premise is that positive social relationships foster a sense of social belonging which, in turn, fosters academic engagement (Connell & Wellborn, 1991; Furrer & Skinner, 2003; Wehlage, Rutter, Smith, Lesko, & Fernandez, 1989). In addition, Bollen and Hoyle (1990) suggest that perceived group membership is a prerequisite for following school norms and values.

The social support literature represents a third theoretical stream that has identified students' perceptions of support from teachers and peers as important for promoting development (for a brief review, see Rosenfeld, Richman, & Bowen, 2000). The mechanism through which social support at school influences outcomes remains generally unexplored; however, it is typically hypothesized to be reduction in uncertainty. Supportive communication helps students perceive alternatives and recognize that help is available from others, thereby enabling students to develop a sense of control over stressful circumstances (Albrecht & Adelman, 1987). Despite different theoretical traditions, the core constructs of personal belonging, respect, and support at school are identified as important by each of these streams of research. They are also the core constructs measured by the questions in the Add Health survey.

Measures of school belonging, membership, support, and satisfaction have been demonstrated to be associated with several educational outcomes, including attendance (e.g., Rosenfeld, Richman, & Bowen, 1998); school misconduct, such as cheating, being suspended, and refusing to follow rules (Hawkins, Guo, Hill, Battin-Pearson, & Abbot, 2001; Jenkins, 1997); academic achievement (e.g., Barber & Olsen, 1997); student motivation (e.g., Roeser, Eccles, & Strobel, 1996); and early school dropout (Battin-Pearson et al., 2000). These measures have also been linked to health risk behaviors, in particular substance use (Battistich & Hom, 1997; Hawkins et al., 2001; Resnick et al., 1997), but also sexual intercourse (e.g., Hawkins et al., 2001), mental health (e.g., Roeser et al., 1998), and violence and delinquency (Battistich & Hom, 1997; Hawkins et al., 2001; Resnick et al., 1997).

Complicating the review of the literature is the inconsistent use of terminology. For example, Moody and Bearman (2001) measure school attachment with Bollen and Hoyle's (1990) three-item measure of social belonging. In contrast, Jenkins (1997) measures school attachment with a nine-item scale developed from responses to questions about whether the students have positive relationships with their teachers. Hawkins and colleagues (2001) combine three subscales: commitment to school, attachment to teachers, and attachment to school, the latter of which is very similar to Bollen and Hoyle's social belonging measure. Moreover, it is not clear from previous research, which is primarily cross-sectional, whether connection to school actually promotes these positive outcomes. It is possible that connection to school is merely a correlate, and both connection to school and positive outcomes are produced by a third factor. It is also possible that causality works in the opposite direction, in particular for the academic outcomes. Positive feelings about school may be a result of academic success rather than its cause (Coleman & Collinge, 1993).

Add Health

The current study identifies and evaluates two new measures of school connectedness using data from Add Health, a nationally representative sample of American adolescents in grades 7–12 in 1995. The primary sampling frame for Add Health was U.S. high schools. A stratified sample of 80 high schools was selected with probability proportional to the school's enrollment. A single feeder school was selected for each high school with probability of selection proportional to the percentage of the high school's entering class that came from the feeder school. Schools varied in size from less than 100 to more than 3,000 students. Add Health includes private, religious, and public schools from communities located in urban, suburban, and rural areas of the country (Tourangeau and Shin, 1999; Udry, 1998;).

All students in the eligible grade range at the participating schools were asked to complete in-school questionnaires during the 1994–1995 academic year. Based on rosters of students from each school and the in-school questionnaires, students were selected for Wave 1 in-home data collection. The response rate was 78.9%, yielding a sample of 20,745 youth completing in-home questionnaires. Of these, 1,821 cases were not assigned sampling weights. A second interview was conducted during the following academic year for all students except the 12th graders and a few select subsamples. The Wave 2 response rate was 88.2% ($n = 14,738$).

The present analysis uses two samples. For the psychometric analyses, I use the Wave 1 in-home weighted sample ($n = 18,924$) because it includes the 12th graders and is representative of the full 7th- to 12th-grade age range. To test the predictive validity of the indicators, I restrict the sample to those students who responded to both Wave 1 and Wave 2 surveys and who were assigned survey weights at Wave 2 ($n = 13,570$).

Measures of School Connectedness

Three different measures of school connectedness have been developed from the Add Health data. Resnick et al. (1997) used an eight-item scale (Cronbach's alpha $= .78$) that included the adolescent's perceptions of belonging, feeling cared for and respected by teachers, having trouble getting along with teachers and fellow students, and feeling safe at school. McNeely, Nonnemaker, and Blum (2002) used a five-item measure ($\alpha = .79$, in-school survey) that included the adolescent's perception of belonging, being treated fairly by teachers, and the perception of feeling safe. This same measure was used in a separate sample of 4,773 7th through 12th graders attending public schools (Bonny, Britto, Klosterman, Hornung, & Slap, 2000). Finally, a three-item measure—developed by Bollen and Hoyle (1990) to measure social belonging—was used by Moody and Bearman (2001) in the in-school Add Health sample ($\alpha = .79$).

The study reported here investigated seven Add Health questions that tap aspects of connection to school. Three are the questions developed by Bollen and Hoyle (1990) to measure social belonging. Students are asked how much they agree or disagree with the following statements: "You feel close to people at your school," "You feel like you are part of your school," and "You are happy to be at your school." If the survey was administered during the summer, the questions were asked in the past tense. Responses are indicated on a five-item Likert scale ranging from *strongly agree* to *strongly disagree*.

Another three items ask adolescents about their perceptions of their teachers. The first question asks students to report how much they agree or disagree with the statement, "The teachers at your school treat students fairly." Response categories range from *strongly agree* to *strongly disagree*. A second question asks, "Since school started this year, how often have you had trouble getting along with your teachers?" The five response categories are *never, just a few times, about once a week, almost every day*, and *every day*. The third question about teachers appears in a different section of the survey that asks about how much different people in the young person's life care about him or her. The question is, "How much do you feel that your teachers care about you?" The five response categories are *not at all, very little, somewhat, quite a bit*, and *very much*.

A final question that has been used to measure school connectedness is a perception of school safety (e.g., McNeely et al., 2002). Students are asked how much they agree or disagree with the statement, "You feel safe in your school." The five response categories range from *strongly agree* to *strongly disagree*. Responses to six of the seven school connectedness questions were reverse-coded so that a higher score reflected a more positive response.

Psychometric Analysis

To determine if these seven items comprise one or more dimensions of school connectedness, the underlying organization of the variables was examined using zero-order correlations, principal components analysis, and confirmatory factor analysis. Confirmatory factor analysis was used to test a model consisting of two correlated factors: social belonging and relationship with teachers. Confirmatory factor analysis involves specifying a measurement model and then testing the fit of the model. The specified model implies a variance–covariance structure, which is calculated using parameter estimates based on the data, and then compared to the actual variance–covariance structure of the data. If the two variance–covariance structures are similar (within sampling error), the model is taken to fit the data well (Long, 1983). AMOS 4.0 (Arbuckle & Wothke, 1999) was used to calculate parameter estimates.[1]

---

[1] AMOS uses full information maximum likelihood estimation in the presence of missing data to produce the parameter estimates. For the model to be identified, one of the factor loadings was set equal to 1 on each factor, and the variances of both the common and unique factors were set to 0. An additional necessary restriction imposed on the model for identification was that the errors in the observed variables (the unique factors) be uncorrelated with each other. The common factors were allowed to be correlated. In addition, the mean of one indicator was set to the sample mean for each factor loading. This additional constraint was required due to the presence of missing

Table 1. Weighted Principal Components Analysis of School Connectedness Variables: Add Health Wave 1 Grand Sample

	Principal components	
	Social bonding	Student–teacher relationship
1. You feel close to people at your school.	.88	—
2. You feel like you are part of school.	.86	—
3. You are happy to be at your school.	.70	—
4. The teachers at your school treat students fairly.	—	.73
5. Since school started this year, how often have you had trouble getting along with your teachers?	—	.82
6. How much do you feel that your teachers care about you?	—	.66
7. You feel safe in your school.	.45	.28
Cronbach's alpha with "feel safe in your school"	.77	.66
Cronbach's alpha without "feel safe in your school"	.78	.63

The bivariate correlations of the seven items indicate that the three items developed by Bollen and Hoyle (1990) to measure social belonging are highly correlated ($r = .49$ to $.60$). The correlations between these three items and the remaining items are moderate, ranging between $.19$ and $.40$. Table 1 presents results from principal components analysis of the seven items. Using the criteria of retaining factors that have a minimum eigenvalue of 1 and the scree criterion, two factors were retained. The varimax and oblique solutions yielded similar results, and the oblique rotation was selected because of the relatively high interfactor correlation ($r = .40$). The factor structure accounted for 59% of the total variance.

The three social belonging measures loaded on the first factor, whereas the three student–teacher relationship items loaded on the second factor. Students' report of how safe they feel at school had moderate factor loadings on both factors ($.45$ and $.28$, respectively).[2] The Cronbach's alpha coefficients, presented at the bottom of Table 1 for the full sample, demonstrate that inclusion of the feeling-safe-at-school item decreases the internal consistency of a scale derived from the first factor and only minimally increases the internal consistency of a scale derived from the second factor. Since parsimony is an important feature of an indicator, this item was excluded from subsequent confirmatory factor analysis.

The two-factor solution was tested using confirmatory factor analysis. Consistent with the findings from the principal components analysis, the three items

data and the requirement to estimate the saturated model in addition to the model specified above (Arbuckle & Wothke, 1999). The fit of the model was determined by assessing the magnitude of the discrepancy between the sample and fitted covariance matrices using multiple fit indices (Hu & Bentler, 1995).

[2] Maximum likelihood factor analysis produced similar results. Unlike principal components analysis, the scree criterion suggested a one-factor solution, but when two factors were specified, the rotated factor pattern matched the principal components results.

Table 2. Reliability of the Social Belonging and Student–Teacher Relationship Scales by Demographic Characteristics

	Cronbach's alpha	
	Social bonding	Student–teacher relationships
Gender-Ethnicity Groups		
Hispanic females	.76	.55
Hispanic males	.72	.62
White females	.82	.64
White males	.79	.68
African American females	.75	.57
African American males	.68	.62
American Indian females	.88	.50
American Indian males	.79	.66
Asian American females	.64	.44
Asian American males	.71	.50
Other ethnicity females	.92	.62
Other ethnicity males	.75	.70
Age Groups		
11–14	.76	.67
15–19	.79	.62
Family Structure		
Two-parent biological	.78	.64
One-parent biological	.77	.63
Stepfamily	.80	.60
Other family structure	.78	.64

representing social belonging have higher factor loadings (.70 to .80) than the three items representing relationship with teachers (.50 to .66). The correlation between the two latent factors is .62. The null hypothesis for the chi-square test is that the observed covariance structure is equal to the model covariance structure. Therefore, the smaller the chi-square statistic, the better the model fit. If the chi-square statistic divided by its degrees of freedom (χ^2/df) is 5 or less, the model is usually considered an acceptable fit. However, in large samples, a trivial difference between the sample covariance matrix and the fitted model may result in a large chi-square statistic and rejection of the specified model (Hu & Bentler, 1995). Therefore, the chi-square statistic must be compared to other fit indices. Hu and Bentler (1995) suggest that if the CFI is greater than .96 and the RMSEA is less than .10, the data adequately fit the model. The values of the CFI (.997) and the RMSEA (.060) indicate that the model is an acceptable fit, despite the χ^2/df value (76.45).[3]

The internal consistency of the social belonging and relationship with teachers scales is presented in Table 2. The reliability of the social belonging

[3] A one-factor model that excluded the student–teacher relationship factor (not shown) fits the model better than the two-factor model ($\chi^2/df = 1.56$; CFI = 1.00; RMSEA = .005). This is consistent with both the higher intercorrelations between the three social belonging variables.

scale is adequate for all gender-ethnicity groups. In general, the reliability is slightly higher for females than males. It is highest for White and American Indian females and lowest for Asian Americans of both genders. The scale exhibits excellent reliability across both age groups and across all types of family structure.

The student–teacher relationship scale exhibits lower reliability. For all groups, the Cronbach's alpha coefficient is at or below .70. In contrast to social belonging, the scale tends to have slightly higher reliability among males compared to females. It performs poorly (Cronbach's alpha coefficient < .60) for Hispanic, African American, American Indian, and Asian American females. It also performs poorly for Asian American males. The lower internal consistency among females is most likely due to limited variability among females in responses to the question, "How often do you have trouble getting along with your teacher." Across all ethnicities, females were less likely to report any trouble getting along with their teacher. This was particularly true of Asian American females, 95% of whom reported never or just a few times having trouble getting along with their teacher. Eighty-five percent of Asian American males said they never or just a few times had trouble getting along with their teacher. The reliability of the student–teacher relationship scale decreases slightly with age. It does not vary substantially by family structure.

The distributions of the two school connectedness measures demonstrate that they have good variability across all subgroups. The skewness of the distributions across subgroups is minimal, with the negative values indicating a slight skewness to the left (i.e., slightly higher scores). Kurtosis, a measure of the peakedness of the distribution, is near the desired value of 3, which indicates the variables are normally distributed.

Construct and Discriminant Validity

Table 3 examines construct and discriminant validity. The two scales measuring school connectedness are significantly related ($r = .45$),[4] and their intercorrelation is stronger than their correlation with any other variable in Table 3. Of the two dimensions of school connectedness, one would logically expect the student–teacher relationship measure to be more closely related to classroom functioning because it directly involves the teacher. Conversely, one would expect the social belonging measure to be more closely related to measures of peer relationships at school. The correlations between the student–teacher relationship and students' reports of having trouble paying attention in class and having trouble completing homework are in the expected direction and are stronger than the correlation of social belonging with these variables. However, both social belonging and relationship with teachers are equally correlated with the two peer

[4] The correlation between the two factors estimated by confirmatory factor analysis (CFA) is .62; the higher correlation obtained from CFA reflects decreased measurement error resulting from separating the common and unique variance components.

Table 3. Weighted Bivariate Correlations between School Connectedness Items and Other School Variables: Add Health Wave 1 Grand Sample

Variables	Social belonging	Student–teacher relationship
Classroom Functioning		
Trouble paying attention in class	−0.26	−0.41
Trouble completing homework	−0.22	−0.32
Peer Relationships		
Students are prejudiced	−0.16	−0.16
Trouble getting along with students	−0.27	−0.28

variables (perception that students at school are prejudiced and report of having trouble getting along with other students). The associations between the school connectedness measures and perceptions of prejudice are quite modest for all groups except American Indian students and students of other race/ethnicity (results not shown).

Predictive Validity

The predictive validity of the measures was examined by determining whether the school connectedness measures at Wave 1 were associated with school-related and health-related outcomes approximately 1 year later. Two school-related outcomes were selected, grade point average (GPA) and whether the adolescent was suspended from school between the Wave 1 and Wave 2 interviews. *GPA* was measured by the average letter grade for the last grading period for up to four subjects: English or language arts, mathematics, history or social studies, and science. If students received grades in at least two subjects, their GPA was calculated. If they took fewer than two of these subjects, did not receive letter grades, or were not in school at Wave 2, they were excluded from the analysis. *Out-of-school suspension* is a dichotomous variable (yes/no) measured by responses to the question, "During this school year, have you received an out-of-school suspension?" Given that the survey was administered at different times during the school year, the length of time during which students had the opportunity to be suspended varied. It is not known to what extent this variation is nonrandom.

The two health-related outcomes are weapon-related violence and cigarette use. *Weapon-related violence* is a dichotomous variable indicating whether the adolescent committed at least one of the following acts in the year between the Wave 1 and Wave 2 surveys: threatened to use a weapon to get something from someone, pulled a knife or gun on someone, shot or stabbed someone, used a weapon in a fight, or hurt someone badly enough for that person to need bandages or medical care. Thirteen percent of the sample responded affirmatively to at least one of these items. *Cigarette smoking* is measured with an indicator of whether or not the adolescent is a regular smoker, defined as having smoked on 20–30 days in the past 30 days. An additional indicator for whether the adolescent is a nonsmoker at Wave 2 is used to model the probability of quitting.

The relationship between the school connectedness measures and the outcomes was examined using ordinary least squares and logistic regression. For all outcomes except cigarette use, the models include the Wave 1 measure of the outcome, sociodemographic characteristics (gender, age, race/ethnicity), family characteristics (structure, income, size), and individual characteristics (score on an abbreviated version of the Peabody Picture Vocabulary Test). For cigarette use, two models were tested to explore the effect of school connectedness on the initiation of regular smoking and on quitting. First, I modeled the probability that a nonsmoker at Wave 1 becomes a regular smoker by Wave 2. Next I modeled the probability that regular smokers at Wave 1 quit smoking by Wave 2. I did not use factor scores for the school connectedness measures but rather created scales by averaging the items that make up each scale. This method was chosen because it is the method typically used for measuring indicators by state and local departments of health and education. The analyses were done in Stata 6.0 (StataCorp., 1999) using weights and adjusting for the complex sampling design.

The results from the multivariate models examining the relationship between school connectedness and the Wave 2 outcomes are summarized in Table 4. For each outcome, four models are presented. The first model contains just two independent variables, the social belonging measure and the Wave 1 (baseline) measure of the outcome variable. Similarly, the second model contains just the student–teacher relationship and the baseline value of the outcome. The third model contains both school connectedness measures. The final model adds the background (sociodemographic, family, individual) characteristics outlined previously. The models for cigarette use are slightly different in that they model the transition to regular use *conditional* on not smoking, and the transition to not smoking *conditional* on having been a regular smoker in the 30 days prior to the Wave 1 interview.

School-Related Outcomes

Models 1 and 2 in Table 4 show that each school connectedness variable, taken alone, is associated in the expected direction with GPA and out-of-school suspension. However, when social belonging and the student–teacher relationship measure are included in the same model, social belonging is no longer associated with either GPA or out-of-school suspension. The magnitude of the association between student–teacher relationship and the outcomes remains unchanged with the addition of social belonging and the control variables. The strength of the association between the student–teacher relationship and GPA is quite modest. A 1-unit change in the 5-point student-teacher relationship scale is associated with an increase of .04 point in GPA. The association of student–teacher relationship with out-of-school suspension is slightly stronger than for

Table 4. Weighted Coefficients from the Regression of School Belonging and Student–Teacher Relationship on Wave 2 Outcomes: Add Health Wave 2 Grand Sample

	Model 1		Model 2		Model 3		Model 4[a]	
	b	SE	b	SE	b	SE	b	SE
Weapon-Related Violence (logit)								
School belonging	-0.19**	0.04	—	—	-0.04	0.05	-0.05	0.05
Student–teacher relationship	—	—	-0.39**	0.05	-0.37**	0.05	-0.36**	0.05
Weapon-related violence (W1)	2.06**	0.15	1.95**	0.08	1.95**	0.08	1.74**	0.08
N	13,218		13,219		13,218		12,229	
Suspension (logit)								
School belonging	-0.21**	0.05	—	—	0.02	0.05	-0.02	0.06
Student–teacher relationship	—	—	-0.56**	0.05	-0.57**	0.05	-0.55**	0.06
Suspension (W1)	2.03**	0.10	1.88**	0.10	1.88**	0.10	1.68**	0.11
N	12,268		12,269		12,268		11,346	
Grade Point Average (OLS)								
School belonging	0.02*	0.01	—	—	0.01	0.01	0.01	0.01
Student–teacher relationship	—	—	0.05**	0.01	0.04**	0.01	0.05**	0.01
Grade point average (W1)	0.64**	0.01	0.63**	0.01	0.63	0.01	0.57**	0.01
N	11,723		11,724		11,723		10,836	
Transition from "No" (W1) to "Regular" Smoking								
School belonging	-0.37**	0.07	—	—	-0.11	0.08	-0.11	0.08
Student–teacher relationship	—	—	-0.67**	0.09	-0.62**	0.00	-0.63**	0.10
N	9,945		9,947		9,945		9,167	
Transition from "Regular" (W1) to "No" Smoking								
School belonging	0.12	0.10	—	—	0.10	0.10	0.00	0.10
Student–teacher relationship	—	—	0.10	0.11	0.04	0.11	0.17	0.13
N	1,566		1,566		1,566		1,456	

[a] Model 4 includes control variables for sociodemographic characteristics (age, gender, race/ethnicity), family characteristics (structure, income, size), and the respondent's score on an abbreviated version of the Peabody Picture Vocabulary Test.
*$p < .05$. **$p < .001$.

GPA. For each 1-point increase in the student–teacher relationship scale, a student is .58 times as likely ($e^{-.55}$) to receive an out-of-school suspension. An alternative model specification that modeled out-of-school suspension conditional on having never been suspended yielded similar results (not shown).[5]

Weapon-Related Violence

The story for weapon-related violence is the same as for the school-related outcomes. A positive student–teacher relationship at Wave 1 is associated with a lower probability of engaging in weapon-related violence during the subsequent year. Social belonging, however, is not associated with weapon-related violence once the student–teacher relationship is taken into account. The strength of the association between the student–teacher relationship scale and the probability of engaging in weapon-related violence is modest (odds ratio = .70); that is, for each 1-point increase in the student–teacher scale, a student is .7 times as likely ($e^{-.36}$) to engage in weapon-related violence.

Cigarette Use

Once again, the student–teacher relationship—but not social belonging at school—is protective against the initiation of regular smoking. For each 1-point increase in the student–teacher relationship scale, a nonsmoker is .53 times as likely ($e^{-.63}$) to initiate regular smoking. In contrast to the findings for the initiation of regular cigarette use, neither school connectedness variable was associated with smoking cessation.

Conditioning Effects of Demographic Characteristics

To determine whether the association between student–teacher relationship and the health-related outcomes varied by age, gender, or race/ethnicity, interaction terms were included in the model. Specifically, for each outcome, three separate models were estimated, each one containing the two school connectedness measures, the full set of control variables, and an interaction term between student–teacher relationship and age, gender, and race/ethnicity, respectively. The association between student–teacher relationship and weapon-related violence is slightly stronger among Asian American students than among students of other ethnic groups. In contrast, student–teacher relationship is slightly less

---

[5] An examination of potential collinearity between social belonging and student-teacher relationship in the GPA model suggests that collinearity does not explain the lack of association between social belonging and GPA once student-teacher relationship is added to the model. The weighted bivariate correlation between the two variables is .45, the variance inflation factor (VIF) for all variables is 3.5 or less, and the mean VIF is 1.6. Chatterjee, Hadi, and Price (2000) suggest that if the largest VIF is under 10 and the mean VIF is not considerably larger than 1, multicollinearity is not a problem.

protective against being suspended among older students. Finally, the student–teacher relationship is more protective against the initiation of regular cigarette smoking among American Indian students (results not shown). The lack of a clear pattern of findings across outcomes, combined with the fact that only 3 out of 30 statistical tests were statistically significant, suggests that the results are due to sampling distribution. In general, the association between the student–teacher relationship and the outcomes is consistent across demographic subgroups.

Discussion

The goal of this chapter was to take the items available in the Add Health data set and identify one or more indicators of school connectedness. Exploratory and confirmatory factor analysis identified two potential indicators, *social belonging* and *relationship with teachers*. The social belonging measure was based on a scale developed and validated by Bollen and Hoyle (1990) in a sample of college students and a sample of adult community members. My analysis showed that the three items also seem to tap the same underlying construct in this nationally representative sample of middle and high school students.

I have yet to identify the source of the three items measuring the student–teacher relationship and do not know if they were conceptualized to measure a single construct. Together, the items ask about multiple aspects of the student–teacher relationship, including fairness, caring, and discord. Barber (1997) describes three domains of adolescent–adult relationships—connection, regulation, and autonomy granting—each of which makes unique contributions to adolescent development. The student–teacher relationship measure potentially taps two or more of these domains. This would explain the lower interitem correlations, factor loadings, and reliabilities for this scale. The low alpha reliability could also be due to the mixed levels of observation contained within the scale. Two of the questions making up the student–teacher relationship scale ask the respondents about their personal relationship with their teacher, whereas the third asks the respondent to rate how fair the teachers in school are to all students. Nunnally and Bernstein (1994) caution against overinterpreting factor loadings and reliabilities for scales with just three items. Some even argue that it is not legitimate to develop scales with just three items. Therefore, despite the relatively low alpha coefficient for the student–teacher relationship ($\alpha = .63$), it was included in the models exploring predictive validity.

A positive student–teacher relationship at Wave 1 is associated with a lower probability of engaging in risky behaviors, being suspended, and earning poor grades during the subsequent year. Surprisingly, however, social belonging is not associated with these outcomes once the student–teacher relationship is taken into account. This finding is particularly surprising because coefficients for variables measured with error (i.e., low reliability) are biased toward zero, and so one would expect social belonging to have higher predictive validity than the student–teacher relationship.

This finding suggests that the association between student–teacher relationship and the outcomes is not mediated by a sense of social belonging, as suggested by social support models and the theoretical framework of Wehlage and colleagues (1989). This model does not rule out the possibility that the direct effect of social belonging is mediated by a positive student–teacher relationship, but the theoretical argument that a feeling of social belonging fosters a positive relationship with teachers is less compelling. More likely is that the association between student–teacher relationships on student outcomes operates independently of social belonging. Only one study that I am aware of has competed the different aspects of the school social bond against one another (Jenkins 1997). She found that attachment—a measure of the warmth and support students feel from their teachers—predicted nonattendance, school misconduct, and school crime. She also found that the importance of attachment relative to other measures of the school bond (e.g., school motivation and engagement, involvement, and belief in the fairness of school rules) varied across outcomes.

In this study, the student–teacher relationship was more strongly associated with so-called antisocial behaviors of weapon-related violence, being suspended, and becoming a regular smoker. The association with GPA was much smaller, and the association with smoking cessation was nonexistent. It is possible that the student–teacher relationship is more protective for certain outcomes than for others.

By separating school connectedness into two separate albeit related dimensions, this study contributes to specificity of measurement in the burgeoning field of school connectedness. The broader measures of school connectedness that have received the most attention to date (Hawkins et al., 2001; Resnick et al., 1997) combine general feelings about school (e.g., "I like school") with academic motivation (e.g., "I do extra school work on my own"), perceptions of safety, or relationships with teachers. This research suggests that not all aspects of school connectedness are equally protective. Although the measure of social belonging has better psychometric properties than does the student–teacher relationship measure, the longitudinal analyses suggest that the student–teacher relationship is substantively more important for the outcomes measured.

Two limitations of this study should be noted. First, the development of the school connectedness measures was based on the items available in Add Health. Were a more theoretically driven approach used and additional measures available, other dimensions of connectedness might have surfaced. Second, the predictive validity of these items should be interpreted with caution. Although the baseline measures of the outcomes were included in the models, it is quite probable that there are still unmeasured factors that influence both the outcome and a student's perception of her relationship with her teacher. Ramsey's test for omitted variables in the GPA model suggests this is the case, $F(3, 11668) = 74.06$, $p < .001$. Therefore, the relationship between the student–teacher relationship and the health and educational outcomes may be spurious.

In sum, this study identified a measure of student–teacher relationships that is both brief and has good predictive validity, selection issues notwithstanding. The disadvantage of the indicator is its relatively poor psychometric properties.

Nonetheless, as a general measure of the student–teacher relationship, it might merit inclusion as a monitoring tool until the specific domains of school connectedness and their relative importance to both positive and negative aspects of adolescent development are determined.

Author's Note

This research was supported by a William T. Grant Faculty Scholars Award. I thank James Nonnemaker, Bob Cudeck, Melanie Wall, and Jim Connell for their helpful comments and suggestions. Address correspondence to Clea McNeely, Johns Hopkins Bloomberg School of Public Health, 615 North Wolfe Street, Baltimore, MD 21205.

References

Albrecht, T. L., and Adelman, M. B. (1987). Communicating social support: A theoretical perspective. In T. L. Albrecht & M. B. Adelman (Eds.), *Communicating social support* (pp. 18–39). Newbury Park, CA: Sage.

Arbuckle, J. L., & Wothke, W. (1999). *Amos 4.0 User's Guide*. Chicago: SmallWaters Corporation.

Barber, B. K. (1997). Introduction. Adolescent socialization in context: Connection, regulation, and autonomy in multiple contexts. *Journal of Adolescent Research, 12*(2), 173–177.

Barber, B. K. and Olsen, J. A., (1997). Socialization in context: Connection, regulation, and autonomy in the family, school and neighborhood, and with peers. *Journal of Adolescent Research, 12*(2), 287–315.

Battin-Pearson, S., Newcomb, M. D., Abbot, R. D., Hill, K. G., Catalano, R. F., & Hawkins, J. D. (2000). Predictors of early high school dropout: A test of five theories. *Journal of Educational Psychology, 92*(3), 568–582.

Battistich, V. & Hom, A. (1997). The relationship between students' sense of their school as a community and their involvement in problem behaviors. *American Journal of Public Health, 87*(12), 1997–2001.

Bollen, K., & Hoyle, R. H. (1990). Perceived cohesion: A conceptual and empirical examination. *Social Forces, 69*(2), 479–504.

Bonny, A. E., Britto, M. T., Klosterman, B. K., Hornung, R. W., & Slap, G. B. (2000). School disconnectedness: Identifying adolescents at risk. *Pediatrics 106*(5), 1017–1021.

Chatterjee, S., Hadi, A. S., & Price, B. (2000). *Regression analysis by example* (3rd ed.). New York: John Wiley & Sons.

Coleman, P., & Collinge, J. (1993). Seeking the levers of change: Participant attitudes and school improvement. *School Effectiveness and School Improvement, 4*(1), 59–83.

Connell, J., & Wellborn, J. (1991). Competence, autonomy, and relatedness: A motivational analysis of self-system processes. In M. Gunnar & L. A. Sroufe (Eds.), *Minnesota Symposium on Child Development: Vol. 23. Self processes in development* (pp. 43–77). Hillsdale, NJ: Lawrence Erlbaum.

Furrer, C., & Skinner, E. (2003). Sense of relatedness as a factor in children's academic engagement and performance. *Journal of Educational Psychology, 95*(1), 148–161.

Hawkins, J. D., Guo, J., Hill, K. G., Battin-Pearson, S., & Abbot, R. D. (2001). Long-term effects of the Seattle Social Development Intervention on school bonding trajectories. *Applied Developmental Science, 5*(4), 225–236.

Hawkins, J. D., & Weis, J. G. (1985). The social development model: An integrated approach to delinquency prevention. *Journal of Primary Prevention, 6*(2), 73–97.

Hu, L., & Bentler, P. M. (1995). Evaluating model fit. In R. H. Hoyle (Ed.), *Structural equation modeling: Concepts, issues, and applications* (pp. 76–99).Thousand Oaks, CA: Sage.

Jenkins, P. H. (1997). School delinquency and the school social bond. *Journal of Research in Crime and Delinquency, 34*(3), 337–367.

Long, J. S. (1983). *Confirmatory factor analysis.* London: Sage.

McNeely, C. A., Nonnemaker, J. M., & Blum, R. W. (2002). Promoting school connectedness: Evidence from the National Longitudinal Study of Adolescent Health. *Journal of School Health, 72*(4), 138–146.

Moody, J. S., & Bearman, P. (2001) .School attachment. Unpublished manuscript.

Nunnally, J .C., & Bernstein, I. H. (1994). *Psychometric theory.* New York: McGraw-Hill.

Resnick, M. D., Bearman, P. S., Blum, R. W., Bauman, K. E., Harris, K. M., Jones, J. et al. (1997). Protecting adolescents from harm: Findings from the National Longitudinal Study of Adolescent Health. *Journal of the American Medical Association, 278*(10), 823–832.

Roeser, R., Eccles, J., & Strobel, K. (1998). Linking the study of schooling and mental health: Selected issues and empirical illustrations at the level of the individual. *Educational Psychologist, 33,* 153–176.

Rosenfeld, L. B., Richman, J. M., & Bowen, G. L. (1998). Low social support among at-risk adolescents. *Social Work in Education, 20,* 245–260.

Rosenfeld, L. B., Richman, J. M., & Bowen, G. L. (2000). Social support networks and school outcomes: The centrality of the teacher. *Child and Adolescent Social Work Journal, 17*(3), 205–226.

StataCorp. (1999). Stata Statistical Software: Release 6.0. College Station, TX: Stata Corporation.

Tourangeau, R. & Shin, H. (1999). *National Longitudinal Study of Adolescent Health: Grand sample weight.* Chapel Hill: University of North Carolina, National Opinion Research Center and Carolina Population Center. Web site: www.cpc.unc.edu/projects/addhlth/

Udry, J. R. (1998). *The National Longitudinal Study of Adolescent Health (Add Health), Waves I and II, 1994–1996* [Machine-readable data file and documentation]. Chapel Hill: University of North Carolina, Carolina Population Center.

Wehlage, G. G., Rutter, R. A., Smith, G. A., Lesko, N., & Fernandez, R. R. (1989). *Reducing the risk: Schools as communities of support.* New York: Falmer Press.

19 School Engagement

Jennifer A. Fredricks

Connecticut College

Phyllis Blumenfeld and Jeanne Friedel

University of Michigan

Alison Paris

Claremont McKenna College

There is a growing interest in the construct of school engagement. One reason for the interest in engagement is that it is seen as an antidote to low achievement, high levels of student boredom and disaffection, and the high dropout rates in urban areas. Another reason is that engagement is presumed to be malleable and responsive to variations in the environment. In our review of the literature, we found three types of engagement: *Behavioral* engagement draws on the idea of participation, including involvement in academic, social, or extracurricular activities; it is considered crucial for achieving positive academic outcomes and preventing dropping out (Connell, 1990; Finn, 1989). *Emotional* engagement draws on the idea of appeal. It includes positive and negative reactions to teachers, classmates, academics, or school and is presumed to create ties to the institution and influence willingness to do the work (Connell, 1990; Finn, 1989). Finally, *cognitive* engagement draws on the idea of investment; it incorporates being thoughtful and being willing to exert the necessary effort for comprehension of complex ideas and mastery of difficult skills (Corno & Mandinach, 1983; Newmann, Wehlage, & Lamborn, 1992).

Behavioral engagement has been defined in several ways. Some scholars focus on positive conduct, such as following the rules, adhering to classroom norms, and the absence of disruptive behaviors such as skipping school or getting in trouble (Finn, Pannozzo, & Voelkl, 1995; Finn & Rock, 1997). Other definitions emphasize participation in classroom learning and academic tasks and include behaviors such as persistence, effort, attention, and asking questions (Birch & Ladd, 1997; Finn, 1989; Skinner & Belmont, 1993). Finally, others focus on participation in school-related activities such as athletics or school governance (Finn, 1989; Finn et al., 1995).

Definitions of emotional engagement include students' positive and negative affective reactions in the classroom (Connell & Wellborn, 1991; Skinner & Belmont, 1993) and students' emotional reactions to the school and the teacher (Lee & Smith, 1995; Stipek, 2002). Other scholars conceptualize emotional engagement as identification with the school, which includes belonging, or a feeling of being important to the school, and valuing, or an appreciation of success in school-related outcomes (Finn, 1989; Voelkl, 1997).

In regard to cognitive engagement, definitions from the school engagement literature conceptualize it in terms of a psychological investment in learning, a desire to go beyond the requirements of school, and a preference for challenge (Connell & Wellborn, 1991; Newmann et al., 1992; Wehlage, Rutter, Smith, Lesko, & Fernandez, 1989). Definitions from the learning literature view cognitive engagement in terms of being strategic or self-regulating (Corno & Mandinach, 1983; Meece, Blumenfeld, & Hoyle, 1988).

We noted several strengths and limitations of current conceptualizations of behavioral, emotional, and cognitive engagement. First, definitions of engagement encompass a wide variety of constructs that can help explain how children behave, feel, and think in school. For example, behavioral engagement includes doing work and following the rules; emotional engagement incorporates interest, value, and emotions; and cognitive engagement includes motivation, effort, and strategy use. Second, we noted overlap in the definitions across different types of engagement. For instance, effort is included in definitions of behavioral and cognitive engagement, and no distinction is made between effort that reflects a psychological investment in learning and effort that merely demonstrates compliance with the requirements of school. Third, these three types of engagement overlap in many ways with constructs that have been previously studied. The literature on classroom participation, on-task behavior, and student conduct (Finn, 1989; Karweit, 1989; Peterson, Swing, Stark, & Wass, 1984) is similar to the work on behavioral engagement. Further, the research on identification and belonging (Finn, 1989; Goodenow, 1993; Osterman, 2000), interest and values (Eccles et al., 1983), and student attitudes (Epstein & McPartland, 1976; Yamamoto, Thomas, & Karns, 1969) is similar to the conceptualizations of emotional engagement. Finally, the research on metacognition and self-regulation overlaps with cognitive engagement (Pintrich & De Groot, 1990; Zimmerman, 1990).

Many studies of engagement involve one or two types but rarely include all three (behavior, emotional, and cognitive) or deal with engagement as a multifaceted construct (see Fredricks, Blumenfeld, & Paris, in press). Examining the components of engagement separately dichotomizes students' behavior, emotion, and cognition, whereas in reality these factors are dynamically embedded within a single individual and are not isolated processes. Although there are robust bodies of work on each of the components separately, considering engagement as a multidimensional construct provides a rationale for examining antecedents and consequences of behavior, emotion, and cognition simultaneously and dynamically. Some scholars have proposed moving toward a more holistic conceptualization of engagement that integrates all components. For example, Guthrie and Wigfield (2000) developed a model of "engaged reading" that includes aspects of emotional, cognitive, and behavioral engagement.

Common Measures

Behavioral engagement most commonly has been assessed through teacher and student self-report questionnaires and observational methods; emotional engagement has been measured through student self-report surveys. Cognitive engagement has been assessed using self-report questionnaires of strategy use and self-regulation and classroom observations. In addition, parent surveys have been used as general measures of school engagement.

A few measures conceptualize cognitive engagement as a psychological investment in learning. One example is Connell and Wellborn's (1991) measure of cognitive engagement, which contains items about flexible problem solving, preference for hard work, independent work styles, and ways of coping with perceived failure. There are several measures of students' strategy use by scholars who use either the term *cognitive engagement,* the term *self-regulation,* or both interchangeably. Because Wolters, Pintrich, and Karabenick cover self-regulation in chapter 16 of this volume, we do not review the most common measures of strategy use and cognitive engagement in this chapter.

The *Rochester Assessment Package for Schools* (RAPS) is the most common measure of behavioral and emotional engagement (Wellborn & Connell, 1987). There are student, teacher, and parent versions of this survey. The measures of behavioral engagement contain items about effort, attention, classroom participation, and initiative. Sample items from the behavioral engagement scale for the student version include "The first time my teacher talks about a new topic I listen carefully" and "When I am in class, I just act like I am working." Sample items from the teacher version of the behavioral engagement scale are "When in class, the student participates in class discussions" and "When in class this student just acts like he/she is working." The emotional engagement scale includes items about emotional reactions in the classroom, such as being bored, worried, sad, angry, interested, relaxed, and happy. For these items, children were asked to rate the extent to which they felt different emotions in school using three items: "When we start something new in class, I feel...," "When I am in class I feel...," and "When I am working in class, I feel...."

The teacher and student versions of the emotional and behavioral scales have strong reliability (Cronbach's alpha = .79 to .86). The RAPS has been primarily used with elementary school students in a rural and suburban school district (i.e., Connell & Wellborn, 1991; Patrick, Skinner, & Connell, 1993; Skinner & Belmont, 1993; Skinner, Wellborn, & Connell, 1990; Skinner, Zimmer-Gembeck,

& Connell, 1998). A few studies also have used this measure in urban middle school samples (Connell, Halpern-Felsher, Clifford, Crichlow, & Usinger, 1995; Connell, Spencer, & Aber, 1994).

The RAPS items have been used to validate the self-system model (Connell, 1990). This model asserts that behavioral and emotional engagement will be higher in social contexts where students' needs for relatedness, autonomy, and competence are met. The assumption is that engagement will be higher in classrooms in which teachers create a caring and supportive environment that meets students' needs for relatedness; children are given choices that are not determined by external threats, so they feel autonomous; and children feel like they know what it takes to do well and can achieve success, so they feel competent. Connell and his colleagues have provided evidence to support the proposed links between individual needs and engagement. However, the research is stronger for competence and relatedness than for autonomy (Connell, 1990; Connell & Wellborn, 1991; Patrick et al., 1993; Skinner & Belmont, 1993; Skinner et al., 1990). These results need to be replicated across diverse samples and developmental levels to test the validity of the measures and model.

Items from the *Teacher Ratings Scale of School Adjustment* (TRSSA) have been used to assess teachers' perceptions of young children's behavioral and emotional engagement in kindergarten and first grade (Birch & Ladd, 1997; Ladd, Birch, & Buhs, 1999; Valeski & Stipek, 2001). This measure includes four subscales: school liking, school avoidance, cooperative participation, and self-directedness. The school liking scale assesses aspects of emotional engagement. The school avoidance scale assesses children's desire to avoid school. The cooperative participation scale assesses the degree to which children accept the teachers' authority and comply with classroom rules and responsibilities (e.g., "follows teachers directions"), and the self-directedness scale reflects the extent to which children display independent and self-directed behavior in the classroom (e.g., "seeks challenge"). These scales have strong psychometric properties ($\alpha = .74$–$.91$). Scores on these measures of behavioral participation are related to achievement test scores and measures of emotional adjustment including school avoidance, liking, and loneliness (Buhs & Ladd, 2001; Ladd, Buhs, & Seid, 2000). Further research is necessary to confirm whether the relation between behavioral participation and academic and emotional adjustment holds across different developmental levels and populations.

Other studies have used items in the U.S. Department of Education's *National Educational Longitudinal Study* (NELS) to measure engagement (Finn, 1993; Finn & Rock, 1997; Lee & Smith, 1993, 1995). NELS is a large nationally representative longitudinal study of the educational status of students in 8th through 12th grades ($N =$ approximately 24,000 students). The study has a random sample of high school students from all regions of the United States including four racial/ethnic groups: Asian or Pacific Islander, Hispanic, Black, and White. This data set includes student survey information, achievement test data, parent surveys, and school administrator surveys.

Researchers have selected different items from NELS as indicators of behavioral and emotional engagement. Lee and Smith (1993, 1995) measured school engagement with items about affect, school value, adherence to classroom rules, getting in trouble, and level of participation. Finn and his colleagues (Finn, 1993; Finn & Rock, 1997) created several scales to assess different types of classroom and school behavior, including participation, compliance with classroom norms, attendance, preparation, and misbehavior. The NELS data set also has measures of behavioral engagement that reflect the amount of time the student participates in academic- and nonacademic-related activities that are beyond the regular school hours. Sample items include time spent on homework, extracurricular activities, discussing academic issues with school counselor, and discussing academic issues with adults other than parents.

Other scholars have used NELS to measure aspects of emotional engagement. For example, Finn (1993) measured emotional engagement with items about students' feelings of belonging in the school and the extent to which students value school subjects as being important in their future years. Sample items in the belongingness scale include "The only time I get attention in school is when I cause trouble" and "School is one of my favorite places to be." Sample items in the value scale include "School is more important than people think" and "I can get a good job even if my grades are bad." The behavioral and emotional engagement scales correlate in expected ways with achievement measures, behavioral problems, and dropping out (Finn, 1993; Finn & Rock, 1997). Since researchers have selected different items from NELS as measures of behavioral and emotional engagement, there are questions about the validity of these scales and the consistency of the relationships between behavioral and emotional engagement and school related outcomes.

Although most of the measures of engagement are child and teacher measures, the *National Survey of America's Families* (NSAF) is the first large survey to include parent telephone measures of school engagement. NSAF is part of a larger project at the Urban Institute, and Child Trends analyzes the devolution of responsibility for social programs from the federal to state governments. The parent scale of school engagement has also been incorporated in the 1999 Survey of Program Dynamics and the 5-year follow-up of the national Evaluation of Welfare-to-Work Strategies (Ehrle & Moore, 1999). The parent measure of school engagement was adapted from the parent version of the RAPS (Wellborn & Connell, 1987). The school engagement scale includes four questions that ask parents how well each of the statements describes their child: "did schoolwork only when they were forced to," "did just enough schoolwork to get by," "did homework," and "cared about doing well in school" (Ehrle & Moore, 1999).

The parent school engagement scale had strong reliability ($\alpha = .76$) and adequate variation around the mean. Initial analyses of this scale demonstrated strong validity (Ehrle & Moore, 1999). For example, the percentage of students with low school engagement increased with poverty, single parenthood, and low parental education. In addition, a higher percentage of children (ages 6–11) were highly engaged in school as compared to adolescents (ages 12–17). Finally, White children and girls were more highly engaged in school than children in other subgroups.

New Measures of School Engagement

Based on the prior literature, we developed a child survey, teacher survey, and child interview of behavioral, emotional, and cognitive engagement for a study of children's engagement in inner-city schools. This study was conducted in conjunction with the MacArthur Network for Successful Pathways through Middle Childhood. One goal of the study was to use multiple methods to describe the phenomenology of school engagement. Another goal was to examine the links between classroom context and engagement in the elementary school years. For this study, we chose elementary neighborhood schools located in urban high-poverty neighborhoods. We solicited nominations of well-functioning schools from the central office and researchers working in the cities. *Well functioning* means the schools were well run and maintained, safe, had a relatively stable administration, and focused on improving achievement.

We administered surveys and interviews to children over two waves of data collection. At the first wave, the sample included children in five schools in Chicago, Milwaukee, and Detroit. The sample at the first wave included 661 children ($ns = 238$ third graders, 205 fourth graders, and 218 fifth graders). These children were in 55 classrooms ranging in size from 5 to 27 children. Two of the schools had a majority of Hispanic children, two schools had a majority of African American children, and one school served children from a variety of ethnic backgrounds. Over 95% of children in these schools qualified for free and reduced-price lunch.

At the second wave, we followed children in three of the five schools in Chicago and Milwaukee into the fourth and fifth grades. Two schools were dropped because of financial constraints in the study. Since the network was focused on middle childhood, we did not follow the fifth graders into middle school. Two of the schools had a majority of Hispanic children, and one school had a majority of African American children. At Wave 2, the sample included 294 students (151 fourth graders and 143 fifth graders). These children were in 22 classrooms with up to 23 students per class. Since the school did not permit us to ask the students' ethnicity, we are unable to give an exact breakdown by ethnic groups, though we do have an ethnic breakdown at the school level. At Wave 2, we collected information from teachers about whether students were receiving special education services. At this wave, approximately 3% of the sample (22 students) received some type of special education services.

In addition, teachers filled out individual ratings on each student participating in this study. These surveys included questions about a variety of behavioral (pays attention, completes work, tries hard, follows rules), emotional (likes school), and cognitive (thoughtful when doing work) indicators of engagement. All items were on Likert scales from 1 to 5 ($1 = $ *not at all true*, $5 = $ *very true*). Teachers also were asked to rate children's reading and math achievement on a scale from 2 years below achievement level to 2 years above achievement level in each domain. We collected information from children and teachers because we were interested in whether the two groups were assessing behavioral, emotional, and cognitive engagement similarly. We did not collect survey information from the children's parents.

Survey Measures

The child measures included items about student engagement and classroom perceptions. Behavioral, emotional, and cognitive engagement survey items were drawn from a variety of measures (Finn et al., 1995; Pintrich, Smith, Garcia, & McKeachie, 1993; Wellborn & Connell, 1987) and included new items developed for this study. A list of engagement items is presented in the Appendix. All of the items were on Likert scales from 1 to 5 (1 = *never*, 5 = *all of the time*; or 1 = *not at all true*, 5 = *very true*). The surveys also included items about perceptions of the social context (teacher support and peer support), perceptions of the academic context (task challenge and work orientation), competence, value, and school attachment. These items were drawn from a variety of measures of motivation and classroom climate and context (Eccles, Blumenfeld, & Wigfield, 1984; Midgley et al., 1995; Wellborn & Connell, 1987), as well as new items developed for this study. The surveys were read aloud to students in each class. Bilingual adults administered surveys in Spanish in the bilingual classrooms and to students in other classes who requested a Spanish version or whose teachers felt they were not sufficiently proficient in English. The survey took approximately 30 minutes to administer. We piloted the surveys on individual students in order to assess wording and comprehension.

Procedures

To examine the psychometric properties of the three engagement scales, we examined the quality of the data and the reliability and validity of the scales. We present the psychometric properties of survey items from the first and second wave of data collection for emotional and behavioral engagement. We documented a similar pattern of relations between the behavioral and emotional engagement scales, contextual variables, and demographic factors at both waves. Because Wave 2 had stronger measures of behavioral, emotional, and cognitive engagement, the majority of analyses presented focus on this wave.

We made several changes to the cognitive engagement scale from Wave 1 to Wave 2 because of the low reliability at Wave 1 ($\alpha = .55$; three items). The majority of measures of cognitive engagement have been administered with middle school and high school students. At Wave 1, we had fewer measures and limited items assessing self-regulation and strategy use. Therefore, at Wave 2, we added survey items adapted from measures of strategy use with older grades to use with younger children. The addition of these items improved the reliability of this scale ($\alpha = .82$; eight items). Another possible reason for the low reliability at Wave 1 was the inclusion of third graders. At Wave 1, we included children in third through fifth grade; Wave 2 only included children in fourth and fifth grade. The reliability of the cognitive engagement scale was lowest for the third-grade students ($\alpha = .50$), followed by the fourth-grade students ($\alpha = .54$), and the fifth-grade students ($\alpha = .63$). Because of the problems with reliability at Wave 1, we only present psychometric properties for Wave 2 measures of cognitive engagement.

We examined the distribution of the responses to confirm that there was variation. We anticipated that the distribution of responses would be negatively skewed, as we assumed that most elementary school children would report positive behavioral, emotional, and cognitive engagement. The rate of missing data was low and appeared to be completely random. We tested the internal consistency of the items that compose the behavioral, emotional, and cognitive engagement scales using Cronbach's alpha.

We conducted exploratory factor analysis with all scales and examined their demographic patterns, concurrent validity, and prospective validity. We did not collect demographic data from parents, and therefore we were only able to examine the engagement patterns by gender and age. For construct validity, we examined whether aspects of classroom context (teacher support, peer support, task challenge, and work norms) that have been identified in the literature were associated with the three engagement scales at Wave 2. Further, we ran correlations between engagement and measures of school attachment and value. We ran these correlations using both the whole engagement scale and using each individual item. The purpose of these analyses was to examine the strength of the correlation between individual items and the outcome variables in order to determine whether a more parsimonious scale could be developed.

In addition, we ran zero-order correlations between students' reports of engagement and teachers' individual assessment of students' behavior. The purpose of these analyses was to examine whether teachers and students were seeing similar behaviors. We also conducted hierarchical regression analyses to examine the independent contributions of the four contextual variables (teacher support, peer support, task challenge, and work norms) on the three types of engagement, controlling for gender and grade. Finally, we ran correlations to examine the stability of behavioral and emotional engagement from Wave 1 to Wave 2. Because we made changes in the cognitive engagement measure, we did not examine correlations in this measure over time. We did not collect longitudinal outcome data, and therefore we were not able to use our data to examine prospective validity.

Since there are few empirical or theoretical guidelines for establishing cut points in engagement, in our analyses we used the measures as continuous scales, the common method in the literature.

Results

We documented substantial variation for the three scales at both waves. As expected, there was a higher concentration of scores over 3 (indicating that students report higher behavior, affect, and cognitive engagement). Each of the

Table 1. Overall Descriptives

Relationship Scale	M	SD	Skewness	Kurtosis
Behavior engagement, Wave 1	4.00	.76	−.71	.28
Emotional engagement, Wave 1	3.60	1.00	−.51	−.56
Behavior engagement, Wave 2	4.00	.76	−.40	−.60
Emotional engagement, Wave 2	3.76	.85	−.57	.27
Cognitive engagement, Wave 2	3.49	.79	−.30	−.17

Note: Score range = 1–5.

scales was negatively skewed (behavioral engagement, −.565; emotional engagement, −.301; and cognitive engagement, −.391), indicating a distribution toward higher scores.

We conducted exploratory factor analysis, and all items loaded onto the theorized factor (see Appendix). The three factors corresponded to the hypothesized scales: behavioral, emotional, and cognitive engagement. Based on this factor analysis and theoretical considerations, scales were developed to measure behavioral engagement ($\alpha = .72$ [Wave 1]; $\alpha = .77$ [Wave 2]), emotional engagement ($\alpha = .83$ [Wave 1]; $\alpha = .86$ [Wave 2]) and cognitive engagement ($\alpha = .82$ [Wave 1]). The reliability of the scales was also examined by gender and grade. In general, the results were similar for boys and girls. The reliability for the behavioral engagement scale ($\alpha = .67$) was slightly lower for third grade than for fourth ($\alpha = .74$) and fifth grade ($\alpha = .73$). The reliability for emotional engagement was similar across the grades at both waves.

Validity

The means and standard deviations for the whole sample are presented in Table 1. Tables 2 and 3 show the demographic patterns for the three engagement scales at Wave 1 and Wave 2, which were as expected and confirm previous research (Fredricks et al., in press). Girls reported significantly higher behavioral, emotional, and cognitive engagement than did boys (Table 2). In addition, at Wave 1, we found that behavioral, emotional, and cognitive engagement decreased from third to fifth grade (Table 3). We did not document grade differences between the fourth and fifth graders during the second wave of data collection.

Table 2. Gender Differences in Engagement at Wave 2

	Girls		Boys		
Scale	M	SD	M	SD	F
Behavioral	4.18	.68	3.76	.78	25.15***
Emotional	3.89	.80	3.60	.88	8.68**
Cognitive	3.60	.78	3.36	.78	6.59**

*$p \leq .05$. **$p \leq .01$. ***$p \leq .001$.

Table 3. *Grade Differences in Engagement*

	Third		Fourth		Fifth		
	M	SD	M	SD	M	SD	F
Behavioral, Wave 1	4.13	.75	4.01	.78	3.84	.72	8.51**
Emotional, Wave 1	3.84	1.00	3.50	1.00	3.42	.93	12.00***
Behavioral, Wave 2			4.00	.80	4.01	.72	.00
Emotional, Wave 2			3.70	.87	3.79	.83	.54
Cognitive, Wave 2			3.46	.80	3.50	.73	.52

To examine the concurrent validity, we ran simple zero-order correlations between perceptions of the classroom context and the three components of engagement. We included aspects of classroom context (teacher support, peer support, task challenge, and work orientation) that have been identified in the literature as related to engagement (see Fredricks et al., in press). The teacher and peer support measure included items about whether teachers and peers care and create a supportive social environment. The task challenge scale contained items about level of task difficulty and authentic instruction. The work orientation scale included items about work norms and classroom management.

All zero-order correlations were significant and in the expected direction. Perceived teacher support was positively related to behavioral, emotional, and cognitive engagement ($r = .35$ to .49). Perceived peer support had similar correlations with the three engagement scales ($r = .23$ to .41). Work orientation was positively related to behavioral, emotional, and cognitive engagement ($r = .37$ to .42); task challenge was associated with the three constructs ($r = .30$ to .41). Students' reports of engagement were more strongly correlated with teachers' reports of behavior ($r = .29$ to .43) than with teachers' perceptions of emotion ($r = .15$ to .20). The stronger correlation with behavior was not surprising because teachers tend to be better able to observe behavior than to make inferences about students' emotional state. Finally, students' reports of engagement were highly correlated with school attachment ($r = .44$ to .57) and moderately correlated with perceptions of school value ($r = .26$ to .32).

Not surprisingly, the correlations were stronger when we used the full scale than when we correlated each individual item with the outcome variables. In general, the correlations between the individual items and outcome variables were similar, making it difficult to tear apart the scales to pick out the items that were best able to predict the outcome variables. Two exceptions were that children's perceptions of being bored were slightly less strongly correlated with the outcome variables than the other items in the emotional engagement scale, and that children's reports of completing homework on time were slightly less strongly correlated with the outcome variables than the other items in the behavioral engagement scale.

Standardized regression coefficients are presented in Table 4. Work orientation ($\beta = .28$, $p \leq .001$), task challenge ($\beta = .23$, $p \leq .001$), and peer support

Table 4. Standardized Regression Coefficients

	Behavior		Emotional		Cognitive	
	Step 1	Step 2	Step 1	Step 2	Step 1	Step 2
Controls						
Grade	.03	−.03	.06	−.03	.03	−.05
Gender	.29***	.21***	.17*	.05	.15*	.03
Contextual Variables						
Teacher support		.10		.27***		.25***
Peer support		.13*		.13*		.17***
Task challenge		.23***		.29***		.30***
Work orientation		.28***		.33***		.25***
Change in R²		.26***		.49***		.41***
Total R²		.34		.52		.44

Note: $N = 297$. Gender is coded 0 = male and 1 = female.
*$p \le 05$. ** $p \le 01$. *** $p \le .001$.

($\beta = .13$, $p \le .01$) were significant predictors of behavioral engagement. After controlling for other variables in the model, perceptions of teacher support were not related to behavioral engagement. Each of four contextual factors was uniquely associated with emotional engagement. Similarly, aspects of both the social context (teacher and peer support) and academic context (work orientation and task challenge) were significant predictors of cognitive engagement.

Finally, we ran zero-order correlations between the behavioral and emotional engagement measures at Wave 1 and Wave 2. The behavioral ($r = .60$) and emotional ($r = .50$) measures were highly correlated at the two waves, suggesting considerable stability in children's engagement over time.

Interview Data

To take a more qualitative approach to understanding the phenomenology of engagement, we also interviewed a subset of students in great depth. The purpose of the interviews was to examine differences in how students, identified as high or low in engagement based on their survey responses, talked about their classrooms, schools, work, teachers, and peers. We were interested in whether the two groups noticed different aspects of the classroom or whether they told us similar things about their classrooms but responded to these environments differently. The interviews included questions about aspects of the classroom that were assessed in the student surveys. We asked about teachers, peers, academic tasks, work norms, the school, and the family's participation in and help with school activities and assignments. Children also were asked about their behaviors, their emotions, and cognition. The only difference between the interviews at the two waves was that in our efforts to examine change, the interviews in the second wave included more questions about differences in engagement and a comparison of classroom environments that might explain changes in engagement across the years.[1]

The interviews were conducted individually, audiotaped, and took approximately 30–45 minutes. A bilingual interviewer talked with low-English-proficiency students. We used the survey data to initially select individuals to interview in greater depth about their school experiences. The selection criteria differed across the two waves. At Wave 1, we selected children in classrooms with the highest average total engagement and children in classrooms with the most variation in total engagement scores. The total interview sample at Wave 1 was 92 students. At Wave 2, we selected students who exhibited different engagement trajectories; that is, students who increased or decreased fairly significantly in their total engagement on the surveys compared with the rest of the sample. In total, we interviewed 46 children at this wave.

We used several different analytic techniques to compare the survey and interview responses. First, we took a sample of 10 of the high-engagement interviews and 10 of the low-engagement interviews. Research assistants who were blind to the survey scores read each interview and sorted them into either a high- or a low-engagement group. There was perfect correspondence between the interview sorting and the survey scores, demonstrating that it was possible to discriminate reliability between the high- and low-engagement students. Careful notes were taken about students' comments related to work, behavior, peers, and teacher. Overall, the high-engaged students were more positive about their classroom, teacher, and peers than were the low-engaged students.

Next, we rated the interviews in terms of engagement and aspects of classroom context, including teachers, peers, work, and school. After reading the entire interview transcript, we gave each dimension a numerical rating (1–3 rating or 1–5 rating). For example, we rated children on their own behavior and any indication of cognitive engagement in terms of going beyond the requirements or being strategic. Within the larger dimensions of classroom context, we created subcategories based both on what students discussed and distinctions that have been identified in the literature. For example, we rated teachers on a variety of dimensions (e.g., fairness, personal characteristics, and interpersonal support). We ran zero-order correlations between these numerical interview ratings and the survey scales for engagement and classroom context. We found that the numerical ratings of engagement from the interviews were moderately correlated with the survey scales of engagement. Similarly, the interview ratings of classroom context were associated with individuals' perceptions of classroom context. Finally, the engagement survey scales were moderately correlated with the interview ratings of classroom context. These results provide additional evidence for the validity of interview and survey measures.

In addition to the quantitative analyses of the interview data, we examined interviews more holistically for themes that cut across students in the low-engagement group. We found considerable variability in the reasons why

---

[1] The student engagement interview is available from the authors.

students were disengaging from school. For example, some of the students in the low-engagement group were disengaged because of the academic work, either because it was too easy or too challenging, while others were disengaged because of social problems with their teachers and/or peers.

In sum, these results illustrate the benefits of including interview questions in studies of engagement. In the quantitative analyses, we documented correspondence between the interview and survey responses. However, the thematic analyses revealed variability in low-engagement students' perceptions of the work, teachers, peers, and their classroom. These results show that it is important not to assume that all students within one group are similar. The interviews provided in-depth information about what aspects of the school experience were creating low engagement. This information is critical for designing targeted interventions to increase engagement.

Summary and Discussion

One of the strengths of our study is that we included child survey items assessing behavioral, emotional, and cognitive engagement. In general, the three scales have good face validity, adequate internal consistency, and adequate predictive validity. There is variability in the distribution of responses, though students are more likely to answer these survey questions positively as they do in other measures in the elementary school grades. A strength of this study is that it was conducted with inner-city elementary school students of various backgrounds. These scales appear to be reliable measures of engagement in this sample. The Cronbach's alphas suggest that the items in each scale hang together well as a construct. The descriptive analyses suggest that the three scales are valid measures and follow expected patterns by age and gender. The zero-order correlations between engagement and classroom context were in the expected direction.

Nevertheless, there are several limitations with our survey analyses. First, we were unable to test the prospective validity because we had not collected long-term outcome data. Although there is evidence in the research literature of the association between engagement and positive academic outcomes, more research is needed to test the concurrent and prospective validity of these specific items. The age of the students likely impacted the reliability and validity of this construct. Modifications of these measures may be necessary for older children. The psychometric properties of these items need to be tested across wider and more diverse samples before inclusion into national surveys. Finally, in our analysis, we used the scales as continuous variables, a common practice in the literature. More theoretical and empirical work is necessary to determine the minimum level of behavioral, emotional, and cognitive engagement necessary to achieve positive achievement outcomes.

In our review of the research, we noted several problems with measurement that cut across different surveys of engagement (see Fredricks et al., in press, for a more detailed discussion). One problem is that many studies combine behavioral, emotional, and cognitive items into a single scale, which precludes examining distinctions among the various types of engagement. A second problem is that conceptual distinctions are blurred because similar items are used to assess different types of engagement. For example, questions about persistence and preference for hard work are used as indicators of behavioral engagement (Finn et al., 1995) and cognitive engagement (Connell & Wellborn, 1991).

Another concern is that the three types of engagement overlap with other behavioral and motivational constructs. However, because engagement encompasses several constructs that are usually tapped individually, the measures of engagement are less well developed and differentiated than these constructs. For instance, emotional engagement scales typically include one or two items about interest and value along with items about feelings. Other measures that only focus on interest and values include many items that make distinctions within interest, such as intrinsic versus situational interest, and within value, such as intrinsic, utility, and attainment value (Eccles et al., 1983; Krapp, Hidi, & Renninger, 1992).

An additional limitation with current measures is that survey items do not distinguish a target or source of engagement. In some measures the target is quite general, such as "I like school." Furthermore, these measures are rarely attached to specific tasks and situations, yielding information about engagement as a general tendency. This makes it difficult to determine if students are more engaged in certain parts of the classroom, such as the social or academic dimensions; whether they are more engaged in certain tasks, such as working in groups or doing presentations; or whether they are more engaged in some subjects than others.

There also are likely to be developmental differences in the appropriateness of certain measures. One issue is that children at different ages may interpret engagement items differently because of their developmental capacities. For example, participation may mean different things to elementary and high school students. Finally, assessing cognitive engagement in young children is difficult. Thus, there exists an abundance of self-report data on older students (middle school, high school, and college students) but a dearth of studies with younger children (Pintrich, Wolters, & Baxter, 2000).

There are extensive child and teacher measures of behavioral engagement that include adherence to classroom norms and participation in school and out-of-school activities from a variety of surveys that could be included in national databases. These scales have strong psychometric properties and concurrent and prospective validity. In addition, the measures of emotional engagement provide a quick and easy measure that distinguishes between low- and high-engaged students. However, if researchers want to know about the sources of affect, we recommend using more detailed measures designed to tap specific motivational constructs such as interest, value, and flow (Csikszentmihalyi, 1988; Eccles et al., 1983; Schiefele, Krapp, & Winteler, 1992). Researchers who want to know specifically about how students use learning strategies should refer to more detailed measures of strategy use and metacognition (Pintrich et al., 2000). Finally, our measure of cognitive engagement provided a quick measure that is valid for use with elementary school children.

Appendix

Engagement Scales and Factor Loadings

Items	Behavioral	Emotional	Cognitive
I follow the rules at school.	.83		
I get in trouble at school. (REVERSED)	.78		
When I am in class, I just act as if I am working. (REVERSED)	.72		
I pay attention in class.	.72		
I complete my work on time.	.52		
I like being at school.		.79	
I feel excited by my work at school.		.75	
My classroom is a fun place to be.		.73	
I am interested in the work at school.		.72	
I feel happy in school.		.71	
I feel bored in school. (REVERSED)		.67	
I check my schoolwork for mistakes.			.73
I study at home even when I don't have a test.			.72
I try to watch TV shows about things we do in school.			.69
When I read a book, I ask myself questions to make sure I understand what it is about.			.67
I read extra books to learn more about things we do in school.			.66
If I don't know what a word means when I am reading, I do something to figure it out.			.62
If I don't understand what I read, I go back and read it over again.			.58
I talk with people outside of school about what I am learning in class.			.58

References

Birch, S., & Ladd, G. (1997). The teacher–child relationship and children's early school adjustment. *Journal of School Psychology, 35,* 61–79.

Buhs, E. S., & Ladd, G. W. (2001). Peer rejection as an antecedent of young children's school adjustment: An examination of the mediating process. *Developmental Psychology, 37,* 550–560.

Connell, J. P. (1990). Context, self, and action: A motivational analysis of self-system processes across the life-span. In D. Cicchetti (Ed.), *The self in transition: Infancy to childhood* (pp. 61–67). Chicago: University of Chicago Press.

Connell, J. P., Halpern-Felsher, B. L., Clifford, E., Crichlow, W., & Usinger, P. (1995). Hanging in there: Behavioral, psychological, and contextual factors affecting whether African American adolescents stay in school. *Journal of Adolescent Research, 10,* 41–63.

Connell, J. P., Spencer, M. B., & Aber, J. L. (1994). Educational risk and resilience in African-American youth: Context, self, action, and outcomes in school. *Child Development, 65,* 493–506.

Connell, J. P., & Wellborn. J. G. (1991). Competence, autonomy, and relatedness: A motivational analysis of self-system processes. In M. Gunnar & L. A. Sroufe (Eds.), *Minnesota Symposium on Child Psychology: Vol. 23. Self processes in development* (pp. 43–77). Chicago: University of Chicago Press.

Corno, L., & Mandinach, E. (1983). The role of cognitive engagement in classroom learning and motivation. *Educational Psychologist, 18,* 88–108.

Csikszentmihalyi, M. (1988). The flow experience and its significance for human psychology. In M. Csikszentmihalyi & I. S. Csikszentmihalyi (Eds.), *Optimal experience* (pp. 15–35). Cambridge: Cambridge University Press.

Eccles, J., Adler, T. F., Futterman, R., Goff, S. B., Kaczala, C. M., Meece, J. L., et al. (1983). Expectations, values, and academic behaviors. In J. T. Spence (Ed.), *Achievement and achievement motivation* (pp. 75–146). San Francisco: W. H. Freeman.

Eccles, J. S., Blumenfeld, P. B., & Wigfield, A. (1984). *Ontogeny of self- and task beliefs and activity choice.* Funded grant application to the National Institute for Child Health and Human Development (Grant RO1-HD17553).

Ehrle, J., & Moore, K. A. (1999). *1997 NSAF Benchmarking Measure of Child and Family Well-Being: Report No. 6.* Washington, DC: Urban Institute.

Epstein, J. L., & McPartland, J. M. (1976). The concept and measurement of the quality of school life. *American Educational Research Journal, 13,* 15–30.

Finn, J. D. (1989). Withdrawing from school. *Review of Educational Research, 59,* 117–142.

Finn, F. (1993). *School engagement and students at risk.* Report for National Center for Educational Statistics.

Finn, J. D., Pannozzo, G. M., & Voelkl, K. E. (1995). Disruptive and inattentive-withdrawn behavior and achievement among fourth graders. *Elementary School Journal, 95,* 421–454.

Finn, J. D., & Rock, D. A. (1997). Academic success among students at risk for school failure. *Journal of Applied Psychology, 82,* 221–234.

Fredricks, J. A., Blumenfeld, P. B., & Paris, A. (in press). School engagement: Potential of the concept, state of the evidence. *Review of Educational Research.*

Goodenow, C. (1993). Classroom belonging among early adolescent students: Relationship to motivation and achievement. *Journal of Early Adolescence, 13,* 21–43.

Guthrie, J. T., & Wigfield, A. (2000). Engagement and motivation in reading. In M. L. Kamil, P. B. Mosenthal, P. D. Pearson, & R. Barr (Eds.), *Handbook of reading research* (Vol. 3, pp. 403–422). Mahwah, NJ: Lawrence Erlbaum.

Karweit, N. (1989). Time and learning: A review. In R. E. Slavin (Ed.), *School and classroom organization.* Hillsdale, NJ: Lawrence Erlbaum.

Krapp, A., Hidi, S., & Renninger, K. A. (1992). Interest, learning, and development. In K. A. Renninger, S. Hidi, & A. Krapp (Eds.), *The role of interest in learning and development* (pp. 3–25). Hillsdale, NJ: Lawrence Erlbaum.

Ladd, G. W., Birch, S. H., & Buhs, E. S. (1999). Children's social and scholastic lives in kindergarten: Related spheres of influence. *Child Development, 70,* 1373–1400.

Ladd, G. W., Buhs, E. S., & Seid, M. (2000). Children's initial sentiments about kindergarten: Is school liking an antecedent of early classroom participation and achievement? *Merrill-Palmer Quarterly, 46,* 255–279.

Lee, V. E., & Smith, J. B. (1993). Effects of school restructuring on the achievement and engagement of middle-grade students. *Sociology of Education, 66,* 164–187.

Lee, V. E., & Smith, J. B. (1995). Effects of high school restructuring and size on early gains in achievement and engagement. *Sociology of Education, 68,* 241–270.

Meece, J., Blumenfeld, P. C., & Hoyle, R. H. (1988). Students' goal orientation and cognitive engagement in classroom activities. *Journal of Educational Psychology, 80,* 514–523.

Midgley, C., Maehr, M .L., Hicks, L., Urdan, T. U., Roeser, R. W., Anderman, E., et al. (1995). *Patterns of Adaptive Learning Survey (PALS) manual.* Ann Arbor: University of Michigan.

Newmann, F., Wehlage, G. G., & Lamborn, S. D. (1992). The significance and sources of student engagement. In F. Newmann (Ed.), *Student engagement and achievement in American secondary schools* (pp. 11–39). New York: Teachers College Press.

Osterman, K. F. (2000). Students' need for belonging in the school community. *Review of Educational Research, 70,* 323–367.

Patrick, B. C., Skinner, E. A., & Connell, J. P. (1993). What motivates children's behavior and emotion? Joint effects of perceived control and autonomy in the academic domain. *Journal of Personality and Social Psychology, 65,* 781–791.

Peterson, P., Swing, S., Stark, K., & Wass, G. (1984). Students' cognitions and time on task during mathematics instruction. *American Educational Research Journal, 21,* 487–515.

Pintrich, P. R., & De Groot, E. (1990). Motivated and self-regulated learning components of academic performance. *Journal of Educational Psychology, 82,* 33–40.

Pintrich, P. R., Smith, D. A. F., Garcia, T., & McKeachie, W. J. (1993). Reliability and predictive validity of the Motivated Strategies for Learning Questionnaire (MSLQ). *Educational and Psychological Measurement, 53,* 801–813.

Pintrich, P. R., Wolters, C., & Baxter, G. (2000). Assessing metacognition and self-regulated learning. In G. Schraw & J. Impara (Eds.), *Issues in the measurement of metacognition* (pp. 43–97). Lincoln: University of Nebraska, Buros Institute of Mental Measurements.

Schiefele, J., Krapp, A., & Winteler, A. (1992). Interest as a predictor of academic achievement: A meta-analysis of research. In K. A. Renninger, S. Hidi, & A. Krapp (Eds.), *The role of interest in learning and development.* Hillsdale, NJ: Lawrence Erlbaum.

Skinner, E., & Belmont, M. J. (1993). Motivation in the classroom: Reciprocal effect of teacher behavior and student engagement across the school year. *Journal of Educational Psychology, 85,* 571–581.

Skinner, E. A., Wellborn, J. G., & Connell, J. P. (1990). What it takes to do well in school and whether I've got it: The role of perceived control in children's engagement and school achievement. *Journal of Educational Psychology, 82,* 22–32.

Skinner, E. A., Zimmer-Gembeck, M. L., & Connell, J. P. (1998). Individual differences and the development of perceived control. *Monographs of the Society for Research in Child Development, 63.*

Stipek, D. (2002). Good instruction is motivating. In A. Wigfield & J. Eccles (Eds.), *Development of achievement motivation* (pp. 309–332). San Diego: Academic Press.

Valeski, T. N., & Stipek, D. (2001). Young children's feelings about school. *Child Development, 73,* 1198–2013.

Voelkl, K. E. (1997). Identification with school. *American Journal of Education, 105,* 204–319.

Wehlage, G. G., & Rutter, R. A. (1986). Dropping out: How much do schools contribute to the problem? *Teachers College Record, 87,* 374–392.

Wehlage, G. G., Rutter, R. A., Smith, G. A., Lesko, N. L., & Fernandez, R. R. (1989). *Reducing the risk: Schools as communities of support.* Philadelphia: Falmer Press.

Wellborn, J. G., & Connell, J. P. (1987). *Manual for the Rochester Assessment Package for Schools.* Rochester, NY: University of Rochester.

Yamamoto, K., Thomas, E. C., & Karns, E. A. (1969). School-related attitudes in middle-school aged students. *American Educational Research Journal, 6,* 191–206.

Zimmerman, B. J. (1990). Self-regulated learning and academic achievement: An overview. *Educational Psychologist, 21,* 3–17.

V Enacting Positive Values and Behaviors in Communities

20 Community-Based Civic Engagement

Scott Keeter

Pew Research Center and George Mason University

Krista Jenkins

Fairleigh Dickinson University

Cliff Zukin

Rutgers University

Molly Andolina

DePaul University

Adolescents and young adults today are less interested and engaged in politics than their elders (Moore, 2002; MacPherson 2000). Much of the focus of their lives is on the development of social relations and on school, only a small part of which is devoted to preparing them for the responsibilities of citizenship that lie ahead. Youth lack an attachment to the larger political world that is fundamental to fostering interest and engagement in the issues of democracy. Add to that a cynicism toward politics and politicians (National Association of Secretaries of State, 1999), and it is not surprising that many youth seem to be tuned out and disengaged from what's going on around them.

Those who have examined the political engagement patterns of youth today confirm these suggestions. Youth are not engaged in electoral politics and demonstrate relatively little interest in political affairs. Surveys conducted prior to the 2000 election found that only 50% of 18- to 24-year-olds said they were registered to vote, and just 46% said they were "absolutely" certain they would vote in the upcoming election (Kaiser Family Foundation/MTV, 2000). These numbers fall short of the figures for all adults: 75% of adults claimed to be registered to vote, and more than three quarters of registered voters (84%) said they were absolutely certain to vote in the fall (Pew Research Center for the People and the Press, 2000).

Youth are also not inclined to see voting as a duty of citizenship, and they eschew traditional political activities and orientations. They do not view politics as relevant to their daily lives, consider political leaders to be "out of touch," and find government to be "too slow" (National Association of Secretaries of State, 1999). Almost half (46%) of 15- to 24-year-olds never or almost never talk about politics and government or current events with their parents (National Association of Secretaries of State, 1999).

But youth are not equally disengaged from all forms of participation in public affairs. Youth involvement in community and charitable work is greater than it is with election campaigns and other traditional forms of political participation. Community-based civic involvement is a natural and age-appropriate means of activity for many youth, and schools in the United States are increasingly encouraging and facilitating such activity. High rates of volunteering suggest that youth believe they can make more of a difference in the community than in the voting booth. In fact, 58% of 18- to 24-year-olds who weren't certain they would vote in 2000 said that they could make more of a difference through community involvement than in turning out on election day (Kaiser Family Foundation/MTV, 2000). Taking a closer look at these activities among youth calls into question the legitimacy of such labels as "tuned out" and "disengaged."

Part of the reason youth are more active in civic activities than political work is because high schools and colleges increasingly facilitate community involvement among their students. Our research has found that 75% of high school students say their school arranges or offers service activities or volunteer work for students, and 65% of college students report the same thing. Youth are taking advantage of these opportunities to get involved. Close to half (45%) of those who attend high schools where community work is arranged report volunteering in the recent past, and 38% of college students at service-oriented universities are motivated to volunteer.

Although the apparent disconnect among youth between civic and political behavior is troubling, it should not overshadow the importance of the high incidence of civic activity and the possibility that this foreshadows high levels of civic *and* political engagement as youth eventually become more established in their communities. As the larger project from which this research is drawn has shown, *civic* activity is not necessarily *nonpolitical* activity (Jenkins, Andolina, Keeter, & Zukin, 2003). Many adults who engage in volunteering and community problem solving also attempt to influence governmental policy as a part of their work in this arena. Although some of them have rejected or are indifferent to electoral politics as the best way to get problems solved, even these individuals have not necessarily eschewed the use of governmental power and resources. Similarly, youth who are active in their community may become more likely to understand the complexity of public issues and to recognize political solutions to problems. Their community work has the potential to put them in contact with elected officials and to teach them the best means for communicating with such persons. It's reasonable to expect that civic behavior in adolescence and early adulthood will lead to political engagement in later years.

Civic and Political Engagement in Youth

This chapter examines three measures of community-based civic engagement: informal group activity to solve community problems, volunteering, and group membership. Because these concepts are somewhat broad and amorphous, measuring them reliably is a challenge for survey research. *Civic activity* can be viewed as one element of a broader concept of *civic and political engagement*. This broad construct includes the idea of *cognitive engagement*—paying attention to government and public affairs, following the news in newspapers, on television, radio, or the Internet, talking about politics with friends and family, and expressing interest in the subject. It also includes both government and nongovernment organizations as the objects of activity and the arenas in which that activity occurs. Civic engagement, therefore, is typically defined as organized voluntary activity in nongovernmental arenas undertaken by citizens to solve problems and help others in the community. Political participation, on the other hand, is typically defined as actions undertaken by citizens to influence government and public policy.

Concept Controversies

A key debate about the study of *civic engagement*, which includes most of the community-centered activity we focus on in this chapter, is the extent to which it is political in nature. This debate is important because of disagreement about the consequences of civic activity. One perspective fears that civic activities such as volunteering serve as substitutes for political activity, displacing the essential work citizens need to do to keep a democracy healthy. This debate is seen even among proponents of programs explicitly designed to involve youth, such as service-learning. More broadly, the controversy has now evolved into a debate between liberals and conservatives over the degree to which the nonprofit sector can and should take over social welfare activities that the government has performed to one degree or another since the creation of the modern welfare state in the 1930s and 1940s.

Apart from the debate over the proper scope of government, there is a more neutral question regarding the extent to which civic activity has value as an element of the political system. Political scientists in the United States have long observed that groups and associations not only provide important services to their communities but also function as important players in the political game (Bentley, 1908; Truman, 1951). They serve as a means of mobilizing citizens to influence government and a place for the training of citizens in the tools of collective action that can be turned to more explicitly political activity. Especially for youth, who find certain avenues of the political system closed off as a result of age restrictions and cultural norms, civic involvement in the community may be the best and most appropriate means for developing good skills for citizenship. More generally, Verba and his colleagues (1995) have shown that civic institutions are a critical locale for such skill building.

Beyond these theoretical and normative questions, there is the empirical question of the degree to which active citizens engage in both political and civic activities. That is, how correlated are these two dimensions of activity? Data that we present below provide evidence of the multidimensionality of such engagement. Survey items related to electoral politics—voting, donating money to campaigns, trying to persuade others—correlate with one another better than they correlate with other kinds of activities. Similarly, civic activities, defined as organized voluntary activity focused on problem solving and helping others, also cluster together. Other activities that entail the use of what we call "political voice"—things people do to give expression to their political and social viewpoints—correlate with both the electoral and the civic activities but also tend to cluster with one another. And although these dimensions are both theoretically and empirically distinct, the overall picture is not entirely clear.

Measurement Challenges

One difficulty we and other researchers face in developing measures of civic and political engagement is that there are a limited number of key activities in which citizens engage, and these tend to be discrete events. Voting is, for many, the most important activity and perhaps the best example of this problem. Consequently, it is difficult to create a highly reliable measure of civic and political engagement using a battery of indicators. Given low incidences and a phenomenon that is driven partly by factors external to the citizen (e.g., the rise and fall of certain issues), even a relatively large battery of items reflecting a range of activities will not produce a scale with a high degree of internal consistency.

Since highly reliable scales are not likely to be achieved, we focus on developing an index (which is not presumed to have high internal reliability). Because the challenge in developing good measures of civic and political engagement is somewhat different from that faced in other domains of behavior and attitude, *content validity* is especially important. Ensuring that the full range of relevant behaviors is covered is particularly challenging when the focus is on youth, who may be finding or inventing new means of engagement. Our project, for example, devoted several months of exploratory research to map the full range of political and civic activity going on among young people.

Another challenge, faced by all researchers but especially relevant to our work, is the trade-off between greater coverage and perhaps reliability from the use of multiple measures, and the financial costs of a long survey and the accompanying burden to respondents. Our mission was to develop an index that would cover the most important forms of civic and political engagement but that was short enough for use as a tool for needs assessment or evaluation by nonprofit groups, community-based researchers, and academics working with limited budgets. This need for both broad coverage and concision militated against the development of lengthy batteries of indicators.

Developing Measures

Data for the study reported in this chapter were collected during a 2-year project funded by The Pew Charitable Trusts. The research had two principal goals: (a) to develop a reliable but concise set of indicators of civic and political engagement, with a special focus on individuals 15–25 years old and (b) to assess the civic and political health of the nation from a generational perspective. We began the project with exploratory work using a pair of expert panels and a series of focus groups with citizens of various ages during 2001. In the fall of 2001, we conducted several small surveys to test specific items. In winter 2002, we conducted a large national survey among individuals aged 15–25 years.[1] In spring 2002, we conducted a large national telephone survey. Two focus groups to help us provide validation for our measures were held during the summer of 2002, and another national telephone survey in fall 2002 provided additional evidence about the reliability of the indicators. Data used in this chapter come primarily from the spring 2002 national telephone survey. The total sample size was 3,246. Owing to our focus on youth, people aged 15–25 were oversampled ($N = 1,001$). In the study reported here, we focus primarily on the 461 respondents who were 15–19 years old.[2]

Exploratory research and subsequent item testing during 2001 yielded a core set of 19 dichotomous indicators of civic and political engagement.[3] Factor analysis indicated that these items could be sorted comfortably into three dimensions of activity corresponding to the theoretical categories of electoral work, civic work, and political voice. Although the analysis was cleaner for the adult population, a similar pattern was evident with youth ages 15–19 years.

Measures of Community-Based Civic Engagement

The remainder of the chapter focuses on the civic dimension of youth engagement, primarily through three indicators we consider to be most appropriate for assessing youth involvement in their communities: informal group activity to solve community problems, volunteering, and group membership. We

[1] For this survey, we used Knowledge Networks' probability sample of households that have been provided with Web access.

[2] The sample was weighted to reflect national population parameters on sex, age, race, education, and ethnicity.

[3] For complete question wording of all items and a guide to the use of the indicators, see our report titled "A Guide to the Index of Civic and Political Engagement," available at http://civicyouth.org

focus on civic engagement, as opposed to other forms of involvement, because the opportunities for civic engagement are more abundant among youth. Voting is limited to those 18 and older, and contributing money to a political party or candidate is skewed toward older cohorts with greater economic resources. But volunteer activity, working informally with others to solve a problem in one's community, and group activity are not dependent on money and other age-related resources.

Community problem solving is measured with a two-part item asking about informal collective work to solve a problem in the community (see Appendix).[4] The important elements of this item are the informal nature of the work and the 12-month time frame. The informal nature of the work is critical because of the need to "make sure that survey research does not miss those cases where people get together on their own to solve community problems" (Brady, 1999, p. 779). Community problem solving is often accomplished through loose and informal networks of people getting together for a single purpose, rather than through the organized activity of groups or citizen involvement on town boards or city councils.

In addition, the two-part item is used here to help distinguish recent community-centered work from more distant efforts. This also helps reduce social desirability bias, or the tendency for respondents to offer a socially appropriate response even if that is not a true reflection of their behavior. In this case, an individual has an opportunity to say yes to this "gatekeeper" question about informal community work and thus "get credit" for having done this before answering the more important question that anchors the behavior in the more recent past. The 12-month time frame was adopted as a reasonable compromise between the desire to provide a span long enough to include people who do not do this activity on a regular basis and yet short enough that people might reasonably remember having done it.[5]

Regular volunteering for a nonelectoral organization is measured with a three-part item that first asks if the respondent has spent any time in community service or volunteer activity; those saying yes are asked if they have done it in the past 12 months (see the Appendix). If detail about the type of volunteer work is needed, respondents can be asked about volunteer work with a series of types of groups. For each of these, the respondent is asked if they do this work on a regular basis or just once in a while.[6]

This complicated series of questions is needed because volunteering has proved to be a problematic concept. It can include "random acts of kindness" and regular, lengthy, intensive work for organizations or groups. To some extent,

---

[4] The American National Election Studies and the 1990 American Citizen Participation Study both include a variant of this question, although the question wording is slightly different.

[5] Differences in community problem solving between 15–19-year-olds and those 20 and older were not significant.

[6] The volunteering measure can be used effectively without the follow-up items on types of organizations. If detail about the types of groups is not needed, everyone who said they volunteered in the past year can be asked about the regularity of the activity.

the vast array of volunteer opportunities complicates respondents' ability to remember all that they may have done. For example, the context in which the volunteering question is asked in a survey could affect how easily a respondent remembers an activity. Another problem is social desirability bias, since volunteer work is thought to be a praiseworthy activity. Differences in question wording or in survey context may elicit different degrees of overreporting. Thus, it is not surprising that survey estimates of volunteer activity differ greatly.

Our item on volunteering attempts to balance the need to be inclusive with the need to explicitly exclude some types of activities. We offer a definition of what is meant by volunteer activity in order to ensure that respondents do not equate paid work with volunteering. As with our item on informal community work, we opted for a gatekeeper question ("Have you ever volunteered?") to reduce the impact of social desirability bias. But the most critical element of the item is the question asking about the regularity of the activity. Extensive testing suggests that the gatekeeper question, even when limited to 12 months, produces unreliable results (with estimates ranging from 33% to 55% in surveys by highly reputable survey research firms). By contrast, *regular* volunteering appears to be more amenable to reliable measurement. Regular volunteers almost certainly will answer yes to the gatekeeper questions and then need only to judge their degree of regularity. Episodic volunteers may pass the gate but will have little difficulty realizing that they are not regular volunteers. The result is more stable estimates of volunteering from survey to survey. Our spring 2002 survey yielded an estimate of 24% volunteering regularly among those 18 years and older. The same questions on an omnibus survey in August 2002 yielded an estimate of 26% among those 18 years and older. For our younger respondents (age 15–19 years), 25% were regular volunteers. The 1996 National Household Education Survey found 24% regular volunteers among those in grades 9–10, and 32% in grades 11–12.[7]

Active membership in a group or association is measured with a pair of questions: The first asks if the respondent belongs to or donates money to groups or associations (see Appendix). The second asks how active the respondent is in any such groups. This simple approach is the result of extensive testing and some degree of compromise between the need for both efficiency in the survey and comprehensiveness in the measure. It is well documented that providing respondents a long list of group types, rather than a single generic question about "groups," spurs recollection and leads to higher estimates of overall group membership (Walker & Baumgartner, 1988). Going through a long list of groups on a survey, however, is cumbersome and time-consuming. In pretests prior to the spring 2002 national survey and in an experiment embedded within it, we attempted to assess the effectiveness of a shorter method of measuring group activity. We therefore tested a longer list of groups, as well as a single gatekeeper

---

[7] Differences in the rate who report any volunteering in the past year among 15- to 19-year-olds versus those 20 and older were statistically significant; age differences in the rates of *regular* volunteering were not statistically significant.

version of the group membership question. Our measure also probes the level and type of activity in groups in order to differentiate between those who are merely members and those who take a more active role. Active membership is self-defined—those who say they are active members.

The long-form item in our experiment asked about membership in each of seven types of groups (e.g., national or local charities, labor unions, business or professional associations), plus an additional "other" category to capture anything not included in the seven. In the sample as a whole, 78% of those asked the long form of the item indicated they belonged to at least one group; in the short form, 55% did so. In the long form, 39% indicated active membership, while 28% did so in the short form. To evaluate the performance of the long and short versions as indicators of group engagement, we correlated them with an overall index of civic and political participation; there was no significant difference in the correlations for the long and short forms. Thus, we have a classic question of validity: The short form clearly underestimates the incidence of the behavior, but it provides comparable explanatory power in an analysis of the relationship between group activity and other relevant behaviors.[8]

Reliability

Civic and political activity is a peripheral concern for many people. One consequence of this is that measures of community-based civic activity are not as reliable as one would hope. People may have difficulty remembering activities that are not especially salient to them. Moreover, to the extent that people are unsure whether certain activities fit within the definitions stated or implied in survey questions, the measures will be unreliable. These problems may be especially severe with younger respondents whose lives are busy and who have not yet developed the types of mental categories used by the adult population for sorting activities.

We assess reliability in three ways: (a) the extent to which our measures yield similar results with the same population at two different times or by two different survey organizations asking the same questions at the same time; (b) the extent to which our measures yield similar results with the *same individuals* at two different times; and (c) the extent to which our items within the same conceptual domain relate with one another, as measured by Cronbach's alpha.

For the population of greatest interest—youth ages 15–19 years—we have only one survey at one time: the spring 2002 survey. However, our survey work in the fall of 2002, which replicated the spring survey via two different survey organizations, provides an opportunity to examine the consistency of response among all adults and among a comparable group of the youngest respondents,

---

[8] Differences in group membership and active group membership among 15–19-year-olds versus those 20 and older were statistically significant.

those aged 18–29 years. Data from these surveys and from panel surveys we have conducted permit an analysis of the stability of the indicators over time for the same individuals.

Our measure of working with others informally to solve a community problem in the last 12 months provides a reliable estimate of how often this behavior is done. Among respondents aged 18–29 years, 19% reported doing this type of work in the spring 2002 survey. When this question was repeated in fall 2002 by two different survey organizations, they found incidences of 19% and 18%.

As described above, the general question about volunteering produced widely divergent numbers on different surveys. Even the same question with the same respondents produced a relatively low level of consistency in our panel study of New Jersey residents during the fall of 2001. A general question asking about volunteer activity for a civic or community organization found only 62% of respondents providing the same answer three months later. By contrast, 84% gave the same answer to a question about the regularity with which they vote, and 92% gave the same answer in both waves when asked whether they had voted in the 2000 general elections.

Although we did not test the measure of regular volunteering with a panel survey, regular volunteering for a nonelectoral group or organization generates relatively consistent estimates across surveys of independent samples. The spring 2002 survey found 22% of 18- to 29-year-olds saying that they regularly volunteer for nonelectoral groups, with 23% and 25% from the two fall 2002 surveys saying that they do so.

We did not test the reliability of group membership measures with our panel data. But in independent samples from our national surveys, estimates of active membership in a group or organization were relatively stable, with a 23% estimate in the spring 2002 survey and slightly fewer reporting the same in the two fall 2002 surveys (18% and 20%).

Analyses of Items and Indices

An index composed of all 19 indicators of civic and political engagement provides one criterion for assessing the performance of each of the three indicators of community-based civic engagement (data not shown). Overall, this 19-item index has a Cronbach's alpha of 0.69 for the 15- to 19-year-old sample (and 0.76 for those 20 years and older). The item-total correlation[9] for each of the three civic items meets or exceeds the item-total correlations of all of the other items in the index: .36 for active membership in groups, .33 for regular volunteering, and .32 for community problem solving.

For an additive index of just the three civic items, Cronbach's alpha is .58 for the youth sample and .61 for those 20 and older. The relatively low alpha indicates that while these three items are tapping a common dimension,

---

[9] This is the correlation of an item value with the value for the full index.

Table 1. Distribution of Scores on Three-Item[a] Civic
Engagement Index

Score	Frequency	Percentage
Age 15–19 years		
0	262	56
1	111	24
2	56	13
3	32	7
Total	461	100
Age 20+ years		
0	1,419	54
1	696	25
2	392	13
3	239	8
Total	2,746	100

[a] Items = regular volunteer for nonelectoral organization; worked with
others to solve a community problem; active member of a group.

each behavior has distinct elements as well. Adding an additional item for
general fund-raising for charity does not change the alpha of the three-item
index, but adding an item on fund-raising runs or walks reduces the alpha
to .54. Including *both* these fund-raising items increases the alpha marginally
to .59. We see participation in fund-raising as a potential precursor to other
civic behaviors, and thus an activity that may be worth monitoring. But the
case is hardly a compelling one, and the inclusion of these items—as with any
additional survey questions—comes with a cost in terms of increased burden on
respondents.

The additive index of the three civic engagement items is somewhat skewed
in the positive direction, with over half of the cases among both youth and adults
scoring 0 (Table 1). About one quarter receive a score of 1, while only 13% receive
a score of 2. Among youth, 7% get a score of 3 (8% among adults). The mean
score for youth is .71.[10]

Validity

The three-item civic engagement index correlates with several variables to
which it is theoretically related, thus providing evidence of validity. The correlations are not high, a result partly attributable to the skewness of the distribution.[11] Some of these associations, viewed as joint frequency distributions, are
more compelling. Youth who have done any of the three civic activities are more
likely to say that they follow what's happening in public affairs ($r = .25$), to

[10] Differences on the three-item civic index between 15- to 19-year-olds versus those 20 years and
older are not statistically significant.

[11] The correlations are, however, all statistically significant at the .01 level or lower.

Table 2. *Response Percentages on Three-Item[a] Civic Index and Theoretically Relevant Behaviors*

| | Three-Item Civic Index | | | |
	0	1	2	3
Someone in Household Volunteered				
Yes	34	48	57	87
No	66	52	43	13
Total	100	100	100	100
Follow Government and Public Affairs				
Most of the time	13	29	25	52
Some of the time	46	47	51	30
Rarely	30	19	21	14
Never	11	5	3	4
Total	100	100	100	100
Sample size	261	110	56	32

[a] See Table 1 for item definitions.

have grown up in a household where someone volunteered ($r = .29$), to attend religious services at least weekly ($r = .29$), and to feel that they can make a difference in their community ($r = .24$). The differences between youth scores on the three-item civic index and their engagement in the first two of these behaviors are presented in Table 2 and are all statistically significant.

We also have qualitative evidence that supports validity. In the summer of 2002, we conducted focus groups with adults who had done two or more of the activities in a four-item civic scale (using the three core items, plus a single item that includes both general fund-raising for charity and fund-raising runs/walks). One group consisted of individuals who were active on this civic index (scoring 2 or higher), but not active on an index of five electoral activities (scoring less than 2). The other group was composed of "dual activists": people who scored 2 or higher on both indexes. The people in these two groups were clearly engaged and active. Both groups participated actively in the discussions and were reluctant to leave at the end. Individuals in these groups described their civic activities in considerable detail, and it was clear that civic engagement was an integral part of their lives. The civic specialists (those who did not score 2 or higher on the electoral index) tended to reject the electoral sphere as a way to address problems in the community, but they were nevertheless very political. The dual activists were very close to the model of the ideal citizen: highly engaged in both the electoral world and the world of direct action and organizing. Our conclusion from these groups is that the indexes discriminate very well. We have not tried to validate other cut points along the indexes, but we could see clearly that people who scored 2 on the civic dimension were highly engaged in public affairs.

Because these focus groups were made up of adults, the relevance of the findings to 15- to 19-year-olds is uncertain. But there is no reason to believe that youth would differ significantly from adults. Given that these activities may be more difficult in some respects for young people to undertake, the activists on this measure may be even more distinctive.

Conclusions and Recommendations

Community-based civic engagement is an important behavior to foster among young people (as well as their elders), but measuring it reliably poses challenges. There is a reasonable consensus that volunteering and community problem solving are two central ways in which people participate in civic life. Schools increasingly encourage or even require community service, which often involves community problem solving in addition to direct assistance to others. Our work, as well as research by others, indicates that these civic activities during adolescence can have significant political relevance and contribute to the development of well-rounded citizens who are able to contribute to the health of our democracy. There is less consensus that participation in groups per se is a civic activity. Empirically it is clear, however, that much group activity is related to civic participation—or at the least, that it helps individuals develop skills that transfer readily to civic and political work.

In brief, we believe that all three community-based civic activities are worth measuring. But as our analysis has shown, this is not an easy task. Part of the problem is conceptual ambiguity: Bringing greater clarity by narrowing the definitions or specifying certain kinds of activities would increase the reliability of the measures but could reduce the validity by producing an underestimate of the incidence. With long lists of activities, this problem could be minimized, but the cost in terms of lengthening the surveys would be considerable.

Although people who do any one of the three activities are more likely to do the other two, the correlations are not high. Combining the three measures into an additive index provides a reasonable gauge of civic engagement, but the skewed distribution and uncertain reliability of the items make the index less than an optimal tool. In many situations, it may be just as useful to analyze the component items separately as to combine them into an index.

Efforts by schools to promote volunteer activity have been demonstrably successful, and service-learning courses, when properly designed and taught, can help students make the critical linkages between civic life and the broader political world. Although there are many warning signs about the growing disengagement of young people from public life, these measures of civic involvement suggest that the problem may not be as bad as it appears from voting statistics or other indicators of electoral activity. Thus, community-based civic engagement among youth is an activity well worth monitoring.

Authors' Note

This research was supported by a grant from The Pew Charitable Trusts, which bears no responsibility for the analyses or interpretations offered here.

Appendix

Item Wording and Response Percentages, National Random Digit Dial Telephone Survey[a]

Community Problem Solving

Have you ever worked together informally with someone or some group to solve a problem in the community where you live? If yes, was this in the last 12 months, or not?

Percentage who said . . .	Age 15–19 years	Age 20+ years
Yes, within the last 12 months	23	21
Yes, but not within the last 12 months	18	19
No, have not done it	58	60
Don't know	—	—

Volunteering

Have you ever spent time participating in any community service or volunteer activity, or haven't you had time to do this? By volunteer activity, I mean actually working in some way to help others for no pay. If yes, have you done this in the last 12 months?

Percentage who said . . .	Age 15–19 years	Age 20+ years
Yes, within the last 12 months	52	33
Yes, but not within the last 12 months	16	27
No, have not done it	31	40
Don't know	1	1

If yes: I'm going to read a list of different groups that people sometimes volunteer for. As I read each one, can you tell me if you have volunteered for this type of group or organization within the last 12 months? An environmental organization; A civic or community organization involved in health or social services. This could be an organization to help the poor, elderly, homeless, or a hospital; An organization involved with youth, children, or education; Any other type of group.

Thinking about the work for (type of group) over the last 12 months, is this something you do on a regular basis, or just once in a while?

	Age 15–19 years	Age 20+ years
Percentage who reported regular volunteering[a]	25	237

Active Group Membership

Do you belong to or donate money to any groups or associations, either locally or nationally? Are you an active member of this group/any of these groups, a member but not active, or have you given money only?

Percentage who reported . . . [b]	Age 15–19 years	Age 20+ years
Membership in a group or association	36	63
Active membership in a group or association	23	32

Note: N = 461 for 15- to 19-year-olds, N = 2,746 for those 20 years and older.
[a] Respondents are coded as regular if they reported regular activity with any of the types of groups asked about.
[b] Summary measures of short- and long-form group membership questions.

References

Bentley, A. (1908). *The process of government*. Chicago: University of Chicago Press.

Brady, H. E. (1999). Political participation. In J. P. Robinson, P. R. Shaver, & L. S. Wrightsman (Eds.), *Measures of political attitudes* (pp. 737–801). New York: Academic Press.

Jenkins, K., Andolina, M. W., Keeter, S., & Zukin, C. (2003, April). *Is civic behavior political? Exploring the multidimensional nature of political participation*. Paper presented at the annual meeting of the Midwest Political Science Association, Chicago.

Kaiser Family Foundation/MTV. (2000). *Youth, voting, and the 2000 election*. Retrieved September 4, 2003 from www.kff.org

MacPherson, K. (2000, October 22). Big drop in under-30 voters a concern. *Pittsburgh Post-Gazette*, p. A14.

Moore, D. W. (2002, November 5). *Elections could hinge on young voter turnout*. Retrieved September 4, 2003, from www.gallup.com/poll/tb/educayouth/20021105.asp

National Association of Secretaries of States. (1999). *New Millennium Project—phase I: American youth attitudes on politics, citizenship, government and voting* (Report prepared by The Tarrance Group and Lake, Snell, Perry & Associates, Inc). Retrieved September 4, 2003, from www.stateofthevote.org

Pew Research Center for the People and the Press. (2000). *Voter turnout may slip again*. Retrieved September 4, 2003 from people-press.org/reports/display.php3?ReportID=35

Truman, D. (1951). *The governmental process*. New York: Knopf.

Verba, S., Schlozman, K. L., & Brady, H. (1995). *Voice and equality: Civic voluntarism in American politics*. Cambridge, MA: Harvard University Press.

Walker, J. L., & Baumgartner, F. (1988). Survey research and membership in voluntary associations. *American Journal of Political Science, 32*, 908–928.

21 Prosocial Orientation and Community Service

Peter C. Scales and Peter L. Benson

Search Institute

Prosocial orientation and commitment to community service are central aspects of young people's connection to the wider community. These and related constructs such as civic engagement and participation in organized youth activities have been of interest for decades. For example, many of the themes of the current discussion about youth civic engagement are found in the youth participation/youth as resources movement of the late 1960s and early 1980s (Kleinbard, 1997). Youth participation then was defined as the chance for young people to engage in "responsible, challenging action that meets genuine needs, with opportunity for planning and decision making affecting others" (Kleinbard, p. 7). Youth engagement in the life of the community traditionally has been seen as a critical aspect of healthy development. Such engagement may be expressed in terms of "unselfish acts of caring and kindness" (Haynes & Comer, 1997, p. 79), or described as civic activism that addresses societal problems and works toward social change (Wheeler, 2002).

Contributing to community betterment through helping others may be a sign of young people's emerging civic competence. At the same time, however, it is an important means for "youth to develop their identity...not as a self-enclosed individual achievement, but rather as a social identification that transcends a given moment in time" (Youniss et al., 2002, p. 132). That is, in helping to meet the needs of others than themselves, young people start to think of themselves as "partners and stakeholders in society" (Bell, 2002) with an interest in the common good that involves the promotion of democratic values and well-being.

Developmental scholars argue, too, that the bidirectional impact of young people's shaping of society through civic engagement and the shaping of young people by that civil society is an indispensable criterion for youth to be considered thriving and not merely developing adequately (Lerner, Brentano,

Dowling, & Anderson, 2002). Ultimately, not only are such thriving youth contributing to society currently, but through their later adult civic involvements and modeling to the next generations they also are key actors in the cultural transmission of the norms and values of civil society.

There is a need for adequate measurement of all forms of youth connection to community, but this chapter focuses on the measurement of young people's prosocial orientation and their commitment to community service. We do not focus on connection to community as expressed through participation in school clubs or community youth groups, because such activities may, but do not necessarily, involve the nurturing of helping behaviors. Nor do we focus on civic engagement in the sense of young people contributing to collective actions to address social issues. Volunteer and service activities certainly may involve such activist efforts, but they need not. We focus, rather, on the young "citizen as helper."

Walker (2002) notes that a potential problem with this approach is its individualistic bias. Reading to a child, befriending an elderly person, and serving food to the hungry may benefit the recipients and the givers of such help but not necessarily address the broader social and institutional issues that create "needy" persons in the first place. We think there is a need for both measures of youth as helpers—engagement in the sense of reaching out to others, and youth as social activists. But our current measures of youth even as helpers (a broader construct than that of youth as social activists) have some significant weaknesses, as will be explained below. These considerations have led us to focus here on young people's prosocial orientation and service and not on their civic knowledge, competence, or political or collective action.

We suggest in this article that two kinds of measures are needed to get comprehensively but briefly at this particular operationalization of connection to community: an "hours of service" type of measure common in studies of youth community service (*retrospective* behavior report) and a measure of broader prosocial orientation that taps both helping attitudes and intentions to volunteer (attitudes and *prospective* behavior report).

Given the strong positive role that prosocial attitudes and behavior (including volunteering) play in both individual development and the strengthening of civil society, it is important to assess their incidence among American adolescents. Ideally, both the attitudinal and behavioral components of prosocial orientation would be assessed. For a variety of reasons, however, existing measures may not be suitable.

Measures of Prosocial Orientation

With regard to prosocial orientation, for example, one of the more widely used measures is Conrad and Hedin's (1981) Personal and Social Responsibility Scale. The total scale had a reported alpha reliability of .83 (Cronbach's alpha) with seventh graders in the original study, but the full scale includes 12 items across three subscales (social welfare, duty, and efficacy). The social welfare (concern for others) and duty (felt responsibility to help others) subscales, each comprising four items, are perhaps the most relevant for the present purposes. But neither reliability data nor much validity information have been published on the subscales. In addition to limited psychometric information, the items also use a question-and-response format that may be insufficiently precise. The format's general phrasing and limited response options may produce too little variability to be useful in many research settings. Moreover, the scale measures only attitudes and not behaviors.

The Altruistic Behavior Scale was adapted from the original measure of Rushton, Chrisjohn, and Fekken (1981). This nine-item measure has been used with students as young as fourth grade and has reported alpha reliabilities in the .80s. Students are asked whether they have done specific helping acts, such as assisting someone who "fell down" or stopping someone from "hurting an animal." Although the alpha reliability is good and the items are concrete (making the measure useful with younger children, as well as adolescents), it too has a number of drawbacks. The most important one is that only reported behaviors are measured, not attitudes. The concreteness of the items can also be a drawback. Behaviors such as preventing someone from "hurting an animal," for example, may be low-frequency occurrences for most children, a situation that contributes to relatively poor variability of response. Finally, the time referent of "since the start of this school year" is problematic. Students administered the measure earlier in the school year have less likelihood of having done each act, especially low-frequency ones, than students taking the survey more toward the end of the school year.

Penner et al.'s (1995) Prosocial Personality Battery measures "helpfulness," operationally defined as the sum of Personal Distress and Self-Reported Altruism. The five-item Self-Reported Altruism scale has an alpha of .73 with an adult sample. Respondents are asked how often they have done this action "in the past," on a 1-to-5 scale from *never* to *very often*. Although there is a good amount of psychometric information available on this measure, its focus on past experience (rather than current experience or intentions) makes it more suitable for adults than for the adolescents and preadolescents of interest to researchers in the field of positive youth development.

More recently, Carlo, Hausmann, Christiansen, and Randall (2003) reported on the development of the Prosocial Tendencies Measure-Revised (PTM-R), based on a study of 138 middle and high school students. The total measure includes 25 items across six subscales assessing different kinds of prosocial behavior (public, anonymous, helping in dire situations, helping in response to high emotions, being compliant, and altruism). The altruism scale has acceptable 2-week test–retest reliability and internal consistency for middle adolescents, but the reported alpha reliability for early adolescents was only moderate (.59). The PTM-R generally was related in predicted ways to measures of empathy, aggression, and ascription of personal responsibility, suggesting acceptable validity. However, the altruism scale was not significantly related to global prosocial behavior. Thus, although the PTM-R has some promising qualities to be explored in future research, there may also be questions about its use with middle school students and its validity as a predictor of self-reported prosocial behavior.

Measures of Community Service

Current measures directly asking youth about their community *service* do not appear adequate to use alone. At present, most measures of youth's community service or volunteering consist of a single item. For example, in the ongoing Monitoring the Future study of about 16,000 high school seniors (Bachman, Johnston, & O'Malley, 1993), youth are asked how often they have participated in community service or civic affairs: not at all, a couple of times a year, weekly, monthly, or daily.

Similarly, the national evaluation of Learn and Serve America service-learning programs (Melchior, 1997) was a study of 17 programs, and included about 1,000 middle and high school students (60% in service-learning programs and 40% in a comparison group). The measure of volunteering in this study was "During the past six months, how often did you do some volunteer or community service work?" Response options were "I volunteered__days a week," "On average, I volunteered__hours each day," and "I did this for__of the 26 weeks during the last 6 months." In the Youth Development Study, a panel study conducted in late 1980s and early 1990s of 1,000 ninth graders in St. Paul who were followed for 4 years, Johnson, Beebe, Mortimer, and Snyder (1998) measured participation in volunteer work with this two-part item: "Do you currently do any volunteer work (without pay)?" If respondents answered yes, they were then asked how many hours per week they volunteered and what kind of work it was (later coded as face-to-face contact with recipients or not).

Also, in the 1996 National Household Education Survey (Nolin, Chaney, & Chapman, 1997), students in grades 6 through 12 were asked whether they had participated in any community service activity during the current school year. If they responded yes, they were asked whether the activity happened once, twice, or more regularly.

One of the few studies to use a multi-item measure of service or volunteering was by Youniss, McLellan, and Mazer (2001). In their study, 389 suburban Catholic school juniors were asked whether they performed any voluntary community service during the preceding year that was not done for school credit. If they said yes, they were asked what kind: social service, working for a cause, tutoring, coaching, child care, or "functionary" work. "Civic engagement," however, was measured with four factors. *Service intentions* was composed of several items assessing the reported likelihood of doing service in the upcoming summer, in college, and after college. *Political intentions* measured future intentions to work on a political campaign, boycott a product or service, and demonstrate publicly for a cause. *School clubs* asked about students' frequency of participation in the past year in school music, drama, art, or school spirit organizations, and participation in other clubs or student government. Finally, *youth groups* measured students' frequency of participation in church-related youth groups, and in community groups such as 4-H.

In a number of states and cities, single items on volunteering have been added at local discretion to the U.S. Centers for Disease Control and Prevention's *Youth Risk Behavior Survey* (YRBS) (Grunbaum et al., 2002), in order to build a more national database on protective factors. In the 2001 YRBS, for example, Massachusetts youth were asked: "In an average month, how many hours do you spend on volunteer work, community service, or helping people outside of your home without getting paid? (0 hours, 1 to 4 hours, 5 to 9 hours, 10 or more hours)." Similarly, North Carolina's YRBS asked young people: "During the past 30 days, how many times did you perform any organized community service as a nonpaid volunteer (for example, serving meals to elderly, picking up litter, helping out at a hospital, building homes for the poor, etc.)? (0 times, 1 time, 2 or 3 times, 4 or 5 times, 6 or more times)."

Finally, Vermont adolescents were asked: "During an average week, how many hours do you spend helping other people without getting paid (such as helping out at a hospital, daycare center, food shelf, youth program, community service agency, or doing other things) to make your community a better place for people to live? (0 hours, 1 hour, 2 hours, 3–5 hours, 6–10 hours, 11 or more hours)." Vermont used the identical wording as the measure of the "service to others" asset included in the *Search Institute Profiles of Student Life: Attitudes and Behaviors* survey (Benson, Scales, Leffert, & Roehlkepartain, 1999).

This brief review shows that current measures of adolescent service or volunteering largely consist of single items, but service is operationalized in ways that cover a gamut of definitions and time frames. There is still a need for such an item or items in a national system of positive indicators of youth development, but there are several problems with using only a self-report of service frequency. First, what is the best time frame for such recall? All these referents are in use in current service/volunteering items: *currently, over the last month, during the last year, or during an average week.* "Currently" would be freshest in respondents' minds. But since youth volunteering is typically short lived and sporadic, "currently" may be a poor measure of actual volunteer levels. "Average week" gets around that problem but requires the respondent to determine what constitutes an "average" week. Although arguments can be made for any of these referents, to our knowledge there is no empirical evidence to suggest one referent over another. Also, quite different results are obtained depending on the referent.

Second and related to the first issue, how reliable and valid are the measures of recalled hours per week, especially for periods such as the "last year"? With single items predominating, internal consistency reliability is not applicable. Again to our knowledge, test–retest reliabilities for the single items discussed here have not been reported, nor have studies examined the association of these self-reports with actual records of service or volunteer hours.

Perhaps more important, current measures of service/volunteering do not tap prosocial orientation very comprehensively. Differences in students' self-reported hours of service/volunteering may arise from opportunity differences rather than from differences in desire to volunteer or altruistic attitudes. For example, much volunteering/service may be in the context of required school programs—nearly 20% of 6th through 12th graders in one national survey said their schools required community service (Nolin et al., 1997). But young people *required* to contribute service may not have the same attitudinal or value-based perspective on helping others as those who do so voluntarily nor the same commitment to future service. Nor do most existing measures of prosocial orientation seem appropriate. Most are intended for adults, with the language and actions inquired about seeming unsuitable for today's youth. Other measures use problematic formats, have uncertain psychometric quality, or measure either attitudes or retrospective behavior, but not both.

Ultimately, as Youniss et al. (2002) noted, it is not only current connection to the community that is of interest but, even more, whether young people are developing a lifelong commitment to community contribution: "Putting in hours toward . . . a service activity has only limited meaning unless the changes within individuals and groups that lead to *continued* commitment and participation are understood" (p. 129, emphasis added).

Consensus needs to be established on how best to inquire retrospectively about young people's community service. However, a measure that combines items tapping adolescents' prosocial attitudes and their behavioral intentions to contribute volunteer service may conceptually add a more useful supplement to such measures than has as yet been reported. A considerable research literature demonstrates that expressed intentions to do a behavior are significant predictors of the actual subsequent behavior (Azjen, 2001). If a combined attitude-behavioral intention measure of helping others were also found to strongly predict whether an adolescent contributes volunteer service, it might provide more evidence than current measures about that young person's likely *continued* commitment to this form of community connection. It would also have fewer methodological drawbacks than the current modal approach of simply asking a single item about past service frequency. Used with standard wording for eliciting retrospective reports of service, this measure might provide better data for tracking the helping attitudes and behavior of adolescents (i.e., their connection to community) than currently exist.

A New Measure of Prosocial Orientation

The measure of prosocial orientation we discuss in this chapter is taken from the *Youth Supplement Survey* (YS2), which was developed as a companion survey to the *Search Institute Profiles of Student Life: Attitudes and Behaviors* survey (A&B). The A&B survey is the primary research instrument used by Search Institute for collecting data on youth's reports of experiencing developmental assets. Developmental assets are relationships, opportunities, values, self-perceptions, and skills that help young people develop positively (Benson, Scales, & Mannes, 2003). In the YS2, a number of those developmental assets and seven thriving outcomes, including "helping others," are measured with more reliable, multi-item measures than they are in the A&B (Scales, Leffert, & Vraa, 2003).

We analyzed a matched sample of 5,136 6th- to 12th-grade students from Colorado Springs who were administered *both* the A&B and the YS2 in winter 1999. The eligible population was the 15,739 students in grades 6–12 in the district's certified count the fall prior to the survey administration. A "passive" parental consent procedure was used for student participation. Parents were notified prior to the survey administration that they or their children could request that the student not participate, and 781 students or their parents declined (5% of the eligible population). Schools were allowed either to sample all students whose parents gave permission or to use a random sample of those students in their building, based on their concerns about how best to minimize the impact of the surveying on instructional time. Some students were absent for the survey administration, yielding a total of 9,233 surveys for processing. Data quality controls (e.g., more than 40 responses missing; answering yes to use of a fictitious drug) eliminated another 1,000 surveys. Numerous other surveys had to be eliminated because identification numbers on each of the 2 surveys did not match or because grade and gender on each survey did not match. The final sample was the 5,136 students who completed both surveys.

A comparison of these 5,136 students with the 4,097 who had to be eliminated because of various survey matching problems showed that the students eliminated were more likely to be males, students of color, and in 9th or 10th grade (they were also more likely to be older, but this age difference was due to the strong correlation between age and grade). Analyses of variance (available from authors) showed that the eliminated students reported a lower total number of developmental assets, fewer thriving indicators, and more risk behavior patterns and developmental deficits than did the final study sample.

The sample comprised 16% each of 6th, 7th, and 9th graders; 17% of 8th graders; 13% each of 10th and 11th graders; and 8% of 12th graders. Student age ranged from 11 to 19 years, with a mean age of 14. The sample had more females than males (55% versus 45%) and was racially and ethnically diverse. Two thirds of students were White, and the next two largest groups were Multiracial (16%) and Latino/Latina youth (8%). Parental education levels were used as proxies for socioeconomic status, with frequencies indicating a diverse sample. Although 47% of mothers and 52% of fathers were reported to have a college degree or graduate school experience, 29% of mothers and 28% of fathers were reported to have only a high school diploma or less.

Measures

Principal components factor analysis with varimax rotation was used to illuminate the empirical structure of the asset exposure and thriving measures. All items with eigenvalues greater than 1 were allowed to enter, and, for this exploratory construction of the YS2, all items with factor loadings of .30 or greater were retained (Kim & Mueller, 1978).

Prosocial orientation comprised seven items. The seven-item scale had an acceptable alpha reliability of .72, with no significant difference among males and females. Prosocial orientation is a combination of four items that assess youths' attitudes and values about helping others, and three items that tap their intention over the next year to volunteer to help those in need, work to improve their school, or help younger children in formal ways such as tutoring or coaching (see the Appendix). These intention items do not capture the limitless range of activities in which young people can behave prosocially. But they do reflect some common ways in which young people can be connected to society in a "transcendent way" that helps them "participate in a system of meaning" and promotes their long-term civic identity.[1]

Unless otherwise noted, all analyses in this chapter use the continuous version of this construct. A binary version was also created for selected analyses. To be scored as having a prosocial orientation, students needed to average an *agree* (4 on a 5-point scale) across the four attitude items and had to respond with at least *quite likely* (4 on the 5-point scale) to *any one* of the three behavioral intention items. On this basis, 20% of the sample reported a prosocial orientation. Across the total sample, one attitude item and the three behavioral intention items showed good variability. As expected, however, most of the attitude items were skewed to the positive, with from 3 to 9 times as many youth saying they agreed or strongly agreed as said they disagreed or strongly disagreed. On three of the attitude items, about one third of the sample said they were not sure.

The positive skewness of the YS2 prosocial orientation and "helping others" attitude items is similar to that found among this same sample on the A&B survey for an asset measuring the value of "caring." On a 5-point scale from *not important* to *extremely important,* students rated the importance of several things "to you in your life": helping other people, helping to make the world a better place in which to live, and giving time or money to make life better for other people. For each of those "caring" items, as for most of the attitude items, about 2–6 times as many youth said the values were quite or extremely important as said they were not important or only somewhat important. Similar skewness on the "caring" asset was observed in a different sample, an aggregate of more than 217,000 6th–12th graders from more than 300 U.S. communities who took the A&B survey in the 1999–2000 school year (*Developmental assets: A portrait of your youth, 2001*).

Concurrent Validity

Demographic patterns generally are consistent with both theory and previous research. For example, females in this sample more frequently said they had positive attitudes and intentions to help others than did males, $F(1, 4980) = 69.80$, $p \le .0001$. Moreover, for each successive rise in the level of mother's or father's education, there was a corresponding significant increase in reported prosocial orientation. Young people whose mother, $F(2, 4462) = 26.37$, $p \le .0001$,

---

[1] Remarks of James Youniss at Indicators of Positive Youth Development Conference, Washington, DC, March 12–13, 2003.

or father, $F(2, 4227) = 40.74$, $p \leq .0001$, had graduated from college had higher levels of prosocial orientation than those whose parents had just some college or who had a high school diploma or less. Also, those whose parents had just some college reported more prosocial orientation than those with only a high school diploma or less. There were sufficient subgroup cell sizes to compare only White, Latino, Multiracial, and "other" students (the last largely comprising Asian, African American, and Native American students). White and "other" students reported somewhat higher levels of prosocial orientation than Latino students, but not Multiracial students, $F(3, 5068) = 7.79$, $p \leq .0001$. The source of the differences appeared to be in the behavioral intention items more so than in the items measuring attitudes toward helping others.

Developmental assets theory predicts that young people who report experiencing more assets should also report less risk-taking behavior and more thriving dimensions, such as prosocial orientation. Following the procedure in Benson et al. (1999), students were divided into quartiles based on how many of 12 asset domains they reported experiencing (9–12, 6–8, 3–5, or 0–2). Variables were standardized to a mean of 0 and a standard deviation of 1. For each successive increase in asset level, there was a corresponding significant increase in the mean score for prosocial orientation, $F(3, 4625) = 250.83$, $p \leq .0001$.

Risk Behavior and Thriving

As is the case for risk behaviors, positive thriving outcomes also tend to cluster (Benson et al., 2003). Thus, prosocial orientation should be positively correlated with other measures of thriving and negatively correlated with measures of risk behavior.

The continuous version of the prosocial orientation variable was correlated with other thriving outcomes and asset exposure domains from the YS2, as well as with the single-item thriving outcomes and risk behavior patterns from the A&B survey administered at the same time to the same sample of youth. All the correlation coefficients were significant and in the predicted direction (data not shown). Prosocial orientation was positively correlated at moderate levels (.33 to .52) with multi-item, reliable (alphas in the .70s) YS2 measures of positive orientation to schoolwork, belonging to school, valuing diversity, being seen as a leader, active coping, and overcoming adversity. Only for feelings about personal health, a less reliable measure (alphas in the low .60s), was the correlation negligible, albeit in the predicted direction.

As expected, correlations with the single-item thriving measures from the A&B survey were somewhat lower, given the lesser variance likely in using single-item variables. Thus, prosocial orientation was correlated at relatively low to moderate levels (.16 to .36) with resisting danger, valuing diversity, maintaining physical health, delaying gratification, informal helping of friends, exhibiting leadership, overcoming adversity, and succeeding at school.

Also as predicted, prosocial orientation was negatively correlated with all risk behavior patterns measured on the A&B survey. Coefficients ranged from low to moderate (−.14 to −.25) between helping others and problem alcohol use, use of illicit drugs, use of tobacco, gambling, antisocial behavior, violence, school problems, and sexual behavior risk. Only for depression/suicide was the correlation negligible, although in the predicted direction.

To further clarify the predictive validity of the prosocial orientation construct, we included it in stepwise regression analyses predicting a variety of thriving outcomes and risk behavior patterns. Because of the significant differences in the prosocial orientation construct by gender, regressions were run separately for boys and girls. Results for thriving outcomes are displayed in Table 1 (results for risk behavior patterns show similar trends, albeit with lesser amounts of variance explained). The amounts of variance explained (R^2) range from negligible to moderate. However, there were no predictors other than a small number of demographic variables and prosocial orientation (called "Helping others" in Table 1). Thus, the contribution of prosocial orientation was notable.

More important than total amount of variance explained, however, is that prosocial orientation adds a meaningful proportion of explanation, typically more than do demographic variables, to most of the thriving and risk behavior outcomes. Among boys, prosocial orientation adds from 2% (boys' feelings about personal health) to 29% of variance (boys' positive orientation to schoolwork) across the thriving outcomes, and 1% (depression) to 14% (school problems) across the risk behavior patterns. Among girls, prosocial orientation adds 6% (girls' feelings about personal health) to 24% (girls' positive orientation to schoolwork) across the thriving outcomes, and 1% (depression, and gambling) to 18% (sexual behavior risk) across the risk behavior patterns. Among both genders, prosocial orientation seems to be particularly important in explaining a positive orientation to schoolwork, belonging to school, valuing diversity, and active coping. These proportions of variance explained by prosocial orientation in various adolescent outcomes are generally equal to or more than the proportion of variance "community service" explains in similar outcomes in the Monitoring the Future study (Youniss, McLellan, Su, & Yates, 1999). Moreover, in both the current analysis (prosocial orientation) and the Youniss et al. study (service), the service and prosocial orientation predictors typically explain significantly more of those outcomes than do demographics.

Prosocial Orientation and Community Service

Prosocial orientation comprises an attitudinal and behavioral intention component. It should therefore show at least moderate correlations with reports of actual community service and with known predictors of service, such as parents' service activities (Yates & Youniss, 1996). These correlations are all significant and in the predicted direction. Helping others is correlated .36 with students' reported average hours per week of service, as measured on the A&B survey. It is also correlated .33 with student reports of their *parents'* involvement in service (alpha = .73), and .48 with reports of their own participation during the past year in formal service-learning programs or other leadership activities (alpha = .72), as measured on the YS2.

Table 1. Prosocial Orientation as a Predictor of Thriving and Risk Behavior Patterns

Outcomes/Predictors	R^2 Males	R^2 Females	Beta Males	Beta Females
Positive Orientation to Schoolwork				
Demographics	.029	.031		
Grade			−.031	−.023
Race/ethnicity			−.008	−.006
Mother's education			.016	.049
Father's education			.085	.053
Helping others	.286	.244	.513	.472
Valuing Diversity				
Demographics	.011	.006		
Grade			−.011	.048
Race/ethnicity			.070	−.008
Mother's education			.038	−.026
Father's education			−.005	−.016
Helping others	.186	.175	.424	.419
Feelings about Personal Health				
Demographics	.018	.044		
Grade			−.072	−.193
Race/ethnicity			−.026	−.019
Mother's education			.109	.041
Father's education			−.006	.047
Helping others	.022	.061	.071	.136
Being Seen as a Leader				
Demographics	.012	.009		
Grade			.074	.003
Race/ethnicity			−.008	.011
Mother's education			.083	.015
Father's education			−.017	.027
Helping others	.125	.117	.340	.336
Active Coping				
Demographics	.005	.015		
Grade			.038	.037
Race/ethnicity			−.005	−.009
Mother's education			.026	.003
Father's education			−.005	.030
Helping others	.225	.181	.475	.416
Belonging to School				
Demographics	.023	.027		
Grade			.079	.021
Race/ethnicity			−.004	−.031
Mother's education			.070	.027
Father's education			.034	.050
Helping others	.230	.210	.460	.438
Overcoming Adversity				
Demographics	.013	.014		
Grade			.041	.038
Race/ethnicity			.032	.009
Mother's education			.060	−.008
Father's education			.010	.038
Helping others	.199	.188	.436	.426

Because the measure of actual service was highly skewed (half the students reported 0 hours per week and most of the rest just 1 or 2 hours per week), it was dichotomized. Prosocial orientation was also constructed as a binary variable for this analysis. Students who averaged an *agree* (4 on the 5-point scale) to the four attitude items, and who said it was either "quite" or "extremely" likely that they would do any one of the three potential kinds of volunteering over the next year (help the needy, help younger children, work to improve their school), were counted as "having" a prosocial orientation.

Logistic regressions were then run separately for boys and girls to determine the relation of the prosocial orientation construct (which combines attitudes and behavioral intentions) to the self-report of actual service. We examined three different models. Model 1 included demographics and only prosocial orientation. Model 2 included demographics, parents' service activities, and prosocial orientation. Model 3 included demographics, parents' service activities, student reports of exposure over the past year to formal service-learning programs and other leadership activities, and the prosocial orientation variable.

Table 2 shows that in Model 1, with grade, race/ethnicity, and mother's and father's education entered first, both boys and girls who had prosocial orientations were nearly 4 *times* more likely to report actual service than those who did not, by far the most differential variable in the analysis.

Because service is also more likely among those whose parents model service and volunteering, we also examined the role of prosocial orientation in predicting service over and above parental modeling of service. In Model 2, demographics were again entered first, followed by parents' service activities and then prosocial orientation. As expected, students whose parents volunteer are themselves more likely to do so (boys whose parents volunteer are 2.5 times more likely to report service, and girls are nearly 3 times more likely). But for both boys and girls, their attitudes and behavioral intentions regarding helping others are even stronger predictors of service than are parents' service activities. For each, having these prosocial attitudes and behavioral intentions makes it at least 3 times more likely that they report contributing service during an average week.

Finally, on the YS2, we had also asked about young people's frequency during the last year in participating in a community service or service-learning "program," their participation in groups of youths that helped to plan events or activities, or their membership on committees or task forces. Because much of students' reported average weekly service likely comes from participation in formal programs (as contrasted with individual volunteering outside a program context), we wondered whether the role of prosocial orientation in predicting service would lessen once we accounted for differences in exposure to formal service and other leadership activities.

Students were divided into those who said their participation in these kinds of leadership and service roles totaled at least "a few weeks" over the past year, and those whose participation averaged less. In Model 3, demographics were entered first, then parental modeling of service, then student exposure to service and leadership programs for at least a few weeks, and finally prosocial

Table 2. Contribution of Prosocial Orientation to Prediction of Average Weekly Service

	Boys			Girls		
	Coefficient	SE	Odds ratio	Coefficient	SE	Odds ratio
Model 1						
Intercept	−.58	.26		−.10	.22	
Demographics						
Grade	−.11	.10	.89	−.22	.09	.80**
Race	−.14	.05	.87**	−.03	.05	.97
Mother's education	−.04	.07	.96	.07	.06	1.07
Father's education	.25	.07	1.28***	.07	.06	1.07
Prosocial orientation	1.34	.15	3.81****	1.32	.11	3.73****
Model 2						
Intercept	−.80	.26		−.06	.23	
Demographics						
Grade	−.06	.10	.94	−.15	.09	.86
Race	−.13	.06	.88*	−.04	.05	.96
Mother's education	−.08	.07	.92	.06	.06	1.06
Father's education	.24	.07	1.27****	−.00	.06	.99
Parents' service activities	.90	.11	2.47****	1.04	.11	2.82****
Prosocial orientation	1.14	.15	3.11****	1.19	.12	3.30****
Model 3						
Intercept	−.84	.27		.00	.23	
Demographics						
Grade	−.05	.10	.95	−.18	.09	.83*
Race	−.13	.06	.88*	−.04	.05	.96
Mother's education	−.90	.07	.91	.04	.06	1.04
Father's education	.25	.07	1.29****	−.00	.06	.99
Parents' service activities	.85	.12	2.35****	.99	.11	2.70****
Service/leadership programs	1.00	.38	2.71****	1.70	.36	5.49****
Prosocial orientation	1.10	.15	3.02****	1.12	.12	3.10****

N = 5,136 students in 6th through 12th grades.
**** = $p \leq .0005$. *** = $p \leq .008$. ** = $p \leq .01$. * = $p \leq .05$.

orientation. Table 2 shows that for both genders, the expected relation was confirmed of those service and leadership opportunities to reports of "average weekly" service, but the effect is more profound for girls than boys. Girls were 5.5 times more likely to report average weekly service if they had at least a few weeks of formal service/leadership experiences in the last year, whereas boys were only 2.7 times more likely to report service in similar circumstances.

The measure of exposure to service/leadership programs contained three items, one asking about formal community service or service-learning programs, one asking about youth planning groups, and one asking about task forces or committee membership. We conducted a logistic regression among girls, using only the service/leadership program item, entered after demographics, and followed by prosocial orientation. Girls who had at least a few weeks of such exposure were half again as likely as other girls to report average weekly service, but prosocial orientation made a far bigger difference. Girls having prosocial attitudes and intentions were nearly 3 times more likely to report weekly service than girls who did not. Thus, the gender differences in how exposure to formal service/leadership opportunities relates to average weekly service seem less to do with community service or service-learning programs and more to do with the impact that occurs if girls average significant participation across a *range* of leadership roles that include youth event planning groups and issue task forces. In other words, general leadership experience seems more important for girls than for boys in affecting their typical weekly frequency of service.

Summary and Recommendations

Overall, the results of these analyses suggest that the seven-item prosocial orientation variable, comprising both prosocial attitudes and behavioral intentions, is a good measure with acceptable reliability that demonstrates consistent concurrent validity for both male and female adolescents. It may therefore warrant additional examination as a potential measure for inclusion in a system of positive youth development indicators.

Despite those strengths, there are several significant limitations to this measure of young people's prosocial orientation, related to psychometrics, conceptualization, and the politics of social change and diversity. There are three psychometric cautions. First, these results come from a single study of students in one urban school district who received parental permission to participate in the study. Although the sample was large and ethnically and socioeconomically diverse, the nonparticipants generally had higher risk behavior profiles. So it is not clear how well the prosocial orientation measure would have captured this aspect of connection to community for such relatively more vulnerable youth.

Second, both the prosocial orientation measure and all the dependent variables used to examine its validity were student self-reports. Thus, although prosocial orientation consistently showed the expected theoretical relation to risk behavior patterns, thriving indicators, and student service experience, we would expect these relations to be less significant if more objective measures of those dependent variables were used. In addition, all the data are concurrent. We have no prospective validity data, and so longitudinal studies are needed to fill this gap. Moreover, several of the attitude items appear skewed with a positive bias, suggesting that perhaps some rewording would be needed to lessen the likelihood of socially desirable responses and to improve the item-level variability.

Most important, the prosocial orientation measure would not replace, but only supplement, a measure of young people's "actual" amount and kind of community service contributed. Indeed, behavioral intention, although a reasonable proxy for many behaviors, may ultimately prove to be less suitable for assessing connection to community, because youth may not well predict their volunteering much in advance of a personal opportunity to do so. For example, data from Independent Sector surveys on youth volunteering show that youth are 4 times more likely to volunteer if they are asked to do so than if no one requests their help (Hodgkinson & Weitzman, 1996). In the absence of a current request or opportunity, many youth might not be aware of volunteer opportunities they would, in fact, enjoy and be likely to do. They also might be reluctant to take the initiative and offer themselves for volunteer service but be quite willing to accept an invitation to become involved. Specific examinations of how well these behavioral intentions predict actual service in a prospective study are needed to be more confident that this behavioral intention dimension of prosocial orientation has good utility.

Perhaps more fundamentally, this measure, although strong in some traditional respects, still may not validly capture the variety of ways in which young people in differing cultural groups or settings develop and exhibit their "prosocial" orientation. For example, on our surveys done in Minneapolis, Hmong youth typically respond that they contribute no hours of service in a typical week, and perhaps their intention to do so also would be low. Yet in focus groups they indicate they are working at jobs to give their families extra income and that they are helping aunts and uncles take care of the family's younger children. They clearly are engaged in community, but they are not tutoring children through a formal program. For them, we might ask which is the more important developmental experience? The challenge for researchers and policy makers is how to capture such rich variety in young people's expressions of prosocial orientation. Our present measure captures only one kind of prosocial orientation.

Moreover, our interest as *applied* developmental scientists is to create good science that facilitates social change that helps individuals, organizations, communities, and systems more intentionally and effectively build young people's ability to thrive (in this case, specifically to build their connections and contributions to society). Thus, the *process* by which we develop indicators of youth well-being and thriving becomes especially relevant. Our measure of prosocial orientation, despite the strengths that may recommend it, has been developed through the scholarly dialogue of the academy. To promote the widespread adoption and influence of this and other indicators of youth well-being, it would be helpful to have evidence of consensus across the diversities of the American public that this way of thinking about youth connection to society makes good sense.

We have argued that youth reports of their "actual" service carry a number of problems that suggest not relying solely upon those measures to assess adolescent helping behaviors. Those problems range from reliability and validity issues, to questions about the most appropriate time referent to use in such recall, to masking of motivational differences in the likelihood of continued commitment to community contribution. We believe that supplementing that approach with this prosocial orientation variable, even with its own conceptual, psychometric, and political weaknesses, may provide a better continuum of attitudinal, retrospective, and prospective behavior measures. With this continuum, we may better understand not just the current status of contribution to community among the nation's youth but its possible trajectory as well.

Authors' Note

Correspondence should be addressed to Peter C. Scales, Search Institute, 940 Chestnut Ridge Road, Manchester, MO 63021 (scalespc@search-institute.org).

Appendix

Prosocial Orientation Items and Frequencies

	Strongly agree	Agree	Not sure	Disagree	Strongly disagree
A15 Helping others without being paid is not something people should feel they have to do.	10	28	32	21	9
R18 Taking care of people who are having difficulty caring for themselves is everyone's responsibility, including mine.	15	35	35	12	4
R51 Participation in activities that help improve the community is an important job for everyone, even beginners.	17	42	32	7	4
A60 Doing things for other people when they need help is not important to me.	3	5	15	44	33

	Not at all likely	A little likely	Somewhat likely	Quite likely	Very likely
In the next year, how likely is it that you will ...					
A68 Volunteer in programs to help others in need (like food or clothing drives, working at a homeless shelter).	20	26	22	16	15
A69 Actively work to improve your school.	24	26	23	15	11
A70 Volunteer to tutor kids, be a mentor, or coach a team.	31	25	19	14	12

References

Azjen, I. (2001). Nature and operation of attitudes. *Annual Review of Psychology, 52,* 27–58.

Bachman, G.G., Johnston, L.D., & O'Malley, P.M. (1993). *Monitoring the future: A continuing study of the life styles and values of youth.* Ann Arbor: University of Michigan, Survey Research Center.

Bell, D. (2002). Foreword. In D. Wertlieb, F. Jacobs, & R. M. Lerner (Eds.), *Handbook of applied developmental science: Vol. 3. Promoting positive youth and family development—Community systems, citizenship, and civil society* (pp. ix–xii). Thousands Oaks, CA: Sage.

Benson, P. L., Scales, P. C., Leffert, N., & Roehlkepartain, E. C. (1999). *A fragile foundation: The state of developmental assets among American youth.* Minneapolis: Search Institute.

Benson, P. L., Scales, P. C., & Mannes, M. (2002). Development strengths and their sources: Implications for the study and practice of community building. In R. M. Lerner, F. Jacobs, & D. Wertlieb (Eds.), *Handbook of applied developmental science: Vol. 1. Applying developmental science for youth and families: Historical and theoretical foundations* (pp. 369–406). Thousand Oaks, CA: Sage.

Carlo, G., Hausmann, A., Christiansen, S., & Randall, B. A. (2003). Sociocognitive and behavioral correlates of a measure of prosocial tendencies for adolescents. *Journal of Early Adolescence, 23,* 107–134.

Conrad, D. E., & Hedin, D. (1981). National assessment of experiential education: Summary and implications. *Journal of Experiential Education, 4,* 6–20.

Developmental assets: A profile of your youth. (2001). Minneapolis: Search Institute. Unpublished 1999–2000 school year aggregate sample.

Grunbaum, J., Kann, L., Kinchen, S. A., Williams, B., Ross, J. G., Lowry, R., & Kolbe, L. (2002). Youth risk behavior surveillance—United States, 2001. *Journal of School Health, 72,* 313–328.

Haynes, N. M., & Comer, J. P. (1997). Service learning in the Comer School Development Program. In J. Schine (Ed.), *Service learning: Ninety-sixth yearbook of the National Society for the Study of Education* (pp. 79–89). Chicago: National Society for the Study of Education.

Hodkinson, V. A., & Weitzman, M. S. (1996). *Volunteering and giving among teenagers 12 to 17 years of age.* Washington, DC: Independent Sector.

Johnson, M. K., Beebe, T., Mortimer, J. T., & Snyder, M. (1998). Volunteerism in adolescence: A process perspective. *Journal of Research on Adolescence, 8,* 309–332.

Kim, J., & Mueller, C. W. (1978). *Factor analysis: Statistical methods and practical issues.* Newbury Park, CA: Sage.

Kleinbard, P. (1997). Youth participation: Integrating youth into communities. In J. Schine (Ed.), *Service learning: Ninety-sixth yearbook of the National Society for the Study of Education* (pp. 1–18). Chicago: National Society for the Study of Education.

Lerner, R. M., Brentano, C., Dowling, E. M., & Anderson, P. M. (2002). Positive youth development: Thriving as the basis for personhood and civil society. *New Directions for Youth Development, no. 95,* 11–33.

Melchior, A. (1997). *Interim report: National evaluation of Learn and Serve America school and community-based programs.* Washington, DC: Corporation for National Service.

Nolin, M., Chaney, B., & Chapman, C. (1997). *Student participation in community service activity.* Washington, DC: National Center for Education Statistics, 1996 National Household Education Survey (NCES 97-331).

Penner, L. A., Craiger, J. P., Fritzsche, B. A., & Frefeld, T. S. (1995). Measuring the prosocial personality. In J. N. Butcher & C. D. Spielberger (Eds.), *Advances in personality assessment* (Vol. 10, pp. 147–164). Hillsdale, NJ: Lawrence Erlbaum.

Rushton, J. P., Chrisjohn, R. D., & Fekken, C. G. (1981). The altruistic personality and the Self-Report Altruism Scale. *Personality and Individual Differences, 2,* 293–302.

Scales, P. C., Leffert, N., & Vraa, R. (2003). The relation of community developmental attentiveness to adolescent health. *American Journal of Health Behavior, 27*(Suppl. 1), 522–534.

Walker, T. (2002). Service as a pathway to political participation: What research tells us. *Applied Developmental Science, 6,* 183–188.

Wheeler, W. (2002). Youth leadership for development: Civic activism as a component of youth development programming and a strategy for strengthening civil society. In F. Jacobs, D. Wertlieb, & R. M. Lerner (Eds.), *Handbook of applied developmental science: Vol. 2. Enhancing the life contexts of youth and families: Contributions of programs, policies, and service systems* (pp. 491–506). Thousand Oaks, CA: Sage.

Yates, M., & Youniss, J. (1996). A developmental perspective on community service in adolescence. *Social Development, 5,* 85–111.

Youniss, J., Bales, S., Christmas-Best, V., Diversi, M., McLaughlin, M., & Silbereisen, R. (2002). Youth civic engagement in the twenty-first century. *Journal of Research on Adolescence, 12,* 149–158.

Youniss, J., McLellan, J. A., & Mazer, B. (2001). Voluntary service, peer group orientation, and civic engagement. *Journal of Adolescent Research, 16*, 456–468.

Youniss, J., McLellan, J. A., Su, Y., & Yates, M. (1999). The role of community service in identity development: Normative, unconventional, and deviant orientations. *Journal of Adolescent Research, 14*, 248–261.

22 Frugality, Generosity, and Materialism in Children and Adolescents

Tim Kasser

Knox College

It is a psychological truism that as children grow into adulthood, they begin to take on or internalize the various attitudes and values of society. This process of socialization has been relatively well studied for a variety of aspects of culture, including how children come to believe certain things about their gender, their race, the nature of their selves, and multiple other aspects of their identities. There is one key feature common to all cultures that has, however, been relatively ignored by empirical research in psychology. Specifically, all children must be socialized with regards to a culture's economy. For any economy to maintain itself, the next generation must develop the set of economic beliefs, attitudes, and practices that are propounded by that particular economic system; if not, that generation will fail to adequately participate in the economy, which will lead the economy, in turn, to falter (Fromm, 1955; Kasser, Ryan, Couchman, & Sheldon, 2004).

Cultures can espouse a variety of different attitudes about money and its usage that children might internalize to one extent or another. As shown by the historian Shi (1985), U.S. culture has, since colonial times, reflected two conflicting trends regarding the use of money and the material goods it can purchase. At certain times (e.g., the Great Depression, World War II) and in certain subcultures (e.g., Puritans, hippies), people have focused on "plain living and high thinking" and have attempted to live self-sufficiently and frugally. More commonly, however, a materialistic ethos has dominated U.S. culture, suggesting that citizens and consumers should be concerned with the acquisition of more goods and the maximization of profit. A third attitude can also be discerned in U.S. history, as throughout the decades certain sectors of the populace have encouraged the sharing of one's money and possessions (through philanthropy, charitable organizations, etc.).

The prominence of these attitudes of frugality, materialism, and generosity ebbs and flows across time and cultures. Because each attitude has important ramifications not only for people's economic activity but also for their personal well-being, interpersonal relations, the well-being of others, and environmentally relevant behaviors (see below), it is important to be able to measure these three attitudes and track changes in them over time. Unfortunately, there are no brief measures of these three economic attitudes that have been validated for use in samples of children and adolescents. This study therefore set out to develop such measures in the hope that they will be useful for research and survey purposes.

Economic Attitudes

Simply stated, as individuals approach economic behavior, some restrain their purchasing whereas others purchase all they want (i.e., frugality), some share their money and possessions whereas others keep these to themselves (i.e., generosity), and some want to obtain a great deal of money and material possessions whereas others focus on different endeavors (i.e., materialism). Below, I more clearly define each attitude and briefly review some of the existing empirical research concerning each construct.

Frugality

Frugality concerns the extent to which individuals practice self-restraint in their use of money. Individuals high in frugality are rather "tight" with their money, trying to save resources and live with what they have. In contrast, those who are "loose" show little restraint in their purchases. According to a recent review by Lastovicka, Bettencourt, Hughner, and Kuntze (1999), frugality has been essentially ignored in empirical research; the only related empirical work they found was that of DeYoung (1986), who studied people's motivations for being resourceful with their possessions. Lastovicka et al. attempted to correct for this dearth of work by conducting an impressive series of studies to develop and validate a frugality measure for use with adults. In the studies, they found frugal adults were less compulsive in their buying habits, more conscious of a product's price and value, and more likely to engage in restrained consumer use behaviors (e.g., eating leftovers, timing showers, using a clothesline instead of a dryer). Lastovicka et al. only investigated adults, however, so no conclusions can be made about the validity of the frugality measure in samples of children and adolescents.

Generosity

Generosity concerns the extent to which individuals share their money and possessions. Generous people are willing to give away or share their possessions and money, and they make life choices that help other people even if their own personal earnings are diminished. Less generous people, in contrast, share less and care little about the beneficial impact they may have on others. Generosity is clearly related to concepts such as altruism and prosocial behavior, which are more widely studied but concern behaviors beyond those that are financial and economic in nature. Although a couple of scales have been developed to measure generosity, no one measure appears to be widely used. Instead, the construct is most frequently measured among children by providing them with some money or tokens and asking them to donate to others. Work with this methodology suggests that generous children have a more internal locus of control (Fincham & Barling, 1978) and higher self-esteem (Miller, Ginsburg, & Rogow, 1981). Little work has apparently been conducted on generosity in adolescents, where a scale might be more appropriately used.

Materialism

Materialistic individuals expend much energy toward becoming wealthy and owning many possessions, especially those that convey status and the "right" image in one's society (Kasser, 2002); people low in materialism care little for such pursuits. Three types of problems have been associated with strong materialistic tendencies. First, studies in consumer research and psychology have found that materialistic people also report diminished well-being (see Kasser, 2002, for a review). Such results have been documented with a variety of means of measuring well-being, with various age groups, and in several cultures around the world. At least two studies have replicated these findings in older children (Schor, 2004) and early adolescents (Cohen & Cohen, 1996). Second, research also shows that adults who are strongly concerned with material goals report lower quality relationships (Kasser & Ryan, 2001), are more competitive and less co-operative (Sheldon, Sheldon, & Osbaldiston, 2000), and are more Machiavellian (McHoskey, 1999). Parallel findings occur for adolescents, who report more anti-social activities if they score high in materialism (Cohen & Cohen, 1996; Kasser & Ryan, 1993). Finally, materialistic adults act in more ecologically degrading ways, consuming more in resource management games (Sheldon & McGregor, 2000), engaging in fewer materially simple behaviors (Richins & Dawson, 1992), and living lifestyles with higher "ecological footprints" (Brown & Kasser, 2003). To my knowledge, however, the relations of materialism to environmental behaviors have not been investigated in children or adolescents.

The Current Study

The primary purpose of the current study is to develop short, empirically sound measures of each of these three economic attitudes and validate their usage in samples of children and adolescents between the ages of 10 and 18. There currently exist no widely used measures of economic generosity in children, and the one extant frugality scale (i.e., Lastovicka et al., 1999) has not, to my knowledge, been used with children. Regarding materialism, although three scales are widely used (Belk, 1984; Kasser & Ryan, 1993; Richins & Dawson, 1992) and the construct has been measured in children and adolescents (Cohen & Cohen, 1996; Kasser & Ryan, 1993; Schor, 2004), all the existing scales are rather long and unwieldy for use in large-scale surveys of children.

Thus, I integrated and adapted the insights and items from previous research to develop initial drafts of the three economic attitude measures. I then used factor analyses to determine which items held together as a single construct in the total sample, as well as in subsamples divided by gender and age. Once short scales with adequate internal reliability were devised, I attempted to validate them by examining their correlations with each other and with a set of dependent variables that past research suggests should relate to the economic attitudes. Hypotheses are summarized below.

Intercorrelations of the Three Economic Attitudes

Frugality, generosity, and materialism are clearly conceptually distinguishable, but they may be related to each other, as they all concern economic behavior. I therefore examined both their relations to each other and their ability to independently predict outcomes of interest.

In terms of their interrelations, past research suggests that materialism and generosity are at odds with each other (Kasser, 2002; Schwartz, 1996), as it is very difficult to simultaneously obtain a great deal of wealth and possessions while at the same time giving one's wealth away and not caring about money; indeed, Belk (1984) included "non-generosity" as one of the three defining features of materialism. For these reasons, I predicted a negative correlation between materialism and generosity. Regarding the relations of frugality to materialism, Lastovicka et al. (1999) found a significant negative correlation between the two (−.26) in a sample of adults; in contrast, Tatzel (2002) argues that the two are independent. No known work or theory was available to suggest hypotheses concerning the relations of frugality to generosity. For both of these correlations, I therefore predicted no relationships.

Because I expected any intercorrelations between the three economic attitudes to be of moderate size at best, each economic attitude was expected to have its own independent relations to dependent variables. This was tested in a series of analyses in which the dependent variables were simultaneously regressed onto frugality, generosity, and materialism (along with age as a control variable).

Gender and Age

Past research suggests that males are typically more materialistic than females, whereas the converse is true for generosity (Kasser & Ryan, 1993; Weissbrod, 1980). This could of course be due to differential socialization, in which males are still considered to be the primary breadwinners whereas females are supposed to be more concerned with the well-being of others. Concerning frugality, Lastovicka et al. (1999) did not report any gender differences, and we had no reasons to expect any.

Past research has not examined changes in frugality with age. Regarding materialism, Cohen and Cohen (1996) found that desires for money and possessions decreased slightly in boys but increased slightly in girls across adolescence. Some research on generosity suggests no changes during adolescence (Comeau, 1980), whereas other research shows that the desire to be useful and of service to others declines through adolescence (Cohen & Cohen, 1996). Mixed results are reported during childhood (Froming, Allen, & Underwood, 1983; Zarbatany, Hartmann, & Gelfand, 1985). Parallel to this slight and confusing literature, arguments can be made for either positive or negative correlations between age and each of the economic attitudes. On the one hand, as children age from 10 to 18, they develop stronger self-regulatory capacities to restrain impulsive behaviors, and they develop greater capacities for abstract thought that might lead them to care about problems outside of themselves. As such, one might expect age to be positively correlated with frugality and generosity. On the other hand, as they age children are also increasingly exposed to a consumer culture that glorifies material acquisition and impulsive spending to satisfy one's own wants (Kasser et al., 2004). As such, we might expect age to be negatively correlated with frugality and generosity while positively correlated with materialism.

Economic Behavior

As one primary validational test, I examined how well each of the three scales predicted subjects' imagined use of money. Subjects were asked to imagine that they had received an unexpected windfall of $100, and were told that they could divide the money by spending it to buy things for themselves; giving it to church or charity; buying someone a gift; or saving it for the future. I predicted that frugality would correlate negatively with buying things and positively with saving; that generosity would correlate positively with giving to church or charity; and that materialism would correlate positively with the amount spent on oneself and negatively with gifts to charity.

Environmental Resource Conservation

Given that each of the economic attitudes concerns the use of material resources, each should bear relationships to the environmental impact of consumption behaviors. As described above, past research has indeed shown that frugal adults restrain their use of resources (Lastovicka et al., 1999), whereas materialistic adults use more resources (Brown & Kasser, 2003; Sheldon & McGregor, 2000). However, we know very little about whether these same factors will predict the environmentally relevant behavior of children and adolescents. Nonetheless, I predicted that frugality should be positively associated with more resource conservation behavior, as such behavior typically involves saving and reusing what one already has. In contrast, materialism was predicted to be negatively related to positive environmental behavior, as the desire for ever more material goods and wealth often pushes individuals to consume without regard to its impact. I made no predictions about generosity, although I expected that it might relate to more environmental conservation, given that generous individuals care more about the state of the "world at large."

Well-Being

As described above, a growing body of research shows that materialism is associated with lower happiness and greater distress (Kasser, 2002), and this finding has been extended to middle schoolers (Schor, 2004) and teenagers (Cohen & Cohen, 1996). As such, I hoped to provide further validation of the new materialism scale by examining correlations with subjective ratings of happiness, anxiety, and self-esteem.

What work exists on the relationship of generosity to well-being suggests that the two should be positively correlated. For example, children with high self-esteem are more generous (Miller et al., 1981), and adults who feel sad are less likely to be generous (Underwood, 1977). Relatedly, those with strong desires to improve the lives of others generally report greater well-being and less distress (Kasser & Ryan, 1993). We therefore expected generous people to report greater well-being.

Lastovicka et al. (1999) did not explore relations of frugality with happiness, but Tatzel (2002) predicted a quadratic relationship, such that moderate levels of frugality are associated with greater well-being than either high or low levels. I therefore made no predictions about the associations between frugality and well-being, but did explore both linear and quadratic effects.

Risk Behavior

Finally, I examined relations of the economic attitudes to four risk behaviors common in children and adolescents: smoking cigarettes, drinking alcohol, fighting, and getting into trouble at school. Materialism has been related to more risk behaviors (such as smoking and drinking; Williams, Cox, Hedberg, & Deci, 2000) and more conduct problems (Cohen & Cohen, 1996; Kasser & Ryan, 1993) in adolescents, suggesting it should relate positively to each of these risk behaviors. I was unable to find any relevant research on the relationships of generosity to risk behavior, although, theoretically, generous individuals should be less likely to fight and get into trouble at school, given their general concern for the welfare of others. I had two reasons for predicting that frugal individuals would be less involved in risky behaviors. First, the self-restraint implied by frugality might carry over to their actions with other people and with addictive substances. Second, frugal people may be likely to see spending money on cigarettes and alcohol as a "waste" and thus not use their resources in that manner.

Method

Samples and Procedures

Adolescents were recruited from one middle and one high school in a rural western Illinois school district. One hundred sixty packets were distributed at the middle school to approximately 40 students in each of 5th through 8th grades. Similarly, 143 packets were distributed at the high school to approximately 35 students in each of 9th through 12th grades. Students were provided with a parental permission form and the survey packet to take home and fill out at their leisure, and asked to bring both back 2 days later, at which time they were given an honorarium of $3.

Of the 160 packets distributed at the middle school, 94 were returned 2 days later, for a response rate of 58.8%. Two of these packets were missing the first two pages of the survey, so these subjects were dropped from further analyses. Of the 92 middle schoolers returning completed packets, 20 were in the 5th grade, 24 were in the 6th grade, 31 were in the 7th grade, and 17 were in the 8th grade. Of the 143 packets distributed at the high school, 114 were returned 2 days later, for a response rate of 79.7%. Of those returning packets, 31 were in the 9th grade, 24 were in the 10th grade, 32 were in the 11th grade, and 27 were in the 12th grade.

Of the total 206 participants, 114 were male, 91 were female, and 1 subject did not report his/her gender. In terms of ethnicity, 197 were White, 1 was Black, 1 was Hispanic, 1 was Native American, and 6 reported other (mostly mixed) races. Age ranged from 10 to 18 (mean = 14.2 years, SD = 2.3). Of the 186 who knew their father's education, 18 reported their father as having less than a high school education, 73 as having graduated from high school, 59 as having had some college education, 24 as having received a four-year college degree, and 12 as having some graduate degree. Of the 198 who knew their mother's education, 9 reported their mother as having less than a high school education, 65 as having graduated from high school, 72 as having had some college education, 35 as having received a four-year college degree, and 17 as having some graduate degree.

Measures were administered in the order presented below.

Measures of Economic Attitudes

Frugality

We adapted the 8-item frugality scale developed by Lastovicka et al. (1999), slightly changing items 1, 3, and 6 to make them more understandable to a younger sample of participants. Subjects rated their agreement with each item on a 5-point scale, from *strongly disagree* to *strongly agree*.

Materialism

We developed an 8-item materialism scale by adapting items from a variety of sources, including the financial success domain of Kasser and Ryan's (1996)

Aspiration Index, Richins and Dawson's (1992) materialism scale, Cohen and Cohen's (1996) admiration ratings (materialism subscale), and Schor's (2004) consumer involvement scale. Subjects rated their agreement with each item on a five-point, *strongly disagree* to *strongly agree*, scale.

Generosity

We developed a five-item generosity scale by adapting items from the non-generosity subscale of Belk's (1984) materialism scale and the community feeling subscale of Kasser and Ryan's (1996) Aspiration Index. Subjects rated their agreement with each item on a 5-point, *strongly disagree* to *strongly agree*, scale.

Personal Well-Being Measures

Happiness

We used a single-item measure of happiness, asking students to rate on a 5-point scale how they have felt lately, from *very unhappy* to *very happy*. Similar single-item happiness measures have been useful in other samples (e.g., Fordyce, 1988).

Anxiety

The Revised Children's Manifest Anxiety Scale (Reynolds & Richmond, 1978) asks subjects whether they have experienced 16 different symptoms of anxiety. Subjects simply respond yes or no.

Self-Esteem

The 10-item Rosenberg (1965) self-esteem measure assessed students' self-evaluations. This survey is among the most widely used of self-esteem measures for adolescents. Subjects rated their agreement with items on a 5-point, *strongly disagree* to *strongly agree*, scale.

Risk Behavior

Subjects were asked to think about the past 3 months and rate how often they smoked cigarettes, drank alcohol, got into physical fights, and got in trouble at school. Ratings were made on a 5-point scale, from *almost never* to *most every day*.

Other Validity Measures

Environmental Resource Conservation

Ten items adapted from Lastovicka et al. (1999) and Brown and Kasser (2003) assessed the frequency with which subjects engaged in positive environmental behaviors that save resources. Some sample behaviors include turning off electric lights in unused rooms, recycling, reusing paper, and reusing aluminum foil and plastic baggies. The scale included behaviors that children and adolescents could possibly engage in, as opposed to others (e.g., choice of investments) that are more adult-oriented. Subjects rated the frequency with which they did each behavior in the last few months on a 5-point scale, from *never or almost never* to *always or almost always* (alpha = .67).

Imaginary Windfall

To explore subjects' use of money, they were asked to imagine that they had unexpectedly received $100 and could spend it in any of four ways: "buy stuff I want," "give to charity or church," "spend on gifts for other people," and "save for the future." Subjects were told that they could divide the $100 however they wanted, but to make sure that their use of the money in the four categories totaled $100.

Results

Overview

For all three of the economic attitude scales, I followed the same basic analytic strategy. First, a factor analysis was conducted on the relevant items in the entire sample of subjects, and any items that either formed secondary factors or did not load above .5 on the primary factor were dropped. Remaining items were then submitted to factor analyses in each of four subsamples: girls, boys, middle schoolers, and high schoolers. Items that continued to load strongly on the primary factor in each of these subsamples were retained for the final version of the scale, whereas those showing substantially worse loading in any of the subsamples were dropped. Upon obtaining a stable factor structure, Cronbach's alphas were computed for the entire sample and for each of the four subsamples. After creating a factor-derived scale in this manner, I then examined occurrences of missing data, as well as other descriptive measures, including range, mean, standard deviation, skewness, and kurtosis.

Frugality Scale

Initial factor analyses in the entire sample suggested a two-factor solution, but a clean primary factor emerged that consisted of the items concerning restraint of spending (as opposed to items concerning reuse of resources). As can be seen in Table 1, when factor analyses were conducted with only the four financial restraint items, results were quite comparable across samples.

No missing data were noted for any of the four items composing the final version of the frugality measure. A total frugality score was computed by averaging responses to the four items. This summary variable showed substantial

Table 1. *Item Factor Loadings, Eigenvalues, Percentage of Variance Accounted For, and Cronbach's Alphas of the Frugality Scale in the Entire Sample and Subsamples Split by Gender and Grade Level*

Item	Total	Male	Female	Grades 5–8	Grades 9–12
I believe in being careful in how I spend my money.	.72	.74	.69	.75	.72
I control myself to make sure that I get the most from my money.	.72	.72	.74	.70	.74
I am willing to wait on a purchase I want so that I can save money.	.75	.70	.81	.67	.79
There are things I resist buying today so I can save for tomorrow.	.69	.63	.79	.60	.74
Eigenvalue	2.07	1.95	2.30	1.86	2.25
Percentage variance	51.7	48.7	57.6	46.4	56.2
Cronbach's alpha	.69	.65	.75	.61	.74

range (scores varied from 1 to 5), a mean near the midpoint of the scale ($M = 3.61$), and a standard deviation of .68. The distribution was slightly skewed ($-.44$) and kurtosis equaled $-.03$.

Materialism Scale

Initial factor analyses yielded a two-factor solution; after dropping the two items that formed the second factor, a third item was also discarded that loaded poorly on the primary factor. Analyses in the subsamples suggested the deletion of yet a fourth item. Throughout, however, four items loaded consistently on the primary factor; these are reported in Table 2.

Table 2. *Item Factor Loadings, Eigenvalues, Percentage of Variance Accounted for, and Cronbach's Alphas of the Materialism Scale in the Entire Sample and Subsamples Split by Gender and Grade Level*

Item	Total	Male	Female	Grades 5–8	Grades 9–12
I like to own things that impress other people.	.71	.70	.76	.80	.61
My life would be better if I owned things I don't have right now.	.73	.70	.78	.74	.71
It is important to make a lot of money when I grow up.	.69	.73	.58	.72	.68
When I grow up, I want to have a really nice house filled with all kinds of cool stuff.	.72	.74	.68	.62	.81
Eigenvalue	2.03	2.07	1.98	2.10	2.00
Percentage variance	50.8	51.8	49.5	52.3	49.9
Cronbach's alpha	.68	.69	.66	.70	.66

Table 3. Item Factor Loadings, Eigenvalues, Percentage of Variance Accounted for, and Cronbach's Alphas of the Generosity Scale in the Entire Sample and Subsamples Split by Gender and Grade Level

Item	Total	Male	Female	Grades 5–8	Grades 9–12
I enjoy sharing my things with other people.	.57	.51	.68	.74	.46
I enjoy giving things or money to charity.	.78	.79	.74	.77	.79
So long as the job I have helps people, it doesn't matter how much it pays.	.82	.84	.77	.79	.83
It is really important to me that I work to make the world a better place.	.80	.82	.74	.81	.78
Eigenvalue	2.24	2.27	2.15	2.40	2.12
Percentage variance	56.0	56.7	53.7	60.1	53.1
Cronbach's alpha	.74	.74	.71	.78	.70

Only one person skipped one item, suggesting the participants had little trouble responding to the questions. The four items were averaged to form a summary materialism score, which showed substantial range (varying from 1 to 5), a mean near the scale's midpoint ($M = 3.37$), and a standard deviation of .79. The scale had a slight negative skew ($-.15$), and kurtosis equaled $-.28$.

Generosity Scale

Initial factor analyses showed that one item formed its own second factor, so it was dropped. Later factor analyses with the remaining four items were all consistent across the subsamples (see Table 3).

In terms of missing data, one participant skipped the entire scale, but otherwise no items were omitted. A summary score was computed by averaging the four relevant items. This generosity scale showed a substantial range (scores varied from 1 to 5), a mean near the scale's midpoint ($M = 3.34$), and a standard deviation of .79. The distribution was slightly negatively skewed ($-.37$), and kurtosis equaled .36.

Correlations with Validitational Variables[1]

Intercorrelations

As predicted, materialism was negatively correlated with generosity ($r = -.31$, $p < .01$). Frugality was uncorrelated with materialism ($r = -.08$, ns) and marginally positively correlated with generosity ($r = .12$, $p = .08$).

---

[1] I examined whether the patterns of correlations differed by subjects' gender, but no striking trends emerged.

*Table 4. Pearson Correlations between the Three Economic Attitude Variables
and Dependent Variables*

Variable	Frugality	Materialism	Generosity
Imaginary Windfall			
Stuff	−.25**	.28**	−.28**
Charity	.14*	−.19**	.44**
Gift	−.05	−.10	.15*
Save	.21**	−.17*	−.02
Environmental Behavior	.23**	−.21**	.23**
Well-being			
Happiness	.08	−.22**	.22**
Anxiety	−.11	.27**	−.11
Self-esteem	.19**	−.21**	.25**
Risk Behavior			
Cigarettes	−.25**	.11	−.20*
Alcohol	−.12	.15*	−.37**
Fight	−.15*	.16*	−.21**
School trouble	−.07	.09	−.18**

Note: $+ = p < .10.$ * $= p < .05.$ ** $= p < .01.$

Demographics

Correlations were computed between the three economic variables and subjects' age and grade. Generosity showed significant declines with age ($r = -.25$, $p < .01$) and grade ($r = -.19$, $p < .01$). Frugality showed trends in the same direction ($r = -.13$ with age, $p = .06$; and $r = -.11$ with grade, $p = .11$). Materialism was unrelated to either age or grade (both $ps > .66$).

Next we tested for gender differences. As expected, boys (mean $= 3.19$) were lower in generosity than were girls, mean $= 3.52$; $t(202) = -3.08$, $p < .01$. Boys also reported marginally higher materialism (mean $= 3.46$) than did girls, mean $= 3.26$; $t(203) = 1.82$, $p = .07$. No gender differences were detected for frugality ($p = .61$).

Prediction of Money Use

To test the validity of the three economic attitude measures in an economic situation, each was correlated with how participants reported they would spend the imaginary $100 windfall. As reported in the top portion of Table 4, frugal subjects expected to spend less money buying stuff for themselves, to give more to charity, and to save more. Materialistic subjects expected to spend more money buying stuff, to give less to charity, and to save less. Finally, generous subjects reported that they would buy less stuff, give more to charity, and spend more on gifts for others.

Relations to Environmental Resource Behaviors

The three economic variables also related to positive environmental behaviors (e.g., reusing paper, using less water while showering). Frugality and generosity were each positively correlated with such behaviors, whereas the reverse was true for materialism.

Relations to Personal Well-Being

The economic variables also related to several indices of personal well-being. Generosity was associated with more happiness and higher self-esteem. Materialism related to lower happiness and self-esteem and to more anxiety. Finally, frugality was associated with higher self-esteem; no evidence was found, however, to support Tatzel's (2002) predicted quadratic relationship between frugality and well-being.

Risk Behavior

Frugality was associated with less cigarette smoking and less fighting. Generous students reported less engagement in all four of the risk behaviors (i.e., smoking, drinking alcohol, fighting, and getting into trouble at school). Materialistic subjects reported more use of alcohol and more frequent fights.

Regressions with the Economic Attitude Measures

Finally, to determine whether the three economic attitude measures were redundant with each other or whether they each had independent predictive abilities, each dependent variable was simultaneously regressed onto frugality, materialism, and generosity. Because of the relatively large age range of this sample, age was also entered as a control variable.

These results are reported in Table 5. Frugality was an independent and significant predictor of spending little money on oneself and saving more money in the imaginary windfall; engaging in positive environmental behaviors; having high self-esteem; and not smoking cigarettes. Generosity was independently associated with giving more money to charity in the imaginary windfall; engaging in more positive environmental behaviors; being happier and having higher self-esteem; and less frequent alcohol use, fighting, and trouble at school. Finally, materialism related to a desire to spend more on oneself and to save less in the imaginary windfall; less frequent positive environmental behaviors; lower happiness and self-esteem scores; and greater anxiety.

Discussion

The results of this study suggest that the three measures of economic attitudes developed herein bear promise for future research. Each measure was composed of four items making up a single factor, demonstrated sufficient internal reliability, had relatively normal distributions, and related predictably to a number of variables chosen for the purposes of establishing the measures' construct validity.

Table 5. Simultaneous Regressions of Dependent Variables onto Age, Frugality, Materialism, and Generosity: Betas and R-Squared

Variable	Age	Frugality	Materialism	Generosity	R^2
Imaginary Windfall					
Stuff	.07	−.20**	.20**	−.17	.16**
Charity	−.27**	.05	−.08	.34**	.27**
Gift	.03	−.07	−.06	.14+	.03
Save	.06	.21**	−.17*	−.09	.08**
Environmental Behavior	.01	.20**	−.14*	.16*	.11**
Well-being					
Happiness	−.02	.04	−.16*	.16*	.08**
Anxiety	.04	−.08	.26**	−.01	.08**
Self-Esteem	.01	.15*	−.15*	.19*	.11**
Risk Behavior					
Cigarettes	.23**	−.20**	.05	−.10	.14**
Alcohol	.35**	−.04	.06	−.26**	.26**
Fight	−.18**	−.13+	.09	−.21**	.10**
School trouble	−.18*	−.06	.02	−.22**	.07**

Note: $+ = p < .10.$ * $= p < .05.$ ** $= p < .01.$

Overview of Results

As expected, materialism was associated with less generosity, but frugality was unrelated to either materialism or generosity, supporting their conceptual independence. Further, each economic attitude predicted its corresponding use of money in an imaginary windfall scenario. Those scoring high in frugality restrained themselves by using less money to buy themselves things and by saving more, whereas the reverse pattern was discovered for those scoring high in materialism. Generosity, in contrast, predicted how much individuals were willing to donate to church and charity. These results thus provide both predictive and differential validity for the measures.

Relationships with demographic features also support the measures' validity. Consistent with past research, females were more generous than were males, males were more materialistic than were females, and the genders did not differ in frugality. Concerning age, the results were interesting, and somewhat unsettling. Despite the fact that cognitive maturation should allow for greater financial restraint and concern for others, older children were less frugal and less generous than were younger children. These results may indicate that children are being successfully socialized into the consumer beliefs that one should buy what one wants when one wants it, and that they should keep their possessions to themselves, rather than share them. While this might be good news from the perspective of marketers and those who hope to indoctrinate the next generation into a consumer mentality that will support the growth of the U.S. economy, other results suggest numerous problems associated with such "successful" economic socialization.

Specifically, even after controlling for age and the effects of the other economic attitudes (see Table 5), those low in frugality reported lower self-esteem,
more use of cigarettes, and increased incidences of fighting with others. Those
low in generosity reported being less happy, having lower self-esteem, drinking
more alcohol, and getting into more fights and more trouble at school. Those high
in materialism reported less happiness, more anxiety, and lower self-esteem.

There are additional costs as well. As shown in Table 5, each of the three
economic attitudes bore independent associations with subjects' reports of resource use in the last few months. Subjects low in frugality or generosity, or high
in materialism, were unlikely to engage in relatively simple behaviors such as
turning off electric lights in unused rooms; reusing aluminum foil, plastic baggies, and paper; saving water while bathing or brushing one's teeth; and walking
or bicycling instead of driving a car. Americans currently consume resources at
an unsustainable rate that may be irrevocably damaging the biosphere (Winter,
2004). The present results suggest that the economic attitudes of frugality, generosity, and materialism play at least some role in such activity.

Limitations and Future Research

Results indicate that researchers interested in tracking trends in these three
attitudes, or in better understanding various dynamics concerning individual
differences in frugality, generosity, and materialism, might fruitfully use these
three short measures. However, there are three glaring weaknesses of the present
study that future research would do well to remedy. The first concerns the nature
of the sample. Although its size was adequate for the factor analyses conducted,
and it was heterogeneous with regard to gender, age, and parental education, it
was extremely homogeneous both geographically and racially. All students were
from a rural school district in western Illinois and almost all were Caucasian.
Thus, the structure of the economic attitude measures and/or their relations to
other variables may not hold for children and adolescents who live in urban
or suburban settings, for those outside the Midwest, and for those who are not
Caucasian. Future research should investigate these possibilities.

The second important weakness of the present study is that all measures
were self-report in nature. Future research should use a variety of different methods to explore the validity of the economic attitude measures. Will they predict
actual rather than imagined economic and ecologically relevant behavior? Will
they relate to diary rather than retrospective measures of happiness, drug use,
social behavior, and resource use? Will they agree with informants' assessments
of subjects' economic attitudes? Answering these and other questions will give
social scientists greater confidence in their validity.

The third key weakness of the current study concerns its historical fixity:
All data were collected in the first 2 weeks of January 2003, a particular moment associated with particular economic, global, and local facts. As described
in the introduction, frugality, materialism, and generosity are encouraged and
modeled to differing extents at different historical times (Shi, 1985). As the years

progress, social and economic circumstances will certainly change, and these might have important ramifications for these economic attitudes. For example, research suggests that economic and personal insecurity often increases materialism (Abramson & Inglehart, 1995; Kasser, 2002). Would this also be the case for frugality? Similarly, experimental work suggests that generosity decreases when people feel sad (Underwood, 1977), an emotion that might occur as a result of any number of social events. Further, how might changes in media practices, the increasing commercial use of the Internet, and other unimagined changes in our lives relate to the economic attitudes of children and adolescents? Answers to these questions clearly await tracking how frugality, generosity, and materialism change over time.

References

Abramson, P. R., & Inglehart, R. (1995). *Value change in global perspective*. Ann Arbor: University of Michigan Press.

Belk, R. W. (1984). Materialism: Trait aspects of living in the material world. *Journal of Consumer Research, 12*, 265–280.

Brown, K. W., & Kasser, T. (2003). *Values, happiness, and ecological behavior*. Unpublished manuscript, University of Rochester.

Cohen, P., & Cohen, J. (1996). *Life values and adolescent mental health*. Mahwah, NJ: Lawrence Erlbaum.

Comeau, H. (1980). Changes in self-reported values among students in grades 9–12. *Adolescence, 15*, 143–148.

DeYoung, R. (1986). Encouraging environmentally appropriate behavior: The role of intrinsic motivation. *Journal of Environmental Systems, 15*, 281–291.

Fincham, F., & Barling, J. (1978). Locus of control and generosity in learning disabled, normal achieving, and gifted children. *Child Development, 49*, 530–533.

Fordyce, M. W. (1988). A review of research on the happiness measures: A sixty second index of happiness and mental health. *Social Indicators Research, 20*, 355–381.

Froming, W. J., Allen, L., & Underwood, B. (1983). Age and generosity reconsidered: Cross-sectional and longitudinal evidence. *Child Development, 54*, 585–593.

Fromm, E. (1955). *The sane society*. New York: Fawcett.

Kasser, T. (2002). *The high price of materialism*. Cambridge, MA: MIT Press.

Kasser, T., & Ryan, R. M. (1993). A dark side of the American dream: Correlates of financial success as a central life aspiration. *Journal of Personality and Social Psychology, 65*, 410–422.

Kasser, T., & Ryan, R. M. (1996). Further examining the American dream: Differential correlates of intrinsic and extrinsic goals. *Personality and Social Psychology Bulletin, 22*, 280–287.

Kasser, T., & Ryan, R. M. (2001). Be careful what you wish for: Optimal functioning and the relative attainment of intrinsic and extrinsic goals. In P. Schmuck & K. M. Sheldon (Eds.), *Life goals and well-being: Towards a positive psychology of human striving* (pp. 116–131). Goettingen, Germany: Hogrefe & Huber.

Kasser, T., Ryan, R. M., Couchman, C. E., & Sheldon, K. M. (2004). Materialistic values: Their causes and consequences. In T. Kasser & A. D. Kanner (Eds.), *Psychology and consumer culture: The struggle for a good life in a materialistic world* (pp. 11–28). Washington, DC: American Psychological Association.

Lastovicka, J. L., Bettencourt, L. A., Hughner, R. S., & Kuntze, R. J. (1999). Lifestyle of the tight and frugal: Theory and measurement. *Journal of Consumer Research, 26*, 85–98.

McHoskey, J. W. (1999). Machiavellianism, intrinsic versus extrinsic goals, and social interest: A self-determination theory analysis. *Motivation and Emotion, 23*, 267–283.

Miller, S. M., Ginsburg, H. J., & Rogow, S. G. (1981). Self-esteem and sharing in fourth-grade children. *Social Behavior and Personality, 9*, 211–212.

Reynolds, C. R., & Richmond, B. O. (1978). What I think and feel: A revised measure of children's manifest anxiety. *Journal of Abnormal Child Psychology, 6,* 271–280.

Richins, M. L., & Dawson, S. (1992). A consumer values orientation for materialism and its measurement: Scale development and validation. *Journal of Consumer Research, 19,* 303–316.

Rosenberg, M. (1965). *Society and the adolescent self-image.* Princeton: Princeton University Press.

Schor, J. (2004). *Born to buy: Marketing and the transformation of childhood and culture.* New York: Scribner and Sons.

Schwartz, S. H. (1996). Values priorities and behavior: Applying of theory of integrated value systems. In C. Seligman, J. M. Olson, & M. P. Zanna (Eds.), *The psychology of values: The Ontario Symposium* (Vol. 8, pp. 1–24). Hillsdale, NJ: Lawrence Erlbaum.

Sheldon, K. M., & McGregor, H. (2000). Extrinsic value orientation and the tragedy of the commons. *Journal of Personality, 68,* 383–411.

Sheldon, K. M., Sheldon, M. S., & Osbaldiston, R. (2000). Prosocial values and group assortation in an N-person prisoner's dilemma. *Human Nature, 11,* 387–404.

Shi, D. (1985). *The simple life.* New York: Oxford University Press.

Tatzel, M. (2002). "Money worlds" and well-being: An integration of money dispositions, materialism, and price-related behavior. *Journal of Economic Psychology, 23,* 103–126.

Underwood, B. (1977). Attention, negative affect, and altruism: An ecological validation. *Personality and Social Psychology Bulletin, 3,* 54–58.

Weissbrod, C. S. (1980). The impact of warmth and instructions on donation. *Child Development, 51,* 279–281.

Williams, G. C., Cox, E. M., Hedberg, V. A., & Deci, E. L. (2000). Extrinsic life goals and health risk behaviors in adolescents. *Journal of Applied Social Psychology, 30,* 1756–1771.

Winter, D. D. (2004). Shopping for sustainability: Psychological solutions to overconsumption. In T. Kasser & A. D. Kanner (Eds.), *Psychology and consumer culture: The struggle for a good life in a materialistic world* (pp. 69–87). Washington, DC: American Psychological Association.

Zarbatany, L., Hartmann, D. P., & Gelfand, D. M. (1985). Why does children's generosity increase with age: Susceptibility to experimenter influence or altruism? *Child Development, 56,* 746–756.

Contributors

Eric M. Anderman is director of graduate studies and associate professor in the Department of Educational and Counseling Psychology at the University of Kentucky. His research interests include aspects of adolescent motivation, prevention of risky behaviors during adolescence, academic cheating, and the effects of school transitions on psychological and academic outcomes.

Molly Andolina is an assistant professor of political science at DePaul University in Chicago. A previous survey director at the Pew Research Center, she has published work on public opinion and the Clinton scandal and Generation X in the 2000 election.

Bonnie L. Barber is a professor of family studies and human development at the University of Arizona. Her research interests include adolescent and young adult social relationships across life transitions, long-term benefits of activity participation, and positive development in divorced families. She has also studied the effectiveness of empirically based curricula for divorced mothers with adolescents in the United States and Australia, and collaborated on a U.S. outcome evaluation of programs for youth and families at risk.

Brian K. Barber is a professor of child and family studies at the University of Tennessee. His research focuses on family, peer, school, community, and religious influences in adolescent development, and he has conducted survey and interview studies of these issues in cultures in Asia, Australia, the Balkans, Europe, the Middle East, South America, and among ethnic minorities in the United States. Since 1994, Dr. Barber has also been studying adolescent development in contexts of political violence, comparing youth from the Gaza Strip, Palestine, and Sarajevo, Bosnia.

Peter L. Benson is president of Search Institute in Minneapolis, which provides leadership, knowledge, and resources to promote healthy children, youth, and communities. He has written extensively on adolescent development, altruism, and spiritual development. He serves as principal investigator for Search Institute's initiative on spiritual development in childhood and adolescence, which is supported by the John Templeton Foundation, and is general editor for the Search Institute Series on Developmentally Attentive Community and Society, published by Kluwer Academic/Plenum Publishers.

Alysia Y. Blandon is a graduate student in the developmental program in the Department of Psychology at the University of Michigan. Her research addresses the links between marital relationship quality, parental differential treatment, and sibling adjustment outcomes.

Phyllis Blumenfeld is a professor of education and psychology at the University of Michigan. Her research interests are learning environments, school engagement, and motivation. She has published in *Review of Educational Research, Educational Psychologist,* and *Elementary School Journal.*

Sally C. Curtin is currently a research assistant in the Department of Family Studies at the University of Maryland, College Park. Previously, she worked as a statistician for more than 12 years at the National Center for Health Statistics, helping to compile and analyze vital statistics data on births, marriages, divorces, and infant deaths. Her research interests include studying the family demographics and dynamics of child health and well-being, particularly the role of maternal employment.

Jacquelynne S. Eccles is Wilbert McKeachie Collegiate Professor of Psychology, Women's Studies and Education, as well as a research scientist at the Institute for Social Research at the University of Michigan. Over the past 30 years, she has conducted research on a wide variety of topics, including gender role socialization, teacher expectancies, classroom influences on student motivation, and social development in the family and school context. Dr. Eccles is a member of the MacArthur Foundation Network on Successful Adolescent Development and chair of the MacArthur Foundation on Successful Pathways through Middle Childhood.

Sylvia R. Epps is a doctoral student in human development and family sciences at the University of Texas, Austin. She is a graduate research assistant to Aletha Huston on the New Hope Project, a study of the effects on children and families of parents' participation in a work-based program to reduce poverty. Her research focuses on understanding the pathways whereby poverty impacts parents and children and the effect the alleviation of poverty has on child well-being.

Jennifer A. Fredricks is an assistant professor in human development at Connecticut College. She is a currently a postdoctoral fellow at the Spencer Foundation and National Academy of Education. Her research interests are motivation and school engagement, extracurricular participation, school reform, and gender socialization.

Jeanne Friedel is a doctoral student in education and psychology at the University of Michigan. Her research interests include school engagement and motivation among at-risk students, and community and family influences on motivation.

Sarah B. Garrett is a senior research assistant at Child Trends. She is interested in the effects of social relationships, family structure, parental employment, and family religiosity on children and youth.

Penny Gordon-Larsen is an assistant professor of nutrition in the Schools of Public Health and Medicine at the University of North Carolina. Primarily, her research centers on patterns and determinants of obesity in U.S. adolescents, with a focus on sociodemographic and environmental determinants of physical activity and obesity.

Elizabeth C. Hair is a senior research associate at Child Trends. Her research focuses on the influence of social relationships and skills on children's development, positive youth development, and the links between parental education and children's health and well-being.

Kathleen Mullan Harris is Gillian T. Cell Professor of Sociology at the University of North Carolina at Chapel Hill. Her main areas of research are family, poverty, adolescent development, and health.

Sandra L. Hofferth is a professor in the Department of Family Studies at the University of Maryland, College Park. She is the founding director of the Child Development Supplement of the Michigan Panel Study of Income Dynamics. Dr. Hofferth's research looks at fathers' investments in children, U.S. children's use of time, adolescent childbearing, and public assistance policy.

E. Scott Huebner is a professor and director of the School Psychology Program at the University of South Carolina. His research interests involve the conceptualization, measurement, and implications of positive well-being constructs for the delivery of psychological services to children and youth in schools.

Aletha C. Huston is Pricilla Pond Flawn Regents Professor in Child Development and Family Relationships at the University of Texas, Austin. She is a principal investigator in the New Hope Project, a study of the effects on children and families of parents' participation in a work-based program to reduce poverty.

Krista Jenkins is an assistant professor in the School of History, Political Science, and International Studies at Fairleigh Dickinson University in New Jersey.

Stuart A. Karabenick is a professor of psychology at Eastern Michigan University and currently a visiting professor in the combined program in education and psychology at the University of Michigan. His research focuses on motivation, self-regulation, and achievement, with specific interest in such areas as help seeking, delay of gratification, and personal epistemological beliefs.

Tim Kasser is an associate professor of psychology at Knox College in Galesburg, Illinois. He is the author of numerous scientific articles and book chapters on materialism, values, and goals, among other topics. He is the author of *The High Price of Materialism* (2002) and coeditor, with Allen D. Kanner, of *Psychology and Consumer Culture: The Struggle for a Good Life in a Materialistic World* (2004).

Scott Keeter is associate director of the Pew Research Center for the People and the Press. His publications include research on public opinion, political knowledge, religion and politics, and survey methodology.

Rosalind Berkowitz King is a social science analyst at the National Institute of Child Health and Human Development of the National Institutes of Health (NIH). Her research focuses on adolescent social and physical development, union formation, and fertility.

Akemi Kinukawa is a senior research analyst at Child Trends. She is interested in the effects of social relationships, family structure, parental employment, and family religiosity on children and youth.

Laura H. Lippman is the area director for data and measurement at Child Trends. Ms. Lippman is a demographer who develops positive indicators of child well-being and the social context of families. Her work also includes cross-national analyses on family processes and education outcomes.

Clea McNeely is an associate professor in the Bloomberg School of Public Health at Johns Hopkins University. Her research addresses adolescent sexuality, program evaluation, and how communities and schools influence adolescent health behaviors. Dr. McNeely is a 2002 recipient of the William T. Grant Foundation Scholar Award for the study how the social environment in middle and high schools influences health-related behaviors during the transition to adulthood.

Erik Michelsen was formerly a research analyst at Child Trends. Many of his research interests relate to antecedents of youth civic engagement, including community service participation and political involvement.

Kristin Anderson Moore is president of Child Trends. Dr. Moore is a social psychologist who studies trends in child and family well-being, positive development, the determinants of early sexual activity and parenthood, the consequences of adolescent parenthood, the effects of family structure and social change on children, and the effects of welfare and poverty on children.

Susan A. O'Neill is currently a visiting scholar with the Faculty of Education at Simon Fraser University, Canada. Her research interests include motivation, identity, and gender issues associated with young people's engagement in arts and structured out-of-school activities. Dr. O'Neill is director of the Young People and Music Participation Project funded by the Economic and Social Research Council. She has published widely in the fields of music psychology and music education.

Alison Paris is an assistant professor of developmental psychology at Claremont McKenna College. Her research interests include cognitive development, learning and motivation in educational contexts, school engagement, and early literacy development.

Nansook Park is an assistant professor of psychology at the University of Rhode Island. Using cross-cultural and developmental perspectives, she is interested in investigating the structures, correlates, and consequences of positive experiences, life satisfaction, and character strengths, and especially their role in promoting positive development and resiliency among youth. Her recent work with subjective well-being with children and adolescents has received several honors, including the 1999 APA Dissertation Research Award.

Seoung Eun Park is a graduate student in human development and family sciences at the University of Texas, Austin. Her research focuses on children's electronic media use as a context of family life that both affects and is affected by parenting styles and parent–child interactions.

Helen Patrick is an assistant professor of educational psychology at Purdue University. Her research interests include student motivation and engagement, and their associations with teacher practices and students' perceptions of their classroom environment.

Christopher Peterson is a professor of psychology at the University of Michigan, where he formerly was the director of clinical training and held an appointment as the Arthur F. Thurnau Professor, in honor of his contributions to undergraduate teaching. He has a long-standing interest in personality and adaptation, and his most recent project is a consensual classification of the character strengths and virtues that make possible the psychological good life.

Paul R. Pintrich was a professor in the combined program in education and psychology at the University of Michigan, Ann Arbor. His many empirical and theoretical contributions in the areas of motivation and self-regulated learning made him one of the foremost scholars in his field. Tragically, Paul Pintrich died during the time the chapter he coauthored for this book was being finalized. His coauthors miss him as a scholar and colleague but even more so as a friend.

Marika Ripke is the project director for Kids Count Hawaii at the University of Hawaii's Center on the Family. Among her current work and research initiatives are assessing and evaluating the impacts of poverty, homelessness, and welfare and employment programs on parents' and children's well-being; examining supports and opportunities for positive development during the middle childhood years; and aiding in the development of a statewide strategic plan for early childhood development in conjunction with Hawaii's Department of Health.

Eugene C. Roehlkepartain is director of family and congregation initiatives and senior adviser to the president of Search Institute in Minneapolis.

Robert Roeser is currently an assistant professor of education in the Psychological Studies in Education program at Stanford University. His research focuses on the relation between young people's academic and social-emotional development within the context of school during and across the childhood and adolescent years. He is currently researching issues of culture, motivation to learn, and mental health in ethnically diverse groups of adolescents as they move from middle into high school.

Allison M. Ryan is assistant professor in educational psychology at the University of Illinois, Urbana-Champaign. Her research interests include student motivation, help-seeking beliefs and behaviors, peer relations, adolescent development, and social influences on achievement beliefs and behaviors.

Peter C. Scales is senior fellow in the Office of the President at Search Institute. He is a developmental psychologist widely recognized for his work on adolescent development, family relationships, effective schools, and healthy communities. In addition to more than 250 scientific articles and chapters, Dr. Scales is author or coauthor of more than a dozen books and monographs.

Arturo Sesma Jr. is an applied developmental researcher at Search Institute in Minneapolis. He specializes in the conceptualization and measurement of developmental assets, social development in middle childhood and adolescence, risk and resilience models for children at risk, and developmental theory.

C. R. Snyder is M. Erik Wright Distinguished Professor of Clinical Psychology in the Department of Psychology at the University of Kansas, Lawrence. His books on hope include *The Psychology of Hope: You Can Get There from Here* (1994), *Making Hope Happen* (1999), *The Handbook of Hope* (2000), *The Great Big Book of Hope: Helping Children Reach Their Dreams* (2000), and *Hope for the Journey* (2003).

Margaret R. Stone, an assistant research scientist in the Department of Family Studies and Human Development at the University of Arizona, has been associated with the Michigan Study of Life Transitions since 1998. Her research focuses on adolescent development, especially extracurricular activities and the intersection between adolescent social development, social cognitive development, and intergroup relations. She is particularly interested in the peer "crowd" as an emergent social category through which adolescents forge interpretations of their peer world and of their own social identities.

Shannon M. Suldo recently received a doctorate through the School Psychology Program at the University of South Carolina and also completed a predoctoral internship program at the Kennedy Krieger Institute/Johns Hopkins University School of Medicine. Her research interests include the developmental course of life satisfaction during adolescence, effects of parenting behaviors on adolescent mental health, and positive indicators of children's psychological well-being.

Adriana J. Umaña-Taylor is an assistant professor of human development and family studies at the University of Illinois at Urbana-Champaign. Her research focuses broadly on adolescent development and family resiliency and, more specifically, on ethnic identity formation and positive developmental outcomes among Latino adolescents.

Tim Urdan is an associate professor in the Department of Psychology at Santa Clara University near San Francisco. His research interests include effective methods of educating adolescents, teacher and classroom influences on student motivation, and cultural variations in motivation. He is coeditor, along with Frank Pajares, of *Adolescence and Education: Volume 3, International Perspectives on Adolescence* (2003).

Robert F. Valois is a professor of health promotion, education, and behavior in the Arnold School of Public Health and a professor of family and preventive medicine in the School of Medicine at the University of South Carolina. Dr. Valois's research involves child, adolescent, and school health; adolescent risk behavior; quality of life and positive youth development; and program evaluation.

Brenda L. Volling is an associate professor in the Department of Psychology at the University of Michigan. Her main research interests are the relations between family subsystems, including the marital, parent–child, and sibling dyads. Her most recent work focuses on sibling jealousy and the child and family factors that predict young children's jealous responses.

Allan Wigfield is a professor of human development and Distinguished Scholar-Teacher at the University of Maryland, College Park. He currently is collaborating with John Guthrie on a Natonal Science Foundation–funded study of how two reading programs, Concept Oriented Reading Instruction and Strategy Instruction, influence elementary school–age children's reading motivation and comprehension.

Christopher A. Wolters is an associate professor in the Department of Educational Psychology at the University of Houston. His research focuses on the motivational and metacognitive aspects of self-regulated learning during adolescence. In particular, he has examined the ways in which adolescents regulate their cognitive and motivational processing, and the influence of this self-regulation on academic and psychosocial functioning. His recent work in these areas has appeared in the *Journal of Educational Psychology* and *Educational Psychologist*.

Cliff Zukin is a professor of public policy and political science at the Eagleton Institute of Politics, Rutgers University. He is also director of the Star-Ledger/Eagleton-Rutgers Poll, a quarterly survey of New Jersey residents.

Index

A&B: *see Search Institute Profiles of Student Life*
Ability self-perceptions, 7, 237–248; *see also*
    Academic scales
Academic cognition, 251–254, 262–264; *see also*
    Cognitive achievement
Academic goals: *see* School, goals
Academic motivation: *see* Achievement
    motivation
Academic scales
    ability/expectancy, 246–247
    factor analyses, 239–243, 244–245
    generally, 239–248
    perceived task difficulty, 247
    perceived task value, 247–248; *see also*
        Task values
    validity, 241–243, 245–246
    for younger children, 243–246
Achievement goals: *see* School, goals
Achievement motivation, 251, 253–258,
    262–266
Activities, organized; *see also*
        Michigan Study of Adolescent
        Life Transitions; Outdoor
    activities; Time use; specific activities
    and civic engagement, 143
    gender differences, 138
    measures of involvement, 134–136
    and outcomes, high school, 141–142
    and outcomes, young adulthood, 142–143
    participation in, generally, 5, 133–145
    and peer groups, 134, 140
    and positive development, 133
    and prosocial orientation, 5, 141
    and psychological adjustment, 143
    and self-concept, 140–141
    and social identity, 134
    and task values, 140–141
Add Health: *see* National Longitudinal Study of
    Adolescent Health
Adolescent's Perception of
    Deprivation-Satisfaction Scale, 186
Adult relationships, *see also* Parent–Adolescent
    Relationship Scale
    importance of, 272
    networks of, 34–35
Adult Sibling Relationship Questionnaire, 205

Alcohol use: *see* Risk behaviors
Altruism
    and generosity, 359
    and volunteering, 343–344
Altruistic Behavior Scale, 341
America's Children (2003), 2–3, 9
Anderman, Eric M., 7
Andolina, Molly, 8
Andrews and Withey one-item scale, 45
Annie E. Casey Foundation, 2–3, 9
Anxiety
    and materialism, 369
    and well-being, 364
Art, and time use, 98; *see also* Performing arts
Aspinwall, L. G., 38
Aspiration Index, 364
Assets, developmental: *see* Developmental
    assets
Attainment value, defined, 7
Autonomy, 6, 178

Barber, Bonnie L., 5
Barber, Brian K., 5–6
Behavior Problem Index (BPI), 164–165
Behavior problems, and time use, 107–108;
        see also Risk behaviors
Benson, Peter L., 4, 8, 34n
Blandon, Alysia Y., 6
Blumenfeld, Phyllis, 7–8
BMSLSS: *see* Brief Multidimensional Students'
        Life Satisfaction Scale
Body image, and healthy habits, 5, 113–114, 118,
    124–126
Boundaries, and expectations, as
        developmental assets, 34n
Brief Multidimensional Students' Life
        Satisfaction Scale (BMSLSS), *see also*
        Students' Life Satisfaction Scale
    demographics, 54–55
    factor analysis, 52
    generally, 41–42, 50–56
    reliability, 52
    responses and scoring, 51, 56
    samples, 51
    validity, 52–54
Brother–Sister Questionnaire, 205

CDS: *see* Child Development Supplement
Centers for Disease Control and Prevention, 95, 343
Character strengths
 components and definitions, 13–17
 measures, 13–15
 signature strengths, 20
  and values, 3–4, 13–22; *see also* Values; Values in Action Inventory of Character Strengths for Youth (VIA Youth); Values in Action (VIA) Classification of Strengths
 in very young children, 15
 and virtues, 13–14, 17, 19
 among youth, 17–19
Child Behavior Checklist, 163–164
Child Depression Inventory, 65
Child Development Supplement (CDS), 5, 165–167
 assessments and analysis, 102
 cognitive development, 102
 data and methods, 99–102
 demographics, 102, 105
 generally, 99–102
 math scales, 245–246
 negative indicators, 107
 positive indicators, 107
 reading scales, 245–246
 reliability, 101
 results, 102–108
 time use, measures, 95, 99–109; *see also* Time use
 validity, 101
Child Evaluation of Relationship with Mother/Caregiver measure, 167–168
Child Health Supplement, 164–165
Child–Parent Relationship Scale, 186
Child Trends, 3, 6, 192, 195–198, 309
Children's Hope Scale (CHS), *see also* Hope
 factor analyses, 68
 gender differences, 4, 67, 69
 generally, 4, 63–71
 psychometrics, 64, 69
 racial differences, 4, 69
 responses and scoring, 71
 samples, 63–64, 66–71
 status, 66–71
 validity, 64–66, 69–70
Children's Social Desirability Questionnaire, 65
CHS: *see* Children's Hope Scale
Cigarette smoking: *see* Risk behaviors
Civic engagement, *see also* Community service; Volunteering
 age differences, 334

and citizenship, 326
and cognitive engagement, 327
community-based, 329–332
community problem solving, measured, 330, 337
defined, 327
generally, 8, 325–337
group memberships, 331–332, 333, 337
measures, 327–337
and organized activities, 143
and political engagement, 325–329, 342
and prosocial orientation, 143, 339–340, 342–343
Classrooms: *see* School
Cognition, as learning strategy, 7; *see also* Academic cognition; Cognitive achievement; Cognitive development; Cognitive engagement
Cognitive achievement, and time use, 105, 107; *see also* Academic cognition
Cognitive development, 62, 102
Cognitive engagement, 305–309, 311–315, 319, 327
Community life: *see* Civic engagement; Community service; Volunteering
Community service, *see also* Civic engagement; Volunteering
 gender differences, 351–352
 measures, 342–344
 and prosocial orientation, 8, 339–354
Computers, and time use, 5, 96–97, 108
Conduct Problems Prevention Research Group, 204
Cost value, defined, 7
Curiosity, as character strength, 15
Current Population Survey (1997), 100
Curtin, Sally C., 5

Developmental assets
 categories of, 34n
 and spirituality/religion, 25, 27n, 31–35
Developmental outcomes, *see also* Positive outcomes
 and school, 142–143, 296–300
 and spirituality/religion, 31–35
Diagnostic and Statistical Manual (APA), 15
Diet, and healthy habits, 113, 117–118, 123–124
Diversity, ethnic: *see* Ethnic identity; Race and ethnicity
DOTS-R Mood scale, 45

Eating habits: *see* Diet
Eccles, Jacquelynne S., 5, 7
Eck, Diana, 26

Economic attitudes, *see also* Family income
  age/grade differences, 360–361, 366–367, 370
  and behavior, 361
  demographics, 368, 370, 371
  and environmental behaviors, 357–369
  future research, 371–372
  gender differences, 360–361, 366–367
  generally, 8, 357–372
  imaginary windfalls, 361, 365, 368
  intercorrelations, 360, 367
  measures and studies, 358–360, 363–372
  prediction of money use, 368
  and risk behaviors, 362, 368, 369
Ego and Social Goals scale, 224
EIS: *see* Ethnic Identity Scale
Empathy, and intrapersonal relationships, 148, 158
Empowerment, as developmental asset, 34n
Epps, Sylvia R., 6
Erikson, E. H., 16, 75–78, 89–90
Ethnic identity, and self-esteem, 75, 79, 81–82, 85, 88, 90; *see also* Ethnic Identity Scale; Multigroup Ethnic Identity Measure; Race and ethnicity
Ethnic Identity Scale (EIS)
  generally, 4–5, 75–90
  measures, 79–80
  methodology, 78–80, 89
  psychometrics, 78, 90
  reliability, 80
  responses and scoring, 82–89
  samples, 80, 84, 86–87
  validity, 80–82, 84, 87, 90
Ethnicity: *see* Ethnic identity; Race and ethnicity
Evaluation of Welfare-to-Work Strategies, 309
Exercise, and healthy habits, 5, 112–113, 117, 121–123; *see also* Outdoor activities; Sports

Familial Ethnic Socialization Measure (2001), 78–82, 85–86, 88
Family: *see* Parent–Adolescent Relationship Scale; Sibling Inventory of Behavior
Family and Child Well-Being Research Network, 109
Family income, 4, 142–143; *see also* Economic attitudes; Panel Study of Income Dynamics
Federal Interagency Forum on Child and Family Statistics, 1–3, 9
Fighting: *see* Risk behaviors
Finances and money: *see* Economic attitudes; Family income
Flourishing youth, 1, 9

4-H, 342–343
Fredricks, Jennifer A., 7–8
Friedel, Jeanne, 7–8
Frugality, 8, 357–372

Garrett, Sarah B., 6
General Social Survey (1998), 37
Generosity, 8, 357–372
Goal orientation theory, 231
Goals, *see also* School, goals; specific goals
  agency thinking, 4, 61–62
  and hope, 61–63
  pathways thinking, 4, 61–62
Gordon-Larsen, Penny, 5
"Guide to the Index of Civic and Political Engagement, A," 329n

Hair, Elizabeth C., 6
Happiness, and well-being, 364
Harris, Kathleen Mullan, 5
Hart, Daniel, 20
Healthy habits, *see also* Body image; Diet; Exercise; Sleep
  age differences, 119–128
  gender differences, 118–128
  generally, 5, 111–129
  literature review, 112–115
  measures, 116–119
  and positive development, 111
  race/ethnicity differences, 118–128
  relationships among indicators, 126–128
Hobbies, and time use, 98
Hofferth, Sandra L., 5
Homework: *see* School
Hope
  cognitive building blocks, 62
  and goals, 61–63
  in infants-toddlers, 62–63
  measuring, 4, 61–71; *see also* Children's Hope Scale
  motivation, 61–63
  self-perceptions, 61–63
  as virtue, 19
Hopelessness Scale for Children, 61, 66
Housework, and time use, 5, 9, 98–99, 109
Huebner, E. Scott, 4
Human strengths: *see* Character strengths
Huston, Aletha C., 6

Identity, *see also* Ethnic identity; Positive identity; Social identity
  salience, 75
  and socialization, 357, 370
Identity formation theory, 75–76
Independent Sector surveys, 352–353

Index of Child's Perceptions of Parent's
Dissatisfaction, 186
Indicators of Positive Youth Development
Conference (March 2003), 1–8, 20–21
Interpersonal relationships
and economic attitudes, 358
generally, 5–6, 147–159
with parents, 148, 159; see also Ogden Youth
and Family Project
with peers, 148, 159
social initiative, 148, 158–159
Intrapersonal relationships, 5–6, 147–159; see
also Ogden Youth and Family Project
Intrinsic value, defined, 7

Jenkins, Krista, 8
John Templeton Foundation, 1–2

Kaiser Family Foundation/MTV, 325, 326
Karabenick, Stuart A., 7
Kasser, Tim, 8
Keeter, Scott, 8
Keyes, C. L. M., 1, 9
Kids Count Data Book (2003), 2–3, 9
King, Rosalind Berkowitz, 5
Kinukawa, Akemi, 6
Knowledge Networks, 329n

Learn and Serve America, 342
Learning, see also Motivated Strategies for
Learning Questionnaire; Patterns of
Adaptive Learning Survey; School
commitment to, 34n
and help seeking, 259–261, 266–268
positive attitude/behavior toward, 6–8
self-regulated, 251–268
Learning strategies, 7
Life satisfaction
defined, 41–42
generally, 4, 41–56
research with adults and youth, 42; see also
Brief Multidimensional Students' Life
Satisfaction Scale; Students' Life
Satisfaction Scale
Lifespan Sibling Relationship Scale, 205
Lippman, Laura H., vii
Locus of Control scale, 65
Loneliness and Social Dissatisfaction
Questionnaire, 167

MacArthur Network for Successful Pathways
through Middle School, 310
Manuel D. and Rhoda Mayerson Foundation,
20–21
Mastery, defined, 7

Materialism, 8, 357–372
McNeely, Clea, 7
Media, and time use, 96–97
Michelsen, Erik, 6
Michigan Childhood and Beyond Study, 243
Michigan Study of Adolescent Life Transitions
(MSALT)
design and samples, 135–136
questions asked, 144–145
responses, analyses, 136–139
social activities, participation measures,
135–145
validity, 139–142
Money and finances: see Economic attitudes;
Family income
Monitoring the Future, 27–28
Moore, Kristin Anderson, vii
Moral activity, 14
Motivated Strategies for Learning
Questionnaire (MSLQ)
academic behavior, regulation of, 258–263,
266–268
academic cognition, regulation of, 251–254,
262–264
achievement motivation, regulation of, 251,
254–258, 262–266
age/grade differences, 253
generally, 7, 252–268
Motivation, see also Achievement motivation
and achievement/performance goals, 231,
278
and hope, 61–63
as learning strategy, 7
MSALT: see Michigan Study of Adolescent Life
Transitions
MSLQ: see Motivated Strategies for Learning
Questionnaire
Multidimensional Measure of Children's
Perceptions of Control, 65
Multidimensional Students' Life Satisfaction
Scale (MSLSS), 52–53
Multigroup Ethnic Identity Measure (MEIM),
76–77

National Child Care Study (NHIS), 246
National Council of Teachers of Mathematics,
272
National Educational Longitudinal Study
(NELS), 308–309
National Health Interview Survey (NHIS),
164–165
National Household Education Survey
(NHES), 342
National Institute of Child Health and Human
Development (NICHD), 109, 129, 200, 246

National Institute of Health (NIH), 112
National Institute of Mental Health (NIMH),
        149, 157
National Longitudinal Study of Adolescent
        Health (Add Health)
    demographics, 294, 299–300
    healthy habits measures, 5, 111–112, 115–116
    outcomes, 296–300
    parent–child relationships, 187
    psychometrics, 292–295, 301
    reliability, 294
    religiosity measures, 27
    school connectedness measures, 7, 289–302
    validity, 295–297
National Longitudinal Survey of Youth
        (NLSY1997), 6, 165, 187–200; see also
        Parent–Adolescent Relationship Scale
National Research Council and Institute of
        Medicine, 25
National Science Education Standards, 271–272
National Survey of America's Families (NSAF),
        309
Network and Attachment Loneliness Scale, 65
New Chance study, 165–167
New Hope project, 165–176
New Religious America, A (Eck), 26
NICHD: see National Institute of Child Health
        and Human Development
NLSY1997: see National Longitudinal Survey of
        Youth

Obesity, health consequences of, 112; see also
        Healthy habits
Ogden Youth and Family Project (OYFP), see
        also Interpersonal relationships;
        Intrapersonal relationships
    demographics, 153
    generally, 149–159
    measures, 149
    psychometrics, 149, 151–152
    reliability, 149–153, 156–167
    samples, 156
    validity, 154–155, 157
O'Neill, Susan A., 7
Outdoor activities, 97; see also Exercise; Sports
OYFP: see Ogden Youth and Family Project

PALS: see Patterns of Adaptive Learning Survey
Panel Study of Income Dynamics (PSID), 5, 95,
        99–100, 109, 165–177, 245–256
Parent–Adolescent Relationship Scale, see also
        Adult relationships; Parent–youth
        relationships
    cut point, 189
    demographics, 191–192, 195–199

    generally, 6, 183–200
    measures, 186–189
    methodology, 187–190
    procedures, 189–190
    reliability, 191
    results, 190–197
    samples, 187–188
    validity, 192–194
Parent–youth relationships, and
        communication, 148, 159
Parental Control Measures, 186
Parental Expectations and Perceptions of
        Children's Sibling Relationships
        Questionnaire, 205
Parents, and school engagement, 309
Paris, Alison, 7–8
Park, Nansook, 3–4
Park, Seoung Eun, 6
Patrick, Helen, 7
Patterns of Adaptive Learning Survey (PALS)
    generally, 7, 223–232
    manuals and documentation, 227n
    measures, 224–226
    Personal Goal Orientation Scales, 232
    psychometrics, 229–230
    reliability, 228
    validity, 229
Peer groups
    and interpersonal relationships, 148, 159
    and organized activities, 134, 140
    and school connectedness, 296
Perceived Life Satisfaction Scale, 45
Performance, definitions, 7
Performance avoidance: see School
Performance goals: see School, goals
Performing arts, participation in, 141
Persistence, as character strength, 15
Personal and Social Responsibility Scale,
        340–341
Personal Goal Orientation Scales, 232
Perspective taking, and intrapersonal
        relationships, 148, 158
Peterson, Christopher, 3–4
Pew Charitable Trusts, 329, 336–337
Pew Research Council for the People and the
        Press, 325–326
Physical activity: see Exercise; Outdoor
        activities; Sports
Piers-Harris Happiness subscale, 45
Pintrich, Paul R., 7
Play, 99
Positive behavior: see Positive social behavior
Positive Behavior Scale
    autonomy subscales, 178
    compliance subscales, 178

Positive Behavior Scale (*cont.*)
  demographics, 169–174
  generally, 6, 165–178
  measures, 166–168
  psychometrics, 165
  reliability, 168
  samples, 165–166
  social competence subscales, 177
  validity, 168–174
Positive identity, as developmental asset, 34n
Positive indicators, 1–2, 7, 9, 107
Positive outcomes, 1–3, 9; *see also*
      Developmental outcomes
  and prosocial orientation, 349
  and risk behaviors, 25, 349
  and school, 141–142
Positive social behavior, 5–6, 8, 34n, 163–178; *see*
      also Prosocial orientation; Social
      competencies
Profiles of Student Life: *see* Search Institute
      Profiles of Student Life
Prosocial orientation, *see also* Positive social
      behavior; Social competencies
  and civic engagement, 143, 339–340, 342–343
  and community service, 8, 339–354
  demographics, 346–347
  gender differences, 351–352
  and generosity, 359
  measures, 340–342, 344–346, 354
  and organized activities, 5, 141
  and risk behaviors/thriving indicators,
      347–349
Prosocial Personality Battery, 341
Prosocial Tendencies Measure-Revised, 341–342
PSID: *see* Panel Study of Income Dynamics
Psychological adjustment
  and organized activities, 143
  and sibling relationships, 204
Psychology, and study of psychopathological
      conditions, 41
Psychology of Human Strengths, A (APA), 27
Psychopathological conditions, study of, 41
Public affairs: *see* Civic engagement

Race and ethnicity, *see also* Ethnic identity
  healthy habits, 118–128
  and hope, 4, 69
  measured, 4, 79
  and school social environment, 281–283
  and spirituality/religion, 28–30, 33
RAPS: *see* Rochester Assessment Package for
      Schools
Reading for pleasure, and time use, 5, 97–98,
      108
Religion: *see* Spirituality and religion

Revised Children's Manifest Anxiety Scale, 364
Ripke, Marika, 6
Risk behaviors, *see also* Behavior problems
  and economic attitudes, 362, 368, 369
  and parent–child relationships, 184–185
  and positive outcomes, 25, 349
  and prosocial orientation, 347–349
  and school connectedness, 296–300
  and thriving indicators, 27n, 32–35, 347–349
  and well-being, 364
Rochester Assessment Package for Schools
      (RAPS), 307–308
Roehlkepartain, Eugene C., 4, 34n, 35n
Roeser, Robert, 7
Ryan, Allison M., 7

Scales, Peter C., 4, 8
School, *see also* Learning
  adaptive classrooms, 7, 271–287
  age–grade differences in engagement, 314
  behavioral engagement, 305–309, 311–315
  classroom functioning, 296
  cognitive engagement, 305–309, 311–315, 319,
      327
  connectedness, 7, 289–302
  emotional engagement, 305–9, 311–315, 319
  engagement interviews, 315–317
  engagement/involvement in, 7–8, 142,
      143–44, 278, 305–319
  gender differences, 279, 281, 313
  goals, 7, 223–232, 251–268, 271–285
  grade point average, 143–144, 296–299, 301
  homework/studying, 97–98
  motivation, 231, 278
  mutual respect, promotion of, 271–285
  parent engagement, 309
  and peer relationships, 296
  positive attitude/feelings toward, 6–8, 290
  psychometrics, 311
  and social belonging/bonding, 7, 289–296,
      298, 300–302
  as social environment, 7, 271–287
  studying/homework, 97–98
  suspensions, 184–185, 296–299
  task-related interactions, 271–285
  teachers, and school connectedness, 7,
      292–296, 298, 300–302
  teachers, support by, 271–285
  as work of children, 99
School clubs, 142, 342
School trouble: *see* Risk behaviors
Schwartz, Arthur, 1–2
*Search Institute Profiles of Student Life: Attitudes
and Behaviors* survey 27, 31, 343–48
Search Institute, 8, 27–28, 31, 343

Self, positive formation of, 3–5
Self and Task Perception Questionnaire, 168
Self-concept, and organized activities,
    140–141
Self-consciousness, 272
Self-esteem
    and ethnic identity, 75, 79, 81–82, 85, 88, 90
    and frugality/materialism, 8, 369
    and intrapersonal relationships, 148, 151–152,
        157–158
    and well-being, 364
Self-esteem Scale (1979), 78, 81, 364
Self-Perception Profile for Children, 65
Self-perceptions
    ability and task values, 7, 237–248
    and hope, 61–63
    of spirituality/religion, 37
Self-recognition, and hope, 62
Self-regulated learning: see Learning
Self-reliance, and autonomy, 6
Self-Reported Altruism scale, 341
Self-restraint, and frugality, 362
Self-sufficiency, 357
Sesma, Arturo, Jr., 4
Sexual activity: see Risk behaviors
Shopping, and time use, 5, 98–99, 109
SIB: see Sibling Inventory of Behavior
Sibling Behaviors and Feelings Questionnaire,
    205
Sibling Inventory of Behavior (SIB)
    age differences, 213–214
    descriptive statistics, 210
    design and procedure, 208–209
    future directions, 216–217
    gender differences, 213–214
    generally, 6, 203–217
    limitations, 216–217
    measures, 209–210
    methodology, 207
    reliability, 210–211
    samples, 207–208, 216
    validity, 211–212
    well-being links, 212–213
Sibling Qualities Scale, 205
Sibling Relationship Inventory, 205
Sibling Relationship Questionnaire, 205
Sibling Relationships in Early Childhood
    Questionnaire, 205
Sleep, and healthy habits, 5, 114–115, 117,
    119–121
SLSS: see Students' Life Satisfaction Scale
Smoking: see Risk behaviors
Snacks and snacking: see Diet
Snyder, C. R., 4
Social behavior: see Positive social behavior

Social belonging, and school connectedness, 7,
    292–296, 298, 300–302
Social cognition, and sibling relationships, 204
Social competencies, 34n, 163, 177; see also
        Positive social behavior; Prosocial
        orientation
    and parent–child relationships, 184
    and sibling relationships, 203–204
Social desirability, 14
Social identity, and organized activities, 134
Social identity theory, 75–76
Social initiative, and interpersonal
        relationships, 148, 158–159
Social Skills Rating System (SSRS), 164, 167
Socialization, and economic attitudes, 357, 370
Socioeconomic Index (SEI), 142–143
Spirituality and religion
    during adolescence, 27–31
    adult relationships, network for, 34–35
    age–grade differences, 28, 30
    attendance, 4, 29–32, 35–38
    cultural context, 4, 26–27
    demographics, 27–31, 33
    developmental assets/outcomes, 25, 27n,
        31–35
    gender differences, 28, 30, 33
    generally, 4, 25–38
    multidimensionality, 36–37
    race/ethnicity differences, 28–30, 33
    salience/importance, 4, 28–32, 35–38
    and scientific inquiry, 37
    self-perceptions of, 37
    and sentiment, 37–38
    time use, 5, 99, 108
    vertical/horizontal themes, 4
    as virtue, 19
Sports, participation in; see also Exercise;
        Outdoor activities
    team sports, 141, 144
    and time use, 5, 97, 108
SSRS: see Social Skills Rating System
Stone, Margaret R., 5
Strengths: see Character strengths
Students' Life Satisfaction Scale (SLSS), see also
        Brief Multidimensional Students' Life
        Satisfaction Scale
    correlates, 46–48
    demographics, 49–50
    generally, 41–50, 55–56
    reliability, 44–45
    responses and scoring, 44, 46–48, 56
    samples, 43–44
    validity, 45, 48–49
Studying: see School
Suldo, Shannon M., 4

Support, as developmental asset, 34n
Survey of Program Dynamics (1999), 309

Task values, *see also* Academic scales
  and organized activities, 140–141
  subjective, 7, 237–248
Teacher Ratings Scale of School Adjustment,
  308
Teacher support: *see* School
Television viewing, 5, 95–97, 117, 122–123, 128
Thriving indicators
  and prosocial orientation, 347–349
  and risk behaviors, 27n, 32–35, 347–349
Time use, *see also* Activities, organized; Child
    Development Supplement; specific
    activities
  age differences, 103–104
  and behavior problems, 107–108
  gender differences, 103–104
  generally, 5, 9, 95–109
  leisure time, 96–99, 102–105, 109

Umaña-Taylor, Adriana J., 4–5, 75–90
Urban Institute, 309
Urdan, Tim, 7
Utility value, defined, 7

Valois, Robert F., 4
Values, *see also* Task values; Virtues
  and character strengths, 3–4, 13–22; *see also*
    Character strengths
  and community life, 8
  and flourishing youth, 1
  positive, as developmental asset, 34n
Values in Action Institute, 20–21
Values in Action Inventory of Character
    Strengths for Youth (VIA Youth), 3–4,
    17–20
Values in Action (VIA) Classification of
    Strengths, 15–17, 19–22
"VERB: It's What You Do," 95

VIA: *see* Values in Action Institute; Values in
    Action Inventory of Character Strengths
    for Youth; Values in Action
    Classification of Strengths
Violence: *see* Risk behaviors
Virtues, and character strengths, 13–14, 17, 19;
    see also Values; specific virtues
Volling, Brenda L., 6
Volunteering
  and civic engagement, 330–331, 333, 337
  and community service, 340, 343–344
  generally, 8
Voting, low rates among youth, 8

Weapons-related violence: *see* Risk behaviors
Weight: *see* Body image
Well-being
  and anxiety, 364
  and economic attitudes, 358, 362, 364, 368,
    369
  and happiness, 364
  and materialism, 359
  and parent–child relationships, 184
  and risk behaviors, 364
  and self-esteem, 364
  and sibling relationships, 212–213
  vs. well-becoming, 2
Wigfield, Allan, 7
Wisdom and knowledge: *see* Learning; School
Wolters, Christopher A., 7

YHPS: *see* Youth Happiness with Parent Scale
Youth Development Study, 342
Youth groups, and civic engagement, 342–343
Youth Happiness with Parent Scale (YHPS),
    186–187
Youth Risk Behavior Study (YRBS), 343
Youth Supplement Survey (YS2), 344–346, 350
YS2: *see* Youth Supplement Survey (YS2)

Zukin, Cliff, 8